INSANITY

**Other books by Thomas Szasz
available from Syracuse University Press**

Anti-Freud
The Ethics of Psychoanalysis
Ideology and Insanity
Law, Liberty, and Psychiatry
The Manufacture of Madness
The Myth of Psychotherapy
Our Right to Drugs
Pain and Pleasure
Psychiatric Justice
Schizophrenia
Sex by Prescription
The Theology of Medicine

INSANITY

THE IDEA AND ITS CONSEQUENCES

THOMAS SZASZ

With a New Preface by the Author

Syracuse University Press

For Bandi,
who taught me so much, so long ago

Copyright © 1997 by Thomas Szasz
All Rights Reserved

First Syracuse University Press Edition 1997
98 99 00 01 02   6 5 4 3 2

Originally published in 1987 by John Wiley & Sons, Inc.

The paper used in this publication meets the minimum requirements
of American National Standard for Information Sciences—Permanence
of Paper for Printed Library Materials, ANSI Z39.48-1984. ∞™

Library of Congress Cataloging-in-Publication Data
Szasz, Thomas Stephen, 1920–
Insanity : the idea and its consequences / Thomas Szasz.
p. cm.
Originally published: New York : Wiley, c1987.
Includes bibliographical references and index.
ISBN 0-8156-0460-2 (pbk. : alk. paper)
1. Social psychiatry.   2. Power (Social sciences)   3. Mental
illness. I. Title.
[DNLM: 1. Mental Disorders.   2. Philosophy, Medical.   WM 100
S996i 1987a]
RC455.S927   1997
362.2—dc21
DNLM/DLC
for Library of Congress   96-45524

Manufactured in the United States of America

What a thing means is simply what habits it involves . . . there is no distinction of meaning so fine as to consist in anything but a possible difference of practice.

—Charles S. Peirce[1]

CONTENTS

PREFACE

While the consequences of the thesis I argue in this book are complex, its crux is simple: Absent an agreement on an unambiguous definition of the concept of bodily illness, the concept of mental illness is an empty vessel.*

Since the nineteenth century—when medical science embraced the definition of disease as bodily lesion—the main object of medical research has been to identify *pathology-as-etiology*. Ignaz Semmelweis's demonstration of iatrogenic contagion as the cause of puerperal fever is a classic example. Lacking a demonstrable basis in somatic pathology, psychiatrists have long viewed mental illnesses as brain diseases whose nature remained to be elucidated. The discovery that general paralysis of the insane is a late sequela of syphilis exemplified, and seemingly justified, this premise. The continuing search for, and current claims about, the anatomic, infectious, genetic, and neurochemical bases of mental diseases reflect the same assumption.

The somatopathological criterion of disease constrains people and politicians in ways they do not want to be constrained. If demonstrable bodily lesion is the sole criterion of disease, individuals who feel sick cannot define themselves as having a disease, nor can the state define certain behaviors as diseases. (To be sure, drinking or smoking can cause disease, but the behavior itself is not a disease.) For these and other reasons, people reject the discipline of a medical gold standard. Instead, they opt for *fiat* maladies, *declaring* that certain (unwanted) behaviors—stamped as medical diagnoses—are diseases. Adherence to this *conven-*

---

* The vocabulary of psychiatry is in a permanent state of semantic revision. The conditions called "insanity" in the nineteenth century were renamed "mental illnesses" in the twentieth, and these in turn are now being renamed "neurobiological diseases."

tion is supported by peer pressure and is enforced by the power of the medical profession and the state. So long as people accept *fiat* money, it is "valued" currency; however, when they reject it—for example, the German mark after World War I—it ceases to be (real) money. Similarly, so long as people accept *fiat* malady it is a "valid" disease; however, when they reject it—for example, homosexuality in our time—it ceases to be a (real) disease.

If mental illnesses are brain diseases, then they are diseases of the body, not of the mind. In which case psychiatrists would have to conduct themselves like other physicians, that is, inform the patient of their findings and recommendations and then wait until he consents to, or rejects, further diagnostic or therapeutic interventions. Such limitation of the psychiatrist's *power* would render psychiatry, as we know it, useless. This is why the well-being of the mental health professions and of the society they serve requires conflating and confusing disease and diagnosis, disease and disability, illness and incompetence, lesion and lawlessness, and much else besides.

Dwelling on the bodily basis of mental diseases implies that medicine and psychiatry are fundamentally similar enterprises. Indeed, psychiatry is *defined* as a medical specialty. This is misleading. The history of modern medicine begins with Rudolf Virchow's definition of disease as somatic pathology; whereas the history of modern psychiatry begins with declaring certain persons insane and incarcerating them in madhouses. In short, the insanity defense and civil commitment came first; classifying certain patterns of (mis)behaviors as diseases—to justify excusing and coercing the actors as medical interventions—came later. Because the birth of modern psychiatry antedates Virchow by some 200 years, its principles and practices could not be based—and are not based—on the definition of disease as bodily lesion. Physicians detect/diagnose somatopathology (medical disease)—for example, anemia—by examining *bodies*. Psychiatrists detect/diagnose psychopathology (mental disease)—for example, schizophrenia—by examining *persons*. (No mental illness can be detected by examining only the patient's body.)

As medical science and technology advance, diagnosing medical diseases becomes more accurate, treating medical illnesses more effective, and delivering medical goods and services more costly. Prior to the present century, consumers (or their relatives) paid for medical services (or, if they could not afford to pay, received medical care as a charity or went without it). Today, in contrast, people and politicians alike regard relief from disease as an integral part of the state's obligation to its citizens. These circumstances, each reinforcing the other, render the struggle over the definition of disease and disability of the utmost practical, political-economic consequence. De-linked from the constraints of somatic pathology, defining (mis)behaviors as (mental) diseases and hence (compensable) disabilities becomes a *tactic,* immensely useful not only for would-be patients, but also for relatives, employers, teachers, politicians, and nearly everyone else.* As our society constructs and legitimizes more (mental) diseases—such as attention deficit disorder and false memory syndrome—more people are *diagnosed as sick,* and the escalating number of disabled Americans is then interpreted as proof of the prevalence of mental illnesses.

THOMAS SZASZ

Syracuse, New York
September, 1996

---

* See Richard Vedder, "America the disabled," *Wall Street Journal,* September 4, 1996, p. A14.

PREFACE TO THE ORIGINAL EDITION

Ideas have consequences.

—*Richard Weaver*[1]

Before we can even begin to try to understand what *causes* a baffling and troubling phenomenon, or how we might change or remedy it, we must be sure of what it *is*—in other words, that we have correctly identified its indispensable features. John Selden, a seventeenth-century English jurist and scholar, wisely warned that "The reason of a thing is not to be inquired after, till you are sure the thing itself be so. We commonly are at, *what's the reason of it?* before we are sure of the thing."[2]

No truer words could be spoken about psychiatry and its core concept, mental illness. What is, in Selden's words, *the thing itself* that psychiatrists describe, debate, diagnose, and treat? The psychiatrist says it is *mental illness,* which, he now quickly adds, is the name of *neurochemical lesions* of the brain. I say it is conflict and coercion and the rules that regulate the psychiatrist's powers and privileges and the patient's rights and responsibilities. The former perspective leads to an analysis of psychiatry in terms of illness and treatment, medical theory and therapeutic practice, while the latter perspective leads to an analysis in terms of coercion and contract, the exercise of power and the efforts to limit it, in short, political theory and legal practice.

Accordingly, my aim in this book is to present a critical exposition of the idea of mental illness and its consequences. I do so, first, by situating it in relation to the closely related ideas of bodily illness, the patient role, and crime; second, by exploring the connections among the ideas of mental illness, imitation, intention, and responsibility; and third, by articulating the practical uses of the idea of mental illness, especially as a rhetorical device for interpersonal control and social policy, and as an essential element in contemporary explanations of human behavior.

Actually, anyone—even a person quite unfamiliar with psychiatry—could reason that a disease characterized as *mental* must be something other than a bodily disease. A moment's reflection about the way we use our language reveals the metaphoric nature of the mind. For example, we say that we have blood in our veins and ideas in our minds, but we know that the latter expression is only a figure of speech. Similarly, when an assailant shoots someone, the victim may suffer a gunshot wound of the brain, but not of the mind. In short, the term *mind* refers to an abstract idea and not to an actual object. Although this distinction between the concrete and the abstract, the objective and the fictional is obvious to everyone when the *body anatomic* is contrasted with the *body politic*, it mystifies nearly everyone when an *illness anatomic* is contrasted with an *illness politic* (a term by which I mean any personal and social problem now called a mental disease).

I want to add a few words here about what this book is not: It is not about the value of psychiatry in general or of any psychiatric intervention in particular. If we view mental illnesses and psychiatric interventions as socially constructed and culturally sanctioned ideas and institutions—similar to Christianity or Communism, Prohibition or the War on Drugs—then it is superfluous to find value in them. Were such ideas and institutions devoid of values, they would not come into being and would not become important. I have discussed elsewhere the help or harm—which depends on our values—that may accrue to a person from mental hospitalization, neuroleptic drugs, psychoanalysis, and so forth. Here I want to concentrate on locating, clearly and precisely, the conceptual realm into which mental illness and the entire psychiatric enterprise belong and the practical consequences to which they give rise. Once this is clear, evaluating the helpfulness or harmfulness of various psychiatric ideas and interventions is a relatively simple matter that anyone with a modicum of intelligence and information can undertake for himself.

The problem with psychiatry, it is sometimes said, especially by those critical of it, is that psychiatrists have too much power. True enough. But where does this power come from? It does not come from the barrel of a gun held by an oppressor. Instead, it comes from the beliefs of human beings who prefer to rely on mystifying symbols and paternalistic authorities rather than on themselves. Thus, only when people withdraw their blind faith in mental health and mental illness will they see fit to curb the powers of psychiatry, just as only when they withdrew their blind faith in God and the Devil did they see fit to curb the powers of priestcraft.

Finally, a brief caveat. In this book I use the masculine pronoun to refer to both men and women, and the terms *psychiatrist* and *patient* to refer to all mental health professionals and their clients; I do so because I believe there are more effective ways of advancing the dignity and liberty of women, nonmedical professionals, and psychiatric patients, than by the now-fashionable flaunting of linguistic deformations.

THOMAS SZASZ

Syracuse, New York
September, 1986

ACKNOWLEDGMENTS

To my daughter, Suzy, I owe very special thanks for her mercilessly critical but always constructive help with writing this book. My brother, George, read various drafts of the manuscript and made many excellent suggestions, as usual. Peter Uva, librarian at the SUNY Health Science Center at Syracuse, spared no effort securing references and I am grateful for his devoted assistance.

I should also like to thank Lord Bauer, for the twist in the story of the naked emperor; C. V. Haldipur, David Sillars, Andrew Simon, and Roger Yanow for their useful comments; Sharon Staring, my secretary, for her conscientious and untiring labors; and the van Ameringen Foundation for generously supporting this work.

T.S.

INTRODUCTION

*Men have an all but incurable propensity to try to prejudge all the
great questions which interest them by stamping their prejudices
upon their language.*

—Sir James Fitzjames Stephen (1873)[1]

Virtually all books on mental illness and psychiatry are about what
goes on in the heads of either mental patients or psychiatrists. In the
former class fall the tragedies written by former patients, novelists,
philosophers, and some mental health professionals about what
they—the sufferers or those who sympathize with them—think is
going on in the minds of the mentally ill: these are called the inner
experiences of the insane and the torments inflicted on them by others. In the latter class fall the comedies written by psychiatrists, psychoanalysts, and other professionals about what they—the scientists
and therapists eager to understand and help the helpless—think is
going on in the minds of mental patients and what ought to be done
about it: these are called the scientific theories and therapeutic techniques of psychiatry. Clearly, a person interested in mental illness and
psychiatry needs to be familiar with both of these kinds of plays and
the theaters in which they are performed. But for the real action he
must look elsewhere.

1

WHAT THIS BOOK IS ABOUT

The subjective experiences of the mental patient and the theories and therapies of the psychiatrist are like the covers of a book. The front cover, that first attracts our attention, is what the mental patient says and does. Next we usually examine the back cover, namely, what the psychiatrist says about the patient and does with him or to him. Often people go no further, satisfied that they can judge a book by its cover—or covers. I believe something like this has happened with mental illness and psychiatry. Especially during the past half-century, as more and more books have been written on this subject, the figures of the mental patient and the psychiatrist have become illuminated ever more brightly, casting the stage on which they perform—not to mention the activities going on backstage—in increasingly impenetrable darkness.

Insanity: Mental Illness or Religious Symbol?

Thus, the scene I want to illuminate is not located inside the heads of the mental patient or the psychiatrist, but outside, in the real world, in the beliefs and behavior of ordinary men and women. Instead of viewing the mental patient and the psychiatrist as the stars of the show, as they invariably are viewed, I shall treat them as actors who merely play supporting roles. The star, indeed the superstar—is an *idea*—called *insanity* or *mental illness*. I shall focus on the ways this idea shapes the behavior of family members toward one another, of politicians and legislators toward the citizen, of judge and lawyer toward the criminal, of journalist and writer toward his subject, and, in the end, of every one of us toward everyone else.

Like religious symbols in the Age of Faith, in the Age of Madness[2] psychiatric symbols are so richly meaningful that they cast their shadows on virtually every aspect of our lives. Accordingly, I have chosen to examine our principal psychiatric symbol—mental illness—from different angles, necessitating some repetition but, at the same time, permitting me to so organize the material that each chapter can almost stand by itself and can be read independently from the others.

The character and complexity of the psychiatric enterprise and the relatively subordinate positions of the mental patient and the psychiatrist in it suggest another metaphor for it, namely, music. The psychiatric ideology is like a musical score; the institutions of psychiatry, like symphony orchestras; the patients and psychiatrists, like the musical performers; judges and lawyers, like the conductors who direct them; politicians and psychiatric theorists, like the composers who provide the score for them; and intellectuals, opinion-makers, and the general public, like enthusiastic audiences clamoring for more and better orchestral scores and symphonic performances. Of course, this in no way excuses psychiatrists from responsibility for the evil they do, just as it does not diminish the credit due them for the good they do. It does, however, put the malefactions of the psychiatrist in context and thus points the finger at those who share his guilt.

Mental Illness: Fact or Fiction?

Although insanity is, without doubt, one of the most important modern ideas, the *Dictionary of the History of Ideas* has no entry for it or for any of its synonyms, such as *madness, mental illness, psychiatric illness,* or *psychosis.*[3] This remarkable omission points to an important phenomenon, namely, that insanity is now considered to be a fact, not an idea. By fact I mean simply something like, say, cancer of the colon. That human beings have bowels is a fact. That bowels can become cancerous is also a fact.

Today, everyone—including jurists and politicians, physicians and scientists—takes it for granted that just as bodily illness is an objectively definable and identifiable condition, so too is mental illness. As experts in mental health constantly remind us, mental illness is like any other illness. Moreover, the view that mental illness is not an idea but an illness—a fact—is supported by the very existence of the governmental agency called the National Institute of Mental Health—an institution similar in name as well as ostensible purpose to the National Institutes of Arthritis, Cancer, and Neurological Diseases. Arthritis, cancer, and neurological diseases are, of course, illnesses, not ideas.

The proposition that the term *mental illness* names a bona fide illness is also supported by the American Psychiatric Association (APA). The authors of the Association's official *Diagnostic and Statistical Manual of Mental Disorders* (DSM-III) emphasize that "actually what are being classified [in the Manual] are disorders that individuals *have*" (emphasis added).[4] In an obvious effort to underscore the factual/material existence of mental illnesses, the authors add: "The text of DSM-III avoids the use of such phrases as 'a schizophrenic' or 'an alcoholic,' and instead uses the more accurate, but admittedly more wordy 'an individual with Schizophrenia' or 'an individual with Alcohol Dependence.'"[5] By capitalizing the names of mental diseases, the APA evidently hopes to dispel any lingering doubt that these names refer to something other than real diseases.

At the same time, it is obvious that in contemporary American speech and writing, the words *illness* and *health,* especially in their adjectival forms, have a dual reference—to bodily disease or its absence on the one hand, and to good and bad behavior on the other hand. As a result, terms such as *healthy* and *sane* now do the job that words of praise did in the past, and terms such as *sick* and *insane* do the job that words of condemnation did in the past. "What," writes a perplexed person to Ann Landers, "can a woman do with a husband who refuses to live within his income? He brags to everyone that he is going to buy his daughter a car for graduation when our car isn't paid for yet." Ann Landers' reply: "Your husband is a compulsive buyer, which is a sickness."[6]

There is, let us make no mistake about it, nothing humorous or metaphorical in Miss Landers' diagnosis. She knows, and her readers know, that this man is mentally ill. If, then, nearly everyone believes or does not bother to doubt that mental illness is a fact, how does an author who regards mental illness as only an idea—albeit a very important one—describe and discuss it? Every use of the questionable term only reinforces the seeming reality of its existence. There are ways around this problem, of course, as the following familiar example illustrates. Consider these three different phrasings, any of which might have appeared in an American newspaper or magazine article after Pearl Harbor:

1. "Because of the danger Japanese-Americans pose . . ."
2. "Because of the alleged danger Japanese-Americans pose . . ."
3. "Because of the 'danger' so-called Japanese-Americans pose . . ."

The first phrasing implies that the writer accepts the proposition that Japanese-Americans pose a danger; the second questions that they pose a danger; the third questions both the reality of the danger and the legitimacy of classifying certain Americans as Japanese-Americans.

Because I question and reject many conventional psychiatric ideas and interventions, but want to use conventional language to communicate my ideas, there is a temptation to qualify certain commonly used words—such as *mental illness, schizophrenia, mental hospital, mental patient,* and so forth by inserting *alleged* or *so-called* before them or by putting the word between quotation marks. In order not to clutter the text with such disclaimers, I have resisted this temptation. The context, together with my general position on psychiatric matters, should make my meaning clear.

An author who wants to describe and discuss something that nearly everyone accepts as a fact but which he views merely as an idea has some other problems to contend with as well. For example, how does he arouse and hold the interest of the general reader who *knows* that mental illness is an illness like any other? Or of the psychiatrist, who has a *vested interest*—existentially as well as economically—in mental illness *qua* illness. The former has no need for a different perspective on mental illness, while the latter can ill afford one.

Truth and the State

I feel content in the belief that, as Thomas Jefferson put it, "It is error alone which needs the support of the government. Truth can stand by itself."[7] Since, except for national defense, there is nothing that our government now supports more vigorously than Health, especially Mental Health, anyone who values the truth ought to think twice before embracing the flood of information about mental illness that carries our government's imprimatur.

I am convinced that psychiatric explanations and interventions are fatally flawed and that, deep in their hearts, most people think so too. The evidence for this abounds. If mental illness is common, can strike anyone, and is just like any other illness, as the experts claim, then why do people hardly ever think that they themselves have such an illness? Why are they not more afraid that they will get such an illness? And why, if they themselves are so wonderfully free of mental illness, do they find others so terribly full of it? In all these ways mental illness resembles the Scriptural beam in our own eyes and the mote in our brother's much more closely than it does diabetes or cancer. Mark Twain was right when he observed that "Nothing so needs reforming as other people's habits."[8] While distressing behavior is real enough, and while it is possible to describe it more or less accurately, neither that reality nor its mapping has much to do with mental illness or psychiatry. Why this is so I shall try to clarify in the pages that follow.

Another problem I have had to resolve concerns presenting examples of mental illness or so-called case material. Since I do not believe in mental illness, I can present examples only of persons whom others have diagnosed as, or called, mentally ill. Accordingly, I cite many examples of mental illness, and of acts committed by mental patients, culled for the most part from stories in magazines and newspapers. This not only allows both author and reader the same access to the same material; it also protects the reader from being gulled by distorted, contrived, or fabricated accounts of dramatic mental diseases and psychiatric cures.

PART ONE

ILLNESS

1

DEFINING ILLNESS

All illnesses . . . save those having emotional or functional causes, are expressions of cellular derangements . . . .
—*Stanley L. Robbins, M.D.*[1]

The physician's task is to diagnose and treat disease. The vast literature of medicine catalogs the countless characteristics of diverse diseases and the various methods used for detecting and treating them. Despite the incredible outpouring of human labor devoted to this enterprise, and despite the fact that virtually all medical efforts—diagnostic and therapeutic, epidemiological and investigative—presuppose an understanding of, and agreement about, what constitutes disease, physicians and nonphysicians alike often neglect to define disease—or, worse, tacitly accept some temporarily fashionable definition.

Because the concept of mental illness borrows from, and leans on, the concept of bodily illness, it is impossible to clarify the meaning of the former term without first coming to grips with the meaning of the latter. Accordingly, in this chapter I shall try to systematically articulate what we mean—and, also what, if we want to be precise, we ought to mean— when we speak about illness. (It is often objected that scrutinizing the semantics of illness is a waste of time because it addresses only words and does not affect the reality of diseases. According to this view, widely held today, cancer is an illness and it exists regardless of what we call it; similarly, schizophrenia is an illness and it, too, exists regardless of what

9

we call it. I shall let this objection, which embodies a dangerous fallacy, stand for the moment and refute it gradually as I go along.)

In his everyday work, the practicing physician diagnoses and treats many conditions that do not qualify as *objectively* identifiable or identified diseases. People who consult physicians complain of discomforts that may or may not be the manifestations of abnormal bodily processes. Moreover, if we consider the diseases diagnosed and treated by psychiatrists—who, and this is very important, are physicians—then the definition of disease as a structural or functional abnormality of the human body is obviously too narrow. Actually, physicians attend to a variety of problems: (1) *aches* and *pains*—such as of the head or back; (2) *complaints* about the body's behavior—such as insomnia or constipation; and (3) the *behavior* of the person who owns or inhabits his body—such as eating too much or too little, drinking too much, being pregnant without wanting to be, and so forth. Are these—shall we say *phenomena* (the name is important because it is likely to prejudge our attitude)—also diseases? We shall see. Suffice it to say for now that, in an inquiry such as ours, answering this question prematurely would be a mistake: If we answer yes, we start down the perilous road of elasticizing the concept of disease—so that it becomes monstrously large, as it in fact now is; if we answer no, we merely reemphasize the familiar distinctions between bodily disease and mental disease—without helping us grapple with the ambiguities inherent in both the professional and lay definitions of disease. Hence, it is best to withhold judgment and use the question "Are dis-eases diseases?" as a philosophical and semantic bridge to higher ground from which to survey the pandemonium below.

WHAT IS DISEASE?

The question "What is disease?" may seem stupid because everyone now knows, or thinks he knows, the answer. Everyone can name a particular phenomenon, that, he is quite sure, is a disease: for example, cancer, diabetes, AIDS. These are certainly diseases. But why? To this question the answer is by no means obvious. Many people now say that these conditions are diseases because they disable and kill people. So do terrorism and war. Are they diseases too?

I believe we must begin with a clarification of the idea of *illness* or *disease*—I use these two terms interchangeably—precisely because everyone knows what it is, if only through the notoriously fallible formula: "I know it when I see it." To my mind, there is an alarming similarity between the present popular concept of disease and certain previous popular concepts, such as hell or witch: everyone knew what they were too. Whenever masses of people, especially educated people, know something—and when what they know is something they greatly fear because they believe it affects virtually everything they do or want to do—then most likely we stand in the presence of a vast falsehood.

Why do we construct definitions of concepts and categories? Why the periodic table of *elements?* Why the taxonomy of *plants* and *animals?* Why distinguish between *killing* and *murder? Mutatis mutandis,* why do we define *disease?* Why should we distinguish between *being ill* and *being mentally ill?*

Classification is usually said to serve one or more of three interconnected aims: (1) to help us understand, order, and communicate information; (2) to establish jurisdiction or boundaries—for example, between human beings and animals, what is edible and not edible, what is therapeutic and noxious; and (3) to establish legitimacy and thus facilitate control of the environment, animate as well as inanimate. Only in the hardest of the hard sciences—and only where notation is basically mathematical—do definitions serve the first purpose exclusively. In other academic pursuits, the practical professions, and everyday discourse, definitions serve all three goals. It is precisely this multipurpose character of our definitions and criteria of illness and mental illness that make a clear cataloging of the various meanings of the term *illness* imperative. We must, therefore, begin with an examination of the ways we use this term.

Defining the Class Called *Disease*

To begin with, the word *disease* is the name of a class. And what is a class? It is a group or set of persons, things, or qualities possessing common characteristics. Examples of classes of *persons* are males, females, children, doctors, Americans. Examples of classes of *things* are stones, trees, houses, cars, radios. Examples of classes of *characteristics* are pains, pleasures, discomforts, sufferings.

What kind of class does the word *disease* refer to? Negative answers come more easily to mind than positive ones. Clearly, diseases are not persons. Are they, then, things? Well, some diseases seem to be things: for example, when a person has an unsightly blemish or growth on the surface of his body—say a basal cell carcinoma on his nose—the individual so affected may regard the lesion as a thing. He may ask his doctor, "Can't you take *this thing* off?" Medical students, too, are trained, at least initially, to view diseases as things: they dissect cadavers, which are things; cadavers have diseased organs—cancerous livers, tuberculous lungs—which are also things. Although this is a good way to begin identifying what we mean by disease, it is only a beginning. For, clearly, the class we conventionally call *disease* comprises many members that are not things—at least not in the sense that they are material objects, like bodies or organs. What they are is something much more subtle—which, perhaps, is the source of a good deal of the confusion about this subject. Consider diseases such as diabetes or essential hypertension. These are not material objects that can be seen or touched or removed from the body, like a melanoma of the skin. Instead, they are the names of *processes*—that, because of their *consequences,* we deem to be *abnormal* or *pathological.* Medical scientists now view virtually all diseases as pathological processes—with symptoms, signs, and visible and tangible lesions (such as an abscess) as their consequences.

So far we have identified the sorts of items that comprise the core concept of disease: abnormal bodies, organs, tissues, cells, and physiological processes. I shall call these items *bodily diseases* or *real diseases* or simply *diseases.* These, of course, are the diseases that (nonpsychiatric) physicians diagnose and treat.

As I have noted, some classes are composed of persons, others of things, and still others of qualities. What about the various states of personal discomfort, grief, or suffering that plague mankind? Are these diseases? Or are they diseases only if they are the symptoms of bodily abnormalities, as they sometimes are? Obviously, there is no merit in arguing about definitions. But there is a good deal of merit in being clear about them and honest about their consequences. Kenneth Minogue wisely warns "that whatever taxonomy one may adopt, it cannot profitably be discussed except by taking some fairly decisive steps right at the beginning."[2] Let us honestly identify these steps. Psychiatrists and all those steeped in the psychiatric ideology take the decisive initial step of omitting to define illness in general, or bodily illness in particular, and instead *define mental illness* (whatever they mean by it) *as a member of the class called illness.* I reject this approach. Instead of accepting the phenomena called mental illnesses as diseases, the decisive initial step I take is to *define illness as the pathologist defines it—as a structural or functional abnormality of cells, tissues, organs, or bodies.* If the phenomena called mental illnesses manifest themselves as such structural or functional abnormalities, then they are *diseases;* if they do not, they are *not.* Unless we exercise such candor, we shall stand in perpetual danger of confusing definition with discovery.

WHAT COUNTS AS ILLNESS?

How do we know whether something is or is not an illness? Is alcoholism an illness? Or obesity? Or self-starvation? Is a pregnant woman who wants an abortion sick? Or a young man who commits a sensational crime, ostensibly to impress a movie star? Questions such as these now crowd in on us from every side. Let us therefore continue our attempt to map the entire meaning of disease by making a list of the sorts of persons who are now viewed—by professionals and lay people alike—as having an illness:

1. Persons displaying overt or hidden signs of a bodily abnormality—for example, jaundice or persistently elevated blood pressure
2. Persons complaining of being ill—for example, of persistent headache or progressive weight loss
3. Persons complaining of a troubling condition or propensity—for example, homosexuality or agoraphobia
4. Persons complaining of, or said to be exhibiting, insufficient self-control—for example, the alcoholic or compulsive gambler
5. Persons committing shocking crimes—for example, killing their own children, parents, or spouses

I shall now briefly comment on each of these criteria.

Criteria of Illness

1. *Proven or demonstrated lesion.* The criterion is a lesion that may be obvious to the naked eye, for example, bleeding or jaundice; or it may be demonstrable only with special instruments, for example, a blood count, x-rays, the electrocardiogram. This is the core concept of what constitutes disease.

2. *Putative or suspected lesion.* The criterion is still a lesion, but the lesion is postulated rather than proved. Typically, its presence is inferred from certain "clinical" evidence; as the disease progresses, it is expected to advance to a stage where the presence of a lesion can be proven. Before the advent of modern diagnostic technology, diseases such as neurosyphilis or myocardial infarction could not, in their early stages, be securely diagnosed or differentiated from complaints that merely mimicked their symptoms. The fallacy, popular today, that all conditions to which we now attach *the name of an illness* are putative diseases which will, with the advance of science, turn out to be proven diseases, is based on this historical transformation of suspected diseases into proven diseases.

3. *Suffering, causing suffering, and occupying the patient role.* The criterion is not a lesion but a complaint interpreted as having a bodily (medical) reference. For example, according to authoritative medical opinion today, a pregnant woman who wants to be pregnant is not considered to be ill, whereas a pregnant woman who does not want to be pregnant is, and abortion is considered to be a treatment for her illness. "The basic intellectual fact," writes a physician working in a Colorado abortion center, "is that pregnancy is an illness for which there are various kinds of treatment."[3] Similarly, a homosexual satisfied with his sexual orientation is not considered to be ill, but if he is dissatisfied with his sexual orientation then he is considered to be ill, suffering from a disease called *ego-dystonic homosexuality.* Suffering may also be imputed to an uncomplaining person designated as a patient: for example, to an individual with so-called grandiose delusions—who is then said to be *suffering from schizophrenia.* Occupying the sick/patient role—by assuming it voluntarily or by being assigned to it involuntarily—is the criterion that qualifies the occupant's alleged condition as a bona fide illness. Because suffering, whether self-avowed or imputed, is an especially important criterion of illness, I shall say more about it presently.

   4. *Bad habits, dangerousness (to self).* These criteria are unrelated to the body (except insofar as the body is involved in anything we do, from studying mathematics to playing baseball). Nevertheless, certain personally or socially disapproved behaviors, especially when they eventuate in bodily harm to the individual who engages in them, are now conventionally classified as diseases: for example, Soviet psychiatrists find that persons who cannot—or do not—control their displeasure with the political system of their own country suffer from *creeping schizophrenia,* while American psychiatrists find that persons who do not control their greed when in a casino, suffer from *pathological gambling.* Similarly, an article in *Science* is tellingly titled "Obesity declared a disease,"[4] while another, in *The New York Times Magazine,* explains that alcoholism is an illness: "Alcoholism is generally defined as a disease in which the victim has lost control over drinking . . . although he may want to, he is unable on his own to stop drinking. . . ."[5] Anorexia, bulimia, drug abuse, smoking, and many other contemporary diseases fall into this category.

   5. *Criminality, dangerousness (to others).* The criterion used for diagnosing persons who commit certain sensational crimes as suffering from a bona fide illness (typically a mental illness) is similar to the criterion previously used: instead of being dangerous to himself, the person is (said to be) dangerous to others. That the madman is dangerous is, of course, a time-honored idea. This fear is steadily reinforced by the fact that, as nearly everyone realizes, conscience and civilization form only a fragile shield against the violence that lurks in the human mind. Given this ever-present fear of the Dangerous Other, modern man welcomes the idea of insanity—of mental illness as a disease—as a supposedly scientific explanation of murder and mayhem: this is why, despite its nonsensical character, the view that "only crazy people commit crazy crimes" enjoys a large measure of intellectual respectability. (See Chapter 8.)

Of course, the belief that crazy people who do crazy things suffer from a lesion of the central nervous system rests on nothing more than a leap of faith; that they suffer from a condition not so caused but nevertheless properly called an *illness* rests on a metaphorical use of the term *illness*. This particular extended use of the term *illness* is now amazingly popular in the United States: no longer is only the violent madman considered to be sick, everyone who is violent is now viewed as sick. C. Everett Koop, the Surgeon General of the United States, has declared: "Violence is every bit a public health issue for me and my successors in this century as smallpox, tuberculosis, and syphilis were for my predecessors in the last two centuries."[6] Indeed, the United States Center for Disease Control (CDC) in Atlanta has a division called "Violence Epidemiology Branch," which, according to a story in *American Medical News*, "is giving priority to the issue [murder], considering homicide to be a disease of epidemic proportions."[7]

Obviously, if we accept every one of the foregoing as a legitimate criterion of illness, we inflate the meaning of the word *illness* and its synonyms, such as *disease* and *disorder*—the latter being the latest psychiatric catchword. I shall not belabor this point. However, since psychiatrists often claim that experiencing suffering from almost any cause is, itself, sufficient warranty for regarding the subject as suffering from a disease, I want to offer some additional remarks on this subject.

Suffering as a Criterion of Illness

As a personal experience and social problem, suffering is clearly not a purely medical concern. Indeed, in modern English we use words derived from the ancient Greek term for suffering, *pathos*, to refer not only to certain phenomena conceptualized as diseases but also to certain human experiences. For example, we use terms like *pathetic* or *sympathetic* to talk about matters unrelated to medicine or psychiatry, and terms like *pathology* and *psychopathology* to talk about bodily and mental diseases.

Actually, only in earlier times, when efforts to heal spirit and body were united in an undifferentiated priestly-medical enterprise, were physicians interested in suffering *qua* suffering. Today physicians are interested in suffering only as a symptom pointing to an underlying disease.*

---

*Etymologically, the term *symptom* comes from the Greek, *syn + piptein*, meaning to fall together or to come together by chance, and is unrelated to medical matters; it is now often used as if it implied, or was a synonym for, complaint or suffering. In any case, symptoms are subjective and must be contrasted with objective signs.

Traditionally, the problem of suffering has been the business of priests and religions. In the modern world, it has also become the business of politicians and the State. Revealingly, contemporary textbooks of medicine, surgery, pathology, or even therapeutics do not even mention suffering. References to suffering abound, however, in theological texts and in works about religion. For example, in *Problems of Suffering in Religions of the World,* John Bowker states that "There are few better ways of coming to understand the religions of the world than by studying what response they make to the common experience of suffering."[8] Regarding the role of suffering in Judaism, he writes: "Here is perhaps the supreme contribution of Israel to a human response to suffering, that suffering can be redemptive, that it can be the foundation of better things. . . ."[9] In Christianity, the redemptive role of suffering is raised higher still: "In Paul's experience . . . discipleship of Christ involves suffering . . . . Thus, suffering is an important part of identification with Christ."[10] Although redemptive suffering came initially from God or was self-inflicted, suffering inflicted on others also became redemptive in principle and hence justifiable in practice:

> In the sixteenth century, for example, there were three benefits which it was thought might justify the imposition of suffering on others: the unity of the state, the purity of the Church, and the hoped-for repentance and salvation of those on whom suffering was inflicted.[11]

Clearly, this passage is pregnant with portentous implications for our own day when the task of relieving—and inflicting—suffering belongs to the clinician rather than the clergyman. Moreover, since the clinician is increasingly an agent of the State—receiving not only his license to practice but also his salary from the State (or from third parties under the control of public agencies)—we now find ourselves confronted with an intimate alliance between medicine and the State. Institutional psychiatry, let us not forget, owes its origin and present importance wholly to the State, that is, to the fact that it is a service sought and paid for by persons other than the designated mental patient.[12] (Typically, the service is sought by the designated patient's relatives and is paid for by the taxpayer.) With its progressive removal from the free market, medicine has assumed many of the economic and political features, and problems, that have long characterized psychiatry. This is why diagnosis and therapy are now increasingly politicized, and politics is increasingly medicalized. How has medicine, and especially psychiatry, become so entangled with the State, or, more specifically, with politics *qua* diagnosis and therapy?

Briefly put, the answer to this question lies in the modern, Liberal perspective on government, which instead of seeing the State as a threat to liberty, perceives it as a protection against poverty, disease, and other threats inherent in the vicissitudes of life. As Kenneth Minogue has elegantly described, the Liberal identifies himself with the paternalistic State, wants to help, and therefore needs people who need help. Since no one needs help more than the person who suffers, the Liberal, writes Minogue, "adopts an intellectual device which interpret[s] events in terms of what we may perhaps call suffering situations."[13] Moreover, since for the Liberal suffering situations justify the most far-reaching coercions imposed by agencies of the State, from taxing some to forcing unwanted help on others, he will feel strongly inclined to impute suffering, or at least a "history of suffering," to any person or group he wants to help. The result is the "theory of implied suffering,"[14] exemplified by the psychiatric perspective that purports to see suffering in the behavior of persons who smoke, drink, and gamble, all of which are now officially designated as mental diseases. Marching under the banner of this theory, the contemporary psychiatrist has occupied every nook and cranny of human behavior. Wherever he looks, he sees suffering requiring his ministrations: some people are said to suffer because they say they do and because they seek help; others are said to suffer, although they do not say they do and may even deny suffering and refuse psychiatric or other help, because they exhibit behavior psychiatrists call *cries for help*. It goes without saying that all such cries are directed toward psychiatrists, who are eager to respond, provided the State authorizes them to impose their help on unwilling clients and pays them to do so.

WHO DEFINES DISEASE?

All too often the problem of defining disease is debated as if it were a question of science, medicine, or logic. By doing so, we ignore the fact that definitions are made by persons, that different persons have different interests, and hence that differing definitions of disease may simply reflect the divergent interests and needs of the *definers*.

Language is an instrument or tool. This is why, if an activity such as music or sports interests us, we have a rich vocabulary for it; and if it does not interest us, we have a poor vocabulary for it, or none at all. It is no accident that *mama* and *dada* are among the first words children learn. Similarly, as semanticists like to point out, because snow is very important for the Eskimo, the Eskimo language has many different words for identifying a variety of snowy conditions.[15] For us snow is not so important, and we have only a few words for it. Disease, however, is important for us, and we have many words for it. The list of medical terms identifying different diseases—from alopecia to zoophobia—must run into the thousands, with the names of new diseases constantly being added. As we are a medically minded people who value the diagnosis and treatment of disease, this rich vocabulary is useful to us in much the same way that the rich vocabulary of snow is useful to the Eskimo.

However, in our effort to understand illness in purely medical terms, we have stumbled into a great confusion. We have done so because of a stubborn refusal to see that although the idea of illness is rooted in a medical context, certain nonmedical—for example, moral, economic, and political—factors play a decisive role in imparting meaning to it.

Every profession possesses a specialized language, created by and for the particular professionals, serving their own purposes, and legitimized by the authority they enjoy. To see how the medical, psychiatric, and popular definitions of illness differ, let us first see how, for example, the chemical, economic, and popular definitions of, say, gold differ. If we asked, What is gold? the chemist might say it is an element with certain chemical and physical characteristics whose atomic number is 79; the economist, that it is a precious metal traditionally used as a monetary medium worth so many dollars per ounce; and the man on the street, that it is the material out of which elegant and expensive jewelry is made or perhaps that it is a protection against economic and political uncertainties. In short, for the chemist gold is an element, for the economist, a medium of exchange, and for the man on the street, a thing of beauty or a source of security. For each, the term *gold* has a different meaning.

The idea of illness can likewise be understood only if we are willing to entertain similar distinctions with reference to who uses it and for what purpose. For the pathologist—and for most physicians most of the time—illness is a disordered state or function of the body. If pressed, physicians might specify the anatomical or physiological characteristics of various disorders, such as myocardial infarction or hypertension. For the patient, illness is a feeling of discomfort or the experience of disability, perceived as originating in the body. If pressed, patients might specify the experiential characteristics of various disorders, such as chill, fever, or pain. Thus doctor and patient both tell us what disease is—each from his own perspective. We might say that physicians and medical organizations define and determine what constitute diseases and treatments, while patients and other nonmedical persons define and determine which particular discomforts they consider to be troublesome enough to require medical attention and which treatments they regard as beneficial.

Two Types of Illness: Organic and Psychological

Today, the standard medical criteria for determining what is a disease are of two kinds—deviations from biological norms and deviations from social norms: The former group comprises so-called bodily or physical diseases, such as cancer and heart disease; the latter, so-called mental or psychiatric diseases, such as depression and schizophrenia. The medical criteria for determining what constitutes treatment are likewise of two kinds—physiological or physicochemical, and psychological or sociocultural: The former group comprises the so-called organic methods of treatment, the latter the psychosocial methods. It must be kept in mind that each of these definitions rests on the authority of the person or group that makes them; that each varies with the interpretations and decisions of those who make them; that each serves the purposes of those who make them; and, most importantly for our purposes, that mental illnesses are now *defined* as diseases. In this view, mental diseases are members of the class called *illness.* These definitions are useful partly as guides for helping the sick, and partly as guideposts to the definer's ideas and intentions. For example, although it had long been known that syphilis was a disease, during the early years of the First World War British military physicians defined it as a crime, incurred as a result of deliberately careless or illicit sexual intercourse. On the other hand, although it had long been known that sometimes persons fake the manifestations of illness, and that such counterfeit diseases must be distinguished from real diseases, toward the end of the nineteenth century physicians declared that these imitations were themselves illnesses.

When X Is "Not Really" X

If we keep our eyes and ears open, we encounter problems similar to the problem of what counts or does not count as illness wherever we turn. Claims advanced as if they were reasoned arguments, and framed typically in the form "X is 'not really' X," appear almost daily in the newspapers. In a single two-day period, I came across three typical stories. The first, titled "Daughter disowned after marrying Gentile," is an Associated Press report about a young Jewish-Canadian woman who married a non-Jewish man on August 23, 1984. "A few days later, her parents placed their daughter's obituary in the weekly *Jewish Post* newspaper, requesting that 'no condolences be sent or memorials made'."[16] According to Canadian civil authorities, this woman was very much alive; according to her parents and the Orthodox Jewish community to which they belong, she was quite dead. Is she, *really,* alive or dead?

In the second story, the question is not whether a certain person is alive or not, but whether certain persons are Jews or not. On March 25, 1985, a combined United Press-Associated Press release reported that "Ethiopia has demanded the return of thousands of Ethiopian Jews transported to Israel in a secret airlift, saying they are *not really* Jewish and had been 'abducted'" (emphasis added).[17] According to Israeli authorities, the starving Ethiopians airlifted to Israel are Jews; according to Ethiopian authorities, they are not Jews. Are these people, *really,* Jews or non-Jews?

The third story, appearing in the same paper on the same day, is about a 63-year-old man who divorced his wife of 18 years in preparation for becoming a priest. The report cited Loyola University law professor James Forkins, an authority on family law and the Catholic Church, explaining that the man "got divorced 'just to be sure,' but in the eyes of the church he had never been married because he did not have a church wedding."[18] Clearly, it would be pointless to ask whether this man was ever *really* married.

Controversies of this type are not limited to religious and psychiatric authorities and their civil or legal counterparts. They are ubiquitous and no individual or organization is immune to them. For example, the introduction of new legislation authorizing the execution of criminals sentenced to death by means of a lethal injection of drugs has prompted the American Pharmaceutical Association—whose members ought to know better—to declare that certain drugs are not really drugs. According to a report in *American Medical News* (the American Medical Association's official weekly newspaper), in order to help pharmacists who do not want to participate in executions, the American Pharmaceutical Association's House of Delegates decided "that a drug used for lethal injection is *not really* a drug, because it is not 'a medicine for the treatment, cure, or prevention of disease,'" (emphasis added).[19] Among the nondrugs used for such injections are potassium chloride, succinylcholine, decamethonium, sodium thiopental, and d-Tubocurarine.

Here is one more example to illustrate that no sooner do we define class X by certain descriptive criteria than we decide, typically on purely strategic grounds, that some members of X are *not really* members of that class. (See Chapter 9.) In the United States today, some banks are called *non-banks.* The uncertain legal status of these institutions was settled in January, 1986, when the Supreme Court ruled that non-banks can provide banking services: In a report titled "Fed loses 'non-bank' bank case," *The New York Times* explained that "'non-bank' banks function much like full-service banks but limit their activities in order to skirt the statutory definition of banks and thereby avoid restrictions on interstate banking and other regulations."[20]

In short, whether a certain condition or conduct is viewed as disease—be it diabetes or depression, pellagra or pregnancy—may depend on whether the patient so defines it, whether the physician and the medical profession so define it, or whether the State so defines it. The same goes for treatment—be it penicillin or prayer, circumcision or conversation. However, in ordinary speech and practice we designate all manner of conditions and interventions simply as *illness* and *treatment*, without bothering to identify who defines what and why. For example, at the beginning of this century, some women wanted contraceptive advice and asked other women for it. The voluntary participants in this transaction defined their goal as the preservation of the woman's health from unwanted pregnancies. The government defined it as a crime and prosecuted the dispensers of birth control information. Today, the government offers the same service, and some of those who now object to it call the measure *genocide*. Obviously, it is pointless to ask what birth control *really* is: a crime, a health measure, pregnancy prevention, or genocide? It is each of these, from the point of view of certain persons or groups.

It is possible, of course, to define illness as a condition identified by the patient just as it is possible to define it as a condition identified by the physician. However, the former definition would mean that every individual who asserts that he is ill would (have to) be viewed and treated as ill, and every individual who asserts that he is not ill would (have to) be viewed and treated as not ill—a patently absurd proposition and program. But there is no need to go to such extremes. It is enough to acknowledge who defines what and controls whom. For example, in the typical case of bodily illness, say myocardial infarction, the subject identifies himself as suffering from an illness and so does his physician; whereas in the typical case of mental illness, say schizophrenia, the psychiatrist identifies the subject as ill but the subject does not identify himself as ill. (In the case of malingering the subject identifies himself as ill, an identification the physician rejected in the past but now accepts, qualifying the illness as *mental*.)

Let me run through this once more. I am suggesting that it is one thing to assay a piece of ore for its gold content, and quite another to dictate the value of the gold in it. Likewise, it is one thing to assay the nature of a physicochemical disorder of a human body, and quite another to dictate how its owner should conduct himself with respect to it. The first task requires knowledge or technical competence; whether or not a person possesses knowledge or technical competence is a matter of fact (or opinion). The second task requires power or control over persons; whether or not it is legitimate to use power over people is a matter of ethics and politics. To appreciate the importance of these considerations requires making a clear distinction between an abnormal biological condition of the body called *disease,* and the assumption of the social role of the sick person called *patient,* a subject I shall discuss in the next chapter. The regrettable fact that this distinction is now so confused, especially in the minds of physicians, is not my fault, but the fault of the medical profession. Chemists are satisfied with studying and trying to understand the chemical properties of gold and offering their services to clients who want them; but physicians are not satisfied with studying and trying to understand abnormal bodily processes and offering their services to clients who want them, but also insist on defining the patient role and determining the legitimacy of a host of health-related matters. This is a blunder for which all of us, doctors and patients alike, are paying a heavy price.

To understand and perhaps undo this mistake, we must attend to, and honestly acknowledge, the diverse interests of the various moral agents—physician, patient, politician, judge—who may have the authority to define disease. Yet it seems to me that we ignore that, especially in the United States, judges often determine what counts as a disease. For example, in 1985, the policy of a New Jersey high school requiring all students to submit to urine tests for illegal drug use was ruled unconstitutional on the ground that "drug use is a medical illness like diabetes, cancer, or AIDS."[21] Clearly, the term *medical illness* in this sentence does not refer to a scientific or medical concept. Judges are neither scientists nor doctors. Instead, they are experts on, and arbiters of, legal fictions (see Chapter 11). A judge cannot, does not, and is not expected to determine whether a particular piece of ore is radioactive or whether a particular skin lesion is a melanoma. What a judge can do, does do, and is expected to do is decide which *legal fictions* we must accept as *social realities.* If, then, judges determine—as they often do in the United States, but not necessarily in other countries—what is and what is not a disease, then we must realize that the term *disease* stands, among other things, for one of our important legal fictions. In addition, we must recognize that not only may different parties define disease differently, but that there is a crucial difference between having the *authority to define disease* and *having the power to impose one's definition on someone else*—for example, physicians on patients, patients on family members, judges on physicians or hospitals, legislators on everyone else. Finally, we must distinguish between possessing the expertise to deliver treatment and the means of doing so, from possessing the political power to impose treatment on those who do not want it, or to extract it from those who do not want to give it. These are simple distinctions. If we fail to make them, it is because we prefer to pursue hidden agendas of domination and submission concealed by a rhetoric of disease and treatment.

THE CORE CONCEPT OF DISEASE

As we have seen, the meaning of disease, as this term is commonly used, is so broad and vague that it defies definition. The result is two-fold: one is that instead of clear *criteria* for counting, or not counting, something as a disease, we have endless *exemplifications* of it; the other is that the category called *disease* is perfectly elastic, accommodating virtually anything anyone wants to place in it (including metaphoric diseases; see Chapter 5).

However, if we scrutinize what (nonpsychiatric) medical researchers and specialists do, we see an ever-more sophisticated search for, and identification of, anatomical and physiological lesions, such as those obtained by means of Computerized Axial Tomography (CAT scan) and novel immunological techniques; and a similar search for, and identification of, the physicochemical causes of novel lesions, for example, the bacillus causing Legionnaires' Disease or the virus causing AIDS. Thus, now more than ever before, the core concept of illness is bodily disease. If this were not so, why would psychiatric researchers be looking for the chemical lesions of schizophrenia and the pharmacological cures of mania?

Not surprisingly, while medical researchers press forward in their search for bodily lesions, psychiatric researchers outdo each other in their efforts to obscure what constitutes disease. The following remarks by Samuel Guze, a professor of psychiatry at Washington University in St. Louis, are pertinent in this connection:

> Most medical textbooks do not attempt to define disease, and most physicians never show much interest in the problem, suggesting either that the definition is unimportant or that they intuitively grasp its meaning and can therefore get on with more interesting questions. Because of these observations, it was proposed [by Guze himself] that "any condition associated with discomfort, pain, disability, death, or an increased liability in these states, regarded by physicians and the public as properly the responsibility of the medical profession, may be considered a disease."[22]

This elastic definition of *disease* leads to the "gradual incorporation of many personal and social problems into the concern of medicine," a trend Guze enthusiastically endorses. It is, of course, precisely this process of medicalization that underlies and supports psychiatry as a medical specialty, a subject discussed throughout this book. Suffice it to add here that the socially relativistic and morally uncritical nature of such a definition—which, incidentally, is not at all novel—invites the use of medical rhetoric and justifies resorts to coercive interventions to solve vexing social problems. Thus, about a century and a half ago, the idea of illness Guze now endorses was used to define black slaves who tried to run away to freedom as suffering from a disease called *drapetomania* and to justify their torture as treatment.[23]

Authoritative Definitions of Disease: Dictionaries and Textbooks of Pathology

To identify the core meaning of disease we must, finally, look to two types of authorities and sources: (1) students of language and students of disease, (2) dictionaries and textbooks of pathology. Let us see what they tell us.

Most English dictionaries list *dis-ease* as the first and most general meaning of the word *disease*. Once past this obstacle, they all define disease as a disorder of the *material* structure or function of a *living body*. For example, the *Oxford English Dictionary* (OED) defines disease as "A condition of the body, or some part or organ of the body, in which its functions are disturbed or deranged . . . ." In a subsequent entry, there appears this significant addendum: "*Fig.* A deranged, depraved, or morbid condition (of mind or disposition, of the affairs of the community, etc.)." In other words, the OED explicitly defines mental illness as a figurative, or metaphoric, illness.

The Revised First Edition of *Webster's New International Dictionary of the English Language* (1897) defines disease as follows:

> An alteration in the state of the body or of some of its organs, interrupting or disturbing the performance of the vital functions, and causing or threatening pain and weakness; malady; affection; illness; sickness; disorder; applied figuratively to the mind, to the moral character and habits, to institutions, the state, etc.

Surely, there is no need to belabor this: the medical definition of *disease* is its literal meaning; applying the term to the mind, moral character, habits, and so forth are its metaphorical meanings.

The Third (most recent) Edition of *Webster's New International Dictionary* (1961) defines disease as "An impairment of the normal state of the living animal or plant body or of any of its components that interrupts or modifies the performance of the vital functions . . . ." *Sickness* and *illness* are listed as synonyms. Interestingly, illness is defined as "an unhealthy condition of body or mind."

Stedman's Medical Dictionary defines disease as follows:

> *Morbus;* illness; sickness; an interruption or perversion of function of any of the organs; an acquired morbid change in any tissue of an organism or throughout an organism . . . .[24]

Even more remarkable are the definitions of disease offered by the physicians most specifically concerned with the material basis of disease, namely, pathologists. For example, Stanley L. Robbins, professor of pathology at Boston University School of Medicine—whose *Pathologic Basis of Disease* is one of the standard texts used in medical schools— begins his 1592-page work with these words:

> The emerging physician is told so often—be concerned with the whole patient—that he sometimes forgets that behind every organic illness there are malfunctioning cells. Indeed, it is more correct to say that when a sufficient number of cells becomes sick, so does the patient. All illnesses, then, *save those having emotional or functional causes,* are expressions of cellular derangements (emphasis added).[25]

Note the pathologist's firm disavowal of mental illnesses as real— that is, cellular—diseases. Interestingly, this passage appears only in the First Edition, published in 1974. In the Third Edition, published in 1984, the claim that mental illness is an illness is rejected indirectly rather than explicitly. Pathology, we are told, is the medical discipline that "deals with the study of deviations from normal structure, physiology, biochemistry, and cellular and molecular biology."[26] Psychiatry is conspicuous by its absence from this list.

If I have dwelled unduly on defining disease, it was for a good reason. Since the idea of mental illness borrows from, leans on, and cannot be analyzed independently from the popular and professional uses of the term *illness*, it would be foolish to dive into that subject, head first as it were, without making sure there is water in the pool. Faced with the idea of illness, modern man—despite, or perhaps because of, his desperate dependence on a sophisticated, highly technological medical system—is like a primitive person who has no concept of paternity. Such a person does not understand the role of the male in human procreation and hence cannot understand what the term *father* means. How could one explain to him the differences between two kinds of fathers—that is, between men so called because they have begot children, and men so called because they have become priests? Since such a person does not know what literal fathers are, he cannot know what metaphorical fathers are.

Similarly, so long as we do not know, or do not want to know, what literal illnesses are—because we refuse to define disease in an operationally meaningful way—we cannot know what metaphorical illnesses are (see Chapter 5). Hence, if we want to *understand* the idea of mental illness, we must first establish and agree on what belongs, and what does not belong, in the class called *bodily illness* and why.

2

BEING A PATIENT

Anglo-American law starts with the premise of thoroughgoing self-determination. It follows that each man is considered to be the master of his own body, and he may, if he be of sound mind, expressly prohibit the performance of life-saving surgery.
                                        —*Nathanson v. Kline* (1960)[1]

The term *illness*, as we saw, refers to a *condition* of the *body* or its constituent parts. The term *patient*, on the other hand, refers to a *social role* occupied by a *person*, specifically, the person who defines himself as ill or, more strictly, who stands in some socially recognized relationship to a medical professional or institution.

THE PATIENT ROLE

The concept of role, borrowed from the stage, plays a pivotal part in modern sociological, psychological, and psychiatric theories of behavior. Furthermore, even in everyday life, removed from theorizings about the workings of human personality, the concept of social role plays a very large and obvious part: we often identify ourselves and others in terms of our respective roles, for example, as sons, fathers, husbands, doctors, lawyers, and so forth. Roles are readily classified according to the social context or situation to which they belong, for example, familial, occupational, political, religious, and so forth. In the medical context, we recognize roles such as doctor, nurse, and patient, and their refinements, such as anesthesiologist, operating room nurse, and mental patient.

Among the most important characteristics or functions of a social role are the following: (1) It identifies a comprehensive pattern of attitudes, behavior, and expectations; (2) it is publicly, often formally, identified as an entity; (3) it can be played by different individuals; (4) it is the principal criterion for identifying and situating persons in society; and (5) it often constitutes a strategy for coping with a recurrent type of situation or problem. Terms such as *doctor, psychiatrist, patient,* and *mental patient* all refer to roles in the sense used above.

The fact that a role is a socially identified and recognized ensemble or entity, together with the fact that it can be played by different individuals more or less the same way generates an important problem in everyday life—a problem especially acute in medical practice, and most acute in psychiatry. The problem is that the uniformity of certain patterns which we call a role is only one side of the coin: its other side is that a role hides and indeed obliterates the unique individuality of its occupant who becomes, in the language of the law, *fungible* or exchangeable. We cannot have it both ways: As persons, we are considered to be unique individuals; as the occupants of roles, we are supposed to be like other occupants of the same role. Consider the following example. A man says to his family doctor: "My wife needs a psychiatrist." The statement implies that he would accept anyone his doctor recommends as a psychiatrist for his wife. By contrast, suppose he were to say: "I would not let anyone but Dr. Jones operate on me." This means that he wants one particular person as his surgeon.

The fact is that the same (or similar) treatment of different persons suffering from the same disease is now considered to be the hallmark of rational medicine—so-called individualized treatment smacking of being old-fashioned and unscientific. Here again we face the fact that we cannot have everything in life: As patients, we cannot have both the personal care of the old-fashioned general practitioner and the scientific competence and technical skill of the modern superspecialist; as physicians, we cannot simultaneously play the roles of healer compassionately caring for sick persons and of technician scientifically treating diseases.

Becoming a Patient

Medical and allied texts, as I have remarked earlier, deal with diseases and treatments. They do not deal with how physicians come into the presence of diseases, with what authorizes them to make pronouncements about sick persons, or with whether they may or may not intervene in these persons' lives. This situation reflects the fact that most people understand how a person becomes a physician. They are familiar with the education and certification a person must acquire to transform himself from a layman into a socially acknowledged, licensed, practicing physician. People thus understand that being a doctor and being a healer are two separate things: that some doctors are healers, but others—for example, forensic pathologists—are not; and that some healers are doctors, but others—for example, unorthodox practitioners or quacks—are not.*

However, most people have no comparable understanding of how a person becomes a patient. They do not know, and often do not care to know, what a person must do or undergo to transform himself, and be transformed by others, from a nonpatient into a socially acknowledged, *certified* patient. This is why people do not understand that being ill and being a patient are two separate things: that some patients are ill, but others—for example, healthy persons who go to physicians for routine checkups or because they are afraid they are ill—are not; and that while some nonpatients are healthy, others—for example, sick Christian Scientists who avoid physicians—are ill.

Let me pause here for a moment and reconsider what we mean when we use the term *patient*. According to *Webster's*, a patient is a "person under treatment or care, as by a physician or surgeon, or in a hospital." Of course, the concept of patient, like the concept of illness, may be defined by anyone: a person may feel unwell and consider himself to be a patient; his family may treat him as a patient; a physician may accept him as his patient; or a hospital may admit him as a patient. I use the term *patient*, unless otherwise qualified, as meaning a *social role* legitimized by appropriate medical and legal authorities.

Understanding the transformations of *persons into patients* is crucial for our proper grasp of medicine and allied fields as *practical* endeavors. For only in theory do physicians deal with diseases. In practice they deal with persons, who may or may not be ill and who may or may not be patients. To put it differently, the practicing physician deals with diseases only *through* patients. Sick persons are, as it were, the carriers of diseases, or more specifically, of diseased bodies or body parts. We must therefore now ask: Who owns—a person's or patient's—illness?

---

* The fine points of this distinction deserve special emphasis. While anyone with an M.D. degree, from a recognized medical institution, may properly be called a *physician*, not every such person is a *practicing physician*; in addition, the physician must also be *licensed* and must *practice medicine*—that is, interact with *live patients*. Doctor and patient—like husband and wife or lock and key—are meshing, symmetrical concepts. In 1985, this definition of a practicing physician was reaffirmed when a New York City judge ruled that "performing autopsies was not practicing medicine . . . ."[2] In short, the pathologist—the ultimate *scientific* expert on what constitutes disease—is not a practicing physician.

The patient himself, his family, his physician, or the State? Similarly, if we view treatments not abstractly as chemotherapy or psychotherapy, but concretely as interventions performed by physicians on the bodies or minds of patients, we must ask: Who owns—medical or psychiatric—treatment? The physician himself, his patient, his patient's family, or the State? Although these questions are *about* diseases and treatments, they are *not* medical questions. They are economic, moral, legal, and political questions.

THE ANATOMY OF THE MEDICAL SITUATION

Language not only mirrors experience but also shapes it; it not only reflects experience but also refracts it. Language can thus both stimulate and inhibit experience. In contrast to our rich vocabulary for illness, it is the more remarkable how poor our vocabulary is with respect to identifying various kinds of doctor-patient relationships. This semantic impoverishment clearly is not a manifestation of our disinterest in this matter. Instead, our inability to name, simply and correctly, different dimensions of our experiences of being ill and seeking medical care reflects the mystification of aspects of our lives that are intensely important but are, at the same time, also intensely embarrassing and frightening. The result is that we can describe certain conditions and interventions only with cumbrous circumlocutions and are often unable to identify them accurately. For example, we speak of persons as ill regardless of whether they are ill in body or mind, whether they consider themselves sick or are only so considered by others, whether they undergo treatment voluntarily or involuntarily. Thus, we are faced with a remarkable paradox: On the one hand, our culture displays a high degree of sophistication, both medical and lay, with respect to the diagnosis and treatment of the major bodily diseases; on the other hand, it displays an almost total lack of sophistication, both medical and lay, with respect to the rights and obligations of patients and doctors vis-à-vis themselves, each other, and the State. To remedy this situation, we need not more research, but more courage. The information we need to comprehend the ramifications of the doctor-patient relationship is at hand. What is missing is the willingness to clearly articulate that information by using words honestly and supporting their true meaning legally.

Who Owns the Body?

The view that the body is a biological machine—at once explicit and implicit in the practice of modern medicine—requires a decision about who controls or, so to speak, owns the body. Having to make such a decision presupposes a departure from our Judeo-Christian heritage. Inasmuch as in that religious perspective God is believed to have created and thus own everything, including our bodies and souls, the question of who owns the body is already answered and hence cannot arise. It is this religiously inspired understanding of our proper relations to our *own* bodies (note the verb as adjective) that accounts for traditional prohibitions not only against suicide but also against eating certain foods, engaging in certain sexual acts, and, during a long period of Christianity, even against certain medical treatments other than prayer or other Church-approved methods. After the decline of religion during the Enlightenment, the State assumed many of the powers formerly enjoyed by the Church, including certain powers over the bodies of persons as well as over persons themselves. The upshot is that different political systems impose different limits on self-ownership, theological and totalitarian systems allowing less, and free societies more, room for individual self-determination in matters of health.

It is, indeed, impossible to grasp the historical origin and cultural significance of the idea of insanity without situating it clearly in the context of the medical situation of modernizing free societies. In this context, the role of patient—specifically, the right of a competent adult to seek or reject care—is quintessentially voluntary; and so is the role of physician—specifically, his right to accept or reject a person as his patient.

Clearly, in the social context of a market-oriented society, the medical situation is readily assimilated to the model of a voluntary transaction between buyer and seller, patient and physician. Since the voluntary exchange of goods or services for money is the normal mode of human relatedness in the marketplace, the doctor-patient relationship poses no problems so long as it is mutually consensual. While in a moment I shall suggest that we view the human body as if it were like an automobile, asserting that a person owns his body much as he owns his car would be oversimplifying the situation. Suffice it to emphasize here that in a free society, such as the United States, a sane adult has a virtually unlimited right to reject medical interventions, whether diagnostic or therapeutic. I shall refrain from digressing into a discussion of the vast literature on this subject and will limit myself to citing three authoritative comments illustrating the American legal posture toward the right to reject *medical* interventions. The first is the classic case of *In re Estate of Brooks*, in which the courts upheld, even in an emergency situation, the patient's refusal of treatment.[3] The second is former Chief Justice (then Circuit Judge) Warren Burger's frequently cited opinion concerning the constitutionality of allowing Jehovah's Witnesses to reject blood transfusion, even when the transfusion may be life-saving. Recalling Justice Louis

Brandeis' words about our "right to be let alone," Justice Burger added these decisive words:

> Nothing in this utterance suggests that Justice Brandeis thought an individual possessed these rights only as to *sensible* beliefs, *valid* thoughts, *reasonable* emotions, or *well-founded* sensations. I suggest he intended to include a great many foolish, unreasonable, and even absurd ideas which do not conform, such as refusing medical treatment even at great risk (emphasis in the original).[4]

Finally, Robert M. Bryn, a legal scholar, offers this summary of the situation:

> Every competent adult is free to reject lifesaving medical treatment. This freedom is grounded, depending upon the patient's claim, either on the right to determine what shall be done with one's body or the right of free religious exercise—both fundamental rights in the American scheme of personal liberty.[5]

Although Justice Burger bravely defends our right to hold foolish, unreasonable, and even absurd ideas, Bryn correctly emphasizes that the right to reject medical treatment is contingent on the agent's competence or sanity, a caveat that again underscores the pivotal role insanity plays in all of medicine, not just in psychiatry.[6]

The Doctor-Patient Relationship

As we have seen, the core of the modern concept of illness rests squarely on the view that the body is a biological machine: the body is made in a certain way; it works in a certain way; it requires certain raw materials for its maintenance and proper functioning; it exhibits certain weaknesses and ways of reacting to injury; and, finally, it decays and eventually ceases to function. Meshing with this materialistic, biological idea of illness is the view of the physician as a mechanic diagnosing and fixing the human body, and of the hospital as a garage where such repairs are carried out. This model offers a useful, albeit incomplete, account of the way modern physicians practice their craft. The account is incomplete because while doctors often think, and sometimes like to believe, that they practice their craft on *human bodies,* in fact that is obviously not what they do. Actually, they practice their craft on bodies that are aspects or parts of *human beings* or *persons.* Hence, we must attend to how persons relate to bodies—their own and others'—and to how physicians relate to the bodies and personalities (minds) of persons called *patients.*

Let us, then, in the next few pages, treat the human body *as if* it were like an automobile. Automobiles belong to their owners. If a person chooses not to put oil in the crankcase and burns up the engine, that is his business; if he chooses to overload the car and cracks the frame, that is his business; and whether he chooses to take his car to a garage for a mechanic to fix is also his business.

Furthermore, as the owners of automobiles are free to seek or avoid mechanics, so the adult members of free societies are, as a rule, free to seek or avoid physicians. Also, as a rule, people know equally little about the structure and function of their cars and of their bodies. Only rarely does a person take his car to a mechanic with a clear idea of what is wrong with it or how it should be fixed. Of course, sometimes a person does know, as when a tire goes flat: That is an obvious lesion with equally obvious remedies—repairing the tire or purchasing a new one. More often, however, a person takes his car to a mechanic with no such obvious lesion but rather with obscure complaints—for example, the car stalls in traffic or does not accelerate properly. The mechanic examines the sick car, makes a diagnosis, and prescribes the treatment—a tune-up and new spark plugs. In other words, the owner of the automobile presents the mechanic with his car's symptoms; the mechanic examines the car, diagnoses its disease, and treats the lesion(s) responsible for it. The medical parallel is obvious enough. When a person breaks an ankle skiing, the lesion is evident to both patient and doctor; but when he experiences increasing fatigue and weight loss, the lesion, if any, is likely to be far from obvious, and competent diagnostic studies will be needed to discover it.

The important similarity between these two situations is that, in each case, the relevant differences between the two parties pertain to two distinct issues—namely, their differing expertise about recognizing and repairing defects or diseases, and their differing legal authority over the problematic object. Typically, the owner of a malfunctioning automobile knows much less than his mechanic about the defects of automobiles and how to repair them—but the car belongs to him, not to the mechanic; similarly, the patient usually knows much less than his doctor about diseases and treatments—but he, not the physician, has legal control over his body. Once a defect is discovered, these differences often become relatively unimportant. Both parties are now likely to agree that a lesion exists and should be repaired in a mutually agreeable manner. I schematize this situation in Table 2.1, Row 1: Doctor and patient agree about the nature of the illness and the proper remedy for it.

Obviously, there is not always such an agreement between clients and experts. The parties may disagree about the existence or nature of the lesion as well as about the reparative tactic appropriate or necessary for its relief. For example, although a car may have a poorly tuned

TABLE 2.1. Being Ill and Being a Patient: Conventional Perceptions of the Person's Situation

Bodily Condition	Social Role	Patient-Physician Relationship (If Any)
Illness + No Illness −	Being a Patient + Not Being a Patient −	
1. +	+	The sick person: seeks medical help—assumes the patient role: the standard model of the "good" (sick) patient.
2. +	−	The sick person: does not seek medical help—does not assume patient role: the standard model of the sick nonpatient (denial of illness; the sick Christian Scientist rejecting medical help).
3. −	+	The well person: seeks medical help—assumes patient role: the standard model of the "bad" (nonsick) patient (the malingerer, the neurotic).
4. −	−	The well person: does not seek medical help: the standard model of the healthy person.

engine, its owner might choose—because he is negligent or has no money—to continue driving it in its defective condition.

The corresponding medical situation—comprising all the encounters in which demonstrably ill persons reject the patient role—is, as I have emphasized already, very important. A person may be ill with or without obvious symptoms or signs of illness and yet choose, for many reasons, not to seek or receive medical attention. Whether or not a person can—is allowed to—do so is a legal and political question. Sick prisoners often can; sick children, sometimes; sick psychotics, almost never. The important point, again, is that, in free societies, sick adults—neither imprisoned nor declared insane—have a virtually unqualified right to avoid or reject medical care. Such persons are, of course, ill and may properly be said to have a disease; but they cannot, properly speaking, be said to be patients. This situation is represented in Table 2.1, Row 2: The person is ill but is not a patient.

The opposite situation is equally important, for medicine as well as psychiatry: The car is okay but its owner claims it is not, and wants it repaired; a healthy person claims to be sick and wants to be a patient. Although, for obvious reasons, this situation occurs less often with respect to cars than bodies, it is not something I have contrived or imagined. Just as many people are now more interested in keeping their bodies fit than in doing something interesting or useful with them, so many people are more interested in keeping their cars in perfect shape than in using them. Let us assume that such a person hears his car squeak or rattle—noises no one else can hear—and takes it to his mechanic to have it checked and fixed. We know what will happen. Depending on circumstances, the automobile-hypochondriac may be told that there is nothing wrong with his car—or that it has some defect (which will be appropriately named) and needs fixing. In the latter case, having been provided with an automotive diagnosis and the semblance of fixing the trouble, the car owner will be satisfied—and the mechanic will have made some money.

When this situation occurs in medicine, its consequences are momentous—not just for the patient and his body, but also for medicine as an institution, for psychiatry, and for all of society. Here is the scenario: A person, believing that he is sick, goes to a doctor or clinic, or perhaps a succession of doctors and clinics. The doctors examine him and find nothing wrong with his body. What happens next? The doctor might tell the patient that he can find nothing to account for his symptoms—in short, that he is healthy. In the present cultural and medical climate of opinion, this is not likely to happen; moreover, should it happen, it is unlikely to change the patient's conviction that he is ill. It is more probable that the doctor, though convinced that his patient is healthy, conjures up an impressive-sounding diagnosis, tells the patient that is what ails him, and prescribes treatment with a placebo, mild tranquilizer, or worse. There is a long list of such contrived medical diagnoses and treatments, their popularity subject to changes in fashion. In any case, the diagnosis secures for the patient the proof he is seeking and legitimizes him in the patient role, with its myriad personal, social, and economic consequences; it also permits the physician to practice his craft vis-à-vis a much larger clientele than he could were he to identify such persons as healthy and hence not requiring medical services.

Perhaps the reader is growing impatient, saying to himself something like this: "Obviously, these people are mentally ill. They are hysterics and hypochondriacs who believe they are ill and *that* is their illness." Precisely. This is the crucial step—the decisive leap of faith, the shift in definition, the fatal professional compromise—that physicians took about 100 years ago. They have clung to it and have tried to consolidate its catastrophic consequences ever since.

Ostensibly, the modern scientific physician's professional mandate is to discover and treat bodily diseases. When he discovers evidence of disease, he says so. For example, the pathologist declares that a histological specimen of breast tissue shows evidence of malignancy; when he discovers no evidence of disease, he also says so. However, this rule is followed strictly only in relation to laboratory specimens and objective measurements, such as blood tests, roentgenograms, and so forth. Confronted with persons whom doctors consider to be sick—not because they have demonstrable lesions but because they are called *patients*—the rule doctors follow, indeed are expected to follow, is quite different: it is that such persons must under no circumstances be declared to be, or called, healthy. Faced with a healthy patient, the doctor must make a legitimate-sounding diagnosis: in other words, he must contrive or invent a nonexistent disease. During the past century or so, doctors have invented two different kinds of such nonexistent diseases: bodily and mental. Examples of the former are mythical disorders of the uterus and ovaries especially popular in the United States, and mythical ailments of the liver, especially popular in France; examples of the latter are all of the mental diseases, especially neurasthenia in the past, and the various anxiety and stress disorders today. Finally, both doctor and patient are encouraged to, and may, attribute mental (psychological) disease to bodily (somatic) causes (and vice versa)—the patient convincing himself that he has a real disease, and the doctor that he is treating a real disease. Let me offer a few more remarks on why patients and doctors behave this way.

As scientific advances in medical diagnosis accelerated during the second half of the nineteenth century, the physician confronted by a person complaining of undiagnosable ills faced a very serious dilemma: What should he tell such a person? And what should he tell himself? The most obvious option open to a physician in this situation is to tell both the patient and himself the truth: namely, that with the methods and knowledge presently available to him, he cannot find anything wrong with the patient's body. Such a stance, however, frustrates both patient and doctor: the former, because he wants to be legitimized in the patient role; the latter, because he wants to find disease so that he can prescribe treatment. This is why physicians rarely chose telling the truth in the past, and why, as the medical profession and the public have redefined the rules of the medical game, doing so has ceased to be an option altogether.

The redefinition to which I refer consists of the physician following a new rule: regardless of whether or not he can discover a somatic lesion to account for a patient's complaints, he must view the claimant as a bona fide patient and must declare him to be ill. Thus did doctors simultaneously invent symmetrical pairs of mental (fictitious) diseases and mental (fictitious) treatments for them: for example, "all species of maladies" and "magnetization" (Anton Mesmer); neurasthenia and medically imposed rest (S. Weir Mitchell); grand hysteria and hypnosis (Jean-Martin Charcot); "general neuroses" and faradization (Wilhelm Erb); conversion hysteria and catharsis (Joseph Breuer); actual and transference neurosis and psychoanalysis (Sigmund Freud); and so forth.[7]

Clearly, if disease means bodily disease, then mental diseases are metaphoric diseases, just as priests are metaphoric fathers. But this is precisely what is denied by all contemporary authorities and institutions that define the terms by which we must play the medical game. They unanimously declare that mental diseases are bona fide diseases, that metaphoric diseases are literal diseases. Conceptually, psychiatry (except insofar as it addresses bona fide brain diseases) thus rests on a literalized metaphor (Table 2.1, Row 3).

To complete this survey of the combinations generated by the fact that the abnormal biological condition of a human being called *illness* and the assumption of the sick role called *being a patient* vary independently, we must briefly note the fourth and last situation: the person has a healthy body and does not seek medical attention (Table 2.1, Row 4). This is what we ordinarily mean by a healthy person.

Table 2.1 displays, in condensed form, the four combinations that result from identifying the patient-physician encounter in terms of two variables: physicochemical abnormality of bodily structure or function, or literal illness, and assumption of the sick role, or being a patient. The information in this table rests on and embodies several assumptions or definitions, namely: that a disease is a physicochemical abnormality of the human body; that the presence or absence of disease is determined by the physician; that the role of patient is voluntarily assumed or avoided by the subject; and that the State, in its role as the political authority of society, does not interfere with the physician's judgment about illness or the individual's decision about assuming or rejecting the role of patient. This table highlights the fact that being ill and being a patient go together like love and marriage— that is, rarely. Yet most people now assume that persons who are ill are patients, and that persons called patients have diseases. Actually, most persons who have diseases are not patients—because they do not believe they are ill, are poor, or have no access to medical care; and most patients have no diseases—because communicating personal problems through complaints about the body is the universal language of mankind.

Condition and Role: A Restatement

It is impossible to understand the problems mental illness poses for Americans—individually as potential mental patients, and collectively as a society expected to cope with such patients—without a firm grasp of the differences between literal and metaphorical diseases and between biological conditions and social roles. I have described the core meaning of the idea of illness in the previous chapter and will devote a subsequent chapter to the analysis of mental illness as metaphoric disease. I now want to restate the basic distinction between being sick and being a patient in somewhat different terms.

Today, most educated persons understand the differences between a person having been killed and having been murdered, between a person being a killer and being a murderer; but few people now understand the differences between having a disease and being a patient, between being sick and being in the sick role. Actually, killing and murder stand in the same sort of relation to each other as do having a disease and being a patient. The extent to which this analogy falls flat is a measure of the injury which modern medical thinking has inflicted on our understanding of human rights and responsibilities.

Killing and sickness are facts; being officially categorized as a murderer or patient are ascriptions or roles. Thus, a person may be killed, for example, by lightning, without having been murdered; and a person may be considered to be a murderer, for example, an innocent person convicted of murder, without having killed anyone. Similarly, a person may be sick, for example, suffering from hypertension, without knowing it, and not be a patient; and a person may be considered to be a patient, for example, by faking illness to avoid the draft or obtain damages for alleged injuries, without being ill.

Yet the modern, scientifically enlightened person instinctively rejects the disjunction between illness and the sick role, and insists that everyone who is sick is ipso facto a patient and that everyone who is (called) a patient is sick. This posture, generally regarded as both compassionate and scientific, is manifested by the intense intolerance shown toward persons believed to be physically ill who reject the patient role (and, to some extent, also toward those who play the patient role even though they are believed to be not physically ill).*

---

*Individuals falling into the latter group used to be regarded as malingerers, a concept emblematic of the understanding that a healthy person can play the role of a sick person; now malingerers are regarded as suffering from *factitious illnesses*, a concept emblematic of the rejection of the very possibility of a disjunction between illness and the sick role. For further discussion, see Chapter 5.

THE POLITICS OF THE MEDICAL SITUATION

Why does a person become a patient? Since, for the most part, people do not like being sick, one might be tempted to say that they are *forced* into the patient role. In a sense, that is often true; but it is important that we distinguish between the two radically different senses in which persons are forced into the roles of patient and mental patient.

Choice and the Patient Role

Ordinarily, people avoid doctors and the patient role. It is when a person experiences pain or some other bodily discomfort that the fear of illness and the hope of relief from pain and disease *force* him, as it were, to seek out medical services; the person visits his physician or goes to a hospital emergency room. Actually, such a person *chooses* to enter the role of medical patient, a choice often concealed by the fact that the patient may feel that, in his condition, he has *no choice* but to seek medical help. However, the phrase *no choice* is here a figure of speech: the person has a choice—legally, psychologically, and practically—but it is a choice in which the desire to seek the patient role may far outweigh the desire to avoid it.

People also avoid psychiatrists and the role of mental patient. (I disregard, for the moment, the truly voluntary mental patient, who seeks psychiatric help much as the medical patient seeks medical help.) Since, for the most part, people do not like being mental patients, one might be tempted to say that they, too, are *forced* into that role. Indeed, that is true; however, persons are forced into this role literally—by other people. Typically, the mental patient *does not choose* to enter the role he is in, a *lack of choice* readily concealed by the fact that, confronted with the overwhelming powers aligned against him, he may elect to seek psychiatric care.

In other words, the patient with bodily illness, experiencing suffering, is driven to go to a hospital by pain; whereas the patient with mental illness, making others suffer, is driven to a mental hospital by the police. The similarities and differences between bodily illness and mental illness are like the similarities and differences between the ways the word *driven* is used in these two sentences. This is why I insist that the term *voluntary mental patient* is problematic: the would-be mental patient may have no choice but to accept the role, for if he does not become a mental patient voluntarily, he could, through commitment, be compelled to become one involuntarily. (I shall say more about this later.)

Medicine and the State: From Treating Patients to Treating Diseases

Our vocabulary for describing the medical situation is not only impoverished, it is also one-sided. We are accustomed to defining the sphere of medical action in terms of the organ system or type of patient the doctor treats: for example, we identify doctors as dermatologists, cardiologists, nephrologists, neurologists—or as pediatricians or geriatricians. These distinctions do not help lay people to recognize who controls the medical transaction or how it is controlled. Yet, as medicine is increasingly politicized, both doctors and patients are increasingly imperiled if they overlook the elements of power and control in their relationship to each other and to third parties, especially the State.

In the nineteenth century, the elements of power and control in the medical situation were less problematic, if only because they were more overt. Privately practicing physicians caring for private patients were the agents of the patient. Psychiatrists were the agents of the State. And physicians working in charity hospitals caring for the poor were primarily the agents of medical education and medical science, rendering the patient care only insofar as it did not conflict with that mandate.

Today the situation, especially in the United States, is radically different. Everyone now expects the practicing physician to be the patient's agent, and everyone pretends that he is the patient's agent—although the patient rarely pays the physician directly for his services. The result is the economic, ethical, legal, and political disorder that characterizes the present medical scene. It is not within the scope of this study to address this conundrum. However, I want to offer a few remarks on what is now happening in American medicine, because certain current developments in the (so-called) delivery of health services illuminate the problems of psychiatry, and vice versa.

The distinction between having an illness and being a patient or, more specifically, between treating an illness and treating a patient—which has always bedeviled psychiatry—is now coming to plague medicine as well. However obvious this distinction might be, it has not prevented the most influential men and women concerned with health policy in the United States from constructing a scheme for reimbursing hospitals based on the fictitious principle that doctors treat diseases, not patients. The monster called *psychiatry* is a monument to what happens when physicians are entrusted with treating diseases regardless of what the patients desire, consent to, or are willing to pay for. In collaboration with American politicians, American physicians have now created a similar monster and have called it the *DRGs* (Diagnosis Related Groups). While at the moment this system of reimbursing hospitals applies only to patients covered by Medicare or Medicaid, physicians and hospital administrators expect, and fear, that, in an effort to control costs, other third-party payers—in particular, insurance companies, such as Blue Cross-Blue Shield—will adopt a similar policy.

Although the ostensible aim of the DRG system is to control costs, only an idiot would accept that rationalization. Its real aim is to further bureaucratize and technicalize the system and depersonalize and depower both the patient and the physician. In short, the *DRGs* at once symbolize and sanction a system of medical care in which physicians treat—and are expected to treat, or even must treat—diseases; they do not treat—and cannot treat—patients, clients, customers, or buyers. (See Chapter 4.)

Perhaps this is a case of divine retribution. During recent decades, physicians refused to resist the temptation of feeding at the public trough, unhesitatingly betraying their patients and themselves by offers of largesse from the State. To make more money, all the physician had to do was shift the cost from the patient to the State (taxpayer)—and the dollars poured in. Now the politicians and medical bureaucrats who hold the money bag are tightening the strings. How do they do it? By taking seriously what they have learned. Clearly, doctors have stopped treating patients and have switched instead to treating diseases. But, unlike patients, diseases are similar to one another: like cans of tuna fish, toilet seats, or baseball bats, they are, what the lawyers call, *fungible.* So, why should the government pay, say, $500 for treating Jones' pneumonia, and $5,000 or $50,000 for treating Smith's?

Now doctors are beginning to wake up from the nightmare they have brought on themselves. However, perhaps because they have been asleep too long, they do not see very clearly. Thus, the first thing they do is wail, like frightened children, that they are innocent: in other words, that it is not their fault that different patients suffering from the same disease do not necessarily require the same length of treatment. But the physicians and politicians who have created the DRG system know that. We must therefore look for a more subtle, or repressed, explanation for what has happened.

What I think has happened, briefly put, is this: As patients stopped and third parties started to pay doctors, doctors lost interest in pleasing the patients and became more interested in pleasing those who pay them—that is, insurance companies (regulated by the government) and the State. How do you please a patient? By making him feel better and respecting his wishes. How do you please a bureaucracy? By dramatizing and justifying the great things you are doing for your impersonal beneficiaries. This is how the American people fell into the stupor of believing that doctors treat (and cure!) diseases. Now physicians and patients alike are discovering that that is not so.

"As a cancer specialist," writes a physician in *The New York Times*, "I often see patients who are not candidates for chemotherapy, radiation treatment, or surgery but nonetheless need hospital care. . . . Not treating cancer is one thing, not treating a person is another." Indeed, complains the writer, a physician stupid enough to care for such a patient too conscientiously "can be labeled a 'Medicare abuser.'"[8] It does not seem to occur to this physician—or probably to other physicians and lay people—that there may be a connection between this impending persecution of doctors who want to take care of patients as they think they ought to, and the persecution of ordinary men and women (throughout the world) who want to take care of their own lives as they think they ought to. Physicians have eagerly embraced the practice of labeling people as *drug abusers, wife abusers, child abusers,* and the *abusers* of everything else in sight, even though these persons were not sick, were not their patients, and wanted to have nothing to do with the medical profession. Now it is the physicians' turn to be stigmatized and persecuted for trying to help patients, just as they have stigmatized and persecuted people who have tried to help themselves. After all, can we be sure that helping others by bankrupting the economy is any less dangerous than helping oneself by ingesting chemicals a medical profession prostituted to the State calls *dangerous?* In vain will doctors try to use the word *help* once their adversaries have taken control of the vocabulary.

The doctor's duty is clear: He must ensure that American medicine assumes responsibility for dealing with the plague of *Medicare abuse* threatening the nation. Accordingly, psychiatrists must immediately organize clinics and hospitals for the treatment of patients afflicted with Medicare abuse: Surely, we cannot permit sick doctors—harboring the delusion that their duty is to treat patients instead of diseases—to endanger the health and well-being of the American people.

Toward a More Candid Identification of the Medical Situation

Perhaps the time is approaching when a suggestion I made some 20 years ago might be timely. I then proposed that the psychiatrist's

> social position vis-à-vis his client should be clearly defined: Does he represent the interests of the patient (as defined by the patient) or of others (the patient's family, society, and so forth)? . . . This division of functions would reflect the fact that the practicing psychiatrist is usually the agent of

one party and the antagonist of another. I advocate a clear social recognition and professional codification of this situation.[9]

The psychiatric patient has long been a party in conflict with other parties, but was treated, nevertheless, as if he simply had a disease. (Of course, he is still so treated.) Now the physician is being forced to become a party in conflict with other parties but is expected to act as if he were simply treating diseases. This situation is bound to get worse before it gets better. Why? Because I believe it can get better only if we are willing to recognize what we have not been willing to recognize—namely, who controls the medical transaction, how it is controlled, and what its real aims are. Such recognition would require heretofore unseen candor—as well as genuine medical, economic, and political self-disclosure—on the parts of doctors, insurance carriers, and politicians. Then, and only then, could we articulate and acknowledge certain (already existing) categories of medical practice, such as the following: *scientific medicine,* for medicine under the control of the medical profession; *police medicine,* for medicine in the service of the police; *executionary and military medicine,* for medicine used for killing; *forensic medicine,* for medicine in the interests of litigants and law enforcement; *entrepreneurial medicine,* for medicine as a free trade; *socialized medicine,* for medicine as a State-supported and controlled trade; *professional medicine,* for medicine as a profession (in the traditional sense of that word); and so forth.

After all, it is folly to ignore the proverbial warning that "He who pays the piper, calls the tune." A comparison of human medicine with veterinary medicine makes clear the danger that threatens us. From the descriptive point of view, the difference between the physician and the veterinarian is that the former treats human diseases or sick people, whereas the latter treats animal diseases or sick animals. From the moral and political point of view, the difference between them is that the physician is expected to be the agent of the persons who are his patients, whereas the veterinarian is expected to be the agent of persons who own sick animals. In proportion, then, as the physician becomes the agent of the State and in proportion as the State is totalitarian, the physician becomes, from a moral and political point of view, a veterinarian—that is, the agent of a State that owns its citizens, just as the farmer owns his animals. This is why killing animals is part of the normal function of the veterinarian and why incarcerating people is, and killing them may yet become, a part of the normal function of the physician employed by the Therapeutic State.

PART TWO

INSANITY

3

DEFINING MENTAL ILLNESS

The subject of the following course of lectures will be the Science of Psychiatry, which, as its name implies, is that of the treatment of mental disease. It is true that, in the strictest terms, we cannot speak of the mind as becoming diseased . . . . (Die Wissenschaft, die uns in den folgenden Vorlesungen beschäftigen soll, ist die Seelenheilkunde: ihr Gegenstand sind demnach die Seelenkrankheiten. Allerdings kann man, streng genommen, nicht von Erkrankungen der Seele sprechen . . . .)
—Emil Kraepelin[1]

As physicians diagnose diseases of the body and treat medical patients, so psychiatrists diagnose diseases of the mind and treat mental patients. But what are mental diseases and who are mental patients? How do bodily and mental diseases, medical and mental patients, resemble and differ from each other? In this chapter I shall consider what constitutes mental illness; in other words, I shall examine and catalog the cognitive content of this idea.

In examining the idea of mental illness, we must choose between two approaches and be clear about the premises built into each. One approach is to examine mental diseases as if they were bona fide (literal) diseases: in this view the class called *illness* comprises several

47

subclasses, such as, infectious diseases, metabolic diseases, autoimmune diseases—and mental diseases. The other approach is to examine mental diseases as if they were metaphorical diseases—that is, not diseases at all but only bearing the names of diseases: in this view, the class called *illness* comprises bodily diseases only—and only bodily diseases are (literal) diseases.*

In order to present a clear and cogent, albeit critical, account of what counts as mental illness, it is necessary, it seems to me, to go over this ground first from the conventional, currently accepted point of view and treat mental illnesses as if they were illnesses. This is what I shall do in this chapter. In the next chapter I shall present a similar analysis of the idea of being a mental patient. In a later chapter I shall discuss mental illness as a metaphor.†

WHAT COUNTS AS MENTAL ILLNESS?

Descriptions of mental illnesses as proven or putative brain diseases or as functional illnesses of the personality merely scratch the surface. After all, these are the two time-honored categories of mental illness: the organic and the functional. Max Hamilton, Nuffield Professor of Psychiatry at the University of Leeds, puts it this way:

> *Mental illnesses:* a. The functional psychoses. These are true illnesses in which a sharp break in the personality occurs, probably as a result of a neurophysiological disorder which so far has escaped detection . . . . b. The organic states. These are true illnesses . . . These illnesses can be further classified as physical diseases.[2]

According to this view, both the functional and organic mental illnesses are *physical diseases* and *true illnesses.* Surely we can do better than this. Inasmuch as I devote several chapters to the most important meanings of mental illness, in this chapter I shall simply list and briefly explain its currently accepted criteria (Table 3.1).

---

*The reader desiring to understand the distinction I draw between literal and metaphorical diseases may prefer to skip ahead and read the discussion of mental illness as metaphor in Chapter 5 before returning to this chapter.

†The problem we face here is similar to the problem we face when we try to fill in the content of a religious idea which in the past people thought referred to real or literal beings and things, like witches or hell, but which most people now view as abstractions without referents in the real world. Thus, it would be wrong to try to understand the witch-hunts by viewing witches and demons as nonexistent beings. Before dismissing them as metaphoric beings we must first understand what people who believed in them meant when they spoke of them. Similarly, before we can grasp the metaphoric character of mental illness we must first understand what people who believe in it—that is, in its material existence or in its being *like any other illness*—mean when they speak of it.

TABLE 3.1. Criteria of Mental Illness

Proven brain disease
Putative brain disease
A species of medical disorder
A treatable condition (of brain or mind)
Distress, disability, disadvantage
Normality, unhappiness, suffering
Committability
Nonintentionality
Irrationality
Irresponsibility
Deviance and crime
Other, miscellaneous criteria

Mental Illness as Proven Brain Disease

The brain is an organ and diseases of the brain manifest themselves, *inter alia*, as disturbances of behavior. Until as recently as the Second World War, mental hospitals were full of patients with brain diseases, mostly neurosyphilis. However, diseases of the brain are brain diseases; it is confusing, misleading, and unnecessary to call them mental illnesses.

It is important to keep in mind, in this connection, that neurosyphilis (general paresis) is the historical paradigm of insanity. The fact that many insane persons turned out to suffer from brain diseases has imprinted itself indelibly on the collective memory of psychiatry: As a result, psychiatrists continue to look for the twisted molecule behind every twisted thought—and if they cannot find it today, they are confident they will find it tomorrow. Such faith in science, like faith in God, is unshakeable and it is foolish and unnecessary to try to shake it. Let it suffice to note here, then, that the most advanced thinking in psychiatry today again favors the view that mental illness is, quite simply, brain disease. Some say the brain disease is already proven; others, that it remains to be proven. "People who act crazy," explains Candance Pert, a psychiatric research scientist at the National Institute of Mental Health, "are acting that way because they have too much or too little of some chemicals in their brains. It's just a physical illness!"[3]

This message now reverberates not only through the halls of Congress, where it generates funds for research into mental illness, but also through the consciences of the relatives of mental patients, where (as we shall see later, in Chapters 9 and 10) it generates justifications for incarcerating the innocent and excusing the guilty. In a letter written in response to a newspaper article I wrote with two colleagues, a woman who identifies herself as "the relative of a victim of schizophrenia," first charges me with "closing [my] mind to the important research in biochemical psychiatry that has taken place in the last 10 years," and then articulates the mental-illness-is-brain-disease view as follows:

> There exists an abundance of biochemical and pathological evidence for establishing schizophrenic and affective disorders, for instance, as "real illnesses." Doesn't Szasz recognize the brain can suffer from disease just as the lungs or the heart can suffer from disease? That is what is meant by saying that mental illness is "like any other illness," something he criticizes other psychiatrists for saying.[4]

No doubt about it, this woman is well informed (whether that makes her belief true, is, of course, another matter): In 1981, the APA officially declared that schizophrenia is a "biochemically based disease."[5] In 1984, Frederick Goodwin, a leading research psychiatrist at the NIMH, asserted that "The National Institute of Mental Health remains firmly committed to the overwhelming evidence indicating that chronic schizophrenia is a brain disease."[6] Perhaps these gentlemen protest too much, however. Scientists at the National Heart, Lung, and Blood Institute do not keep telling us that myocardial infarction is a heart disease. Scientists at the National Institute of Neurological and Communicative Diseases and Stroke do not keep telling us that stroke is a brain disease. So, if the scientists at the NIMH are so sure that schizophrenia is a brain disease, why do they keep saying so—especially as that is just what its inventor/discoverer told us 74 years ago?[7] And if schizophrenia is a brain disease, why do the scientists at the National Institute of *Mental Health*, rather than those at the National Institute of *Neurological Diseases*, tell us that?

Lastly, I want to note here that although the claim that mental illness is a brain disease is now touted as if it were a new idea based on, and supported by, recent medical discoveries, this is not the case. For example, in 1901, the president of the American Medico-Psychological Association spoke glowingly about "how the insane emerged from darkness into light, from demonism to human beings afflicted with bodily disease . . . ."[8] More recently, Linus Pauling, one of the foremost scientists of our age and the winner of two Nobel prizes, asserted: "I believe that mental diseases are molecular diseases, the result of a biochemical abnormality in the human body."[9]

Most people may find it a daunting prospect to contemplate that such intellectual and scientific giants could be wrong. However, they might be wrong.[10] It has happened before, and I think, is happening again.*

Mental Illness as Putative Brain Disease

This is the same view as described above, the sole difference between the two being that the proponents of the idea that mental illness is a putative brain disease usually express themselves in slightly more restrained terms. For example, Seymour Kety states: "Our ability to demonstrate and elucidate pathological disturbances is limited by the state of the art, and to assume their absence because they have not been demonstrated is a *non sequitur.*"[12] To assume their presence because they have not been demonstrated is, I presume, Kety's idea of displaying the proper psychiatric-scientific attitude. Kety then cites Henry Maudsley's classic, *The Physiology and Pathology of Mind* (1872), as a refutation of "Szasz and Laing before they were born":

> . . . at present we know nothing whatever of the intimate constitution of nerve element and of the mode of its functional action, and it is beyond doubt that important molecular and chemical changes may take place in those inner recesses to which we have not yet gained access. Where the subtlety of nature so far exceeds the subtlety of human investigation, to conclude from the non-appearance of change to the non-existence thereon could be just as if the blind man were to maintain there were no colours or the deaf to assert there is no sound.[13]

True enough. But I do not maintain that the nonexistence of pathological findings in schizophrenia proves there are none; I maintain only that a promise of such findings is only a promise, until it is fulfilled. More than a century has passed since Maudsley issued his promissory note; it is still unredeemed. If psychiatrists had to pay interest on their promises of pathological lesions, as borrowers must to lenders, the interest alone would have already bankrupted them; instead, they keep reissuing the same notes, undaunted by their perfect record of never meeting their obligations.

---

*Actually, evidence of the psychiatrists' hypocrisy about the nature of mental illnesses is strewn about their writings like the bodies of dead soldiers defeated in a bloody battle. Here is a typical example, from the pen of Paul Chodoff, a clinical professor of psychiatry at George Washington University in Washington, D.C.: "Since its official introduction in 1980, *DSM-III* has been a rousing success. . . . The point of view it espouses . . . has augmented a general trend toward the medicalization of the phenomena of psychiatry."[11] But if the phenomena of psychiatry *are* medical, why is there a need to medicalize them?

Here is another example of mental illness defined as a putative brain disease, offered by Samuel B. Guze, professor of psychiatry at Washington University in St. Louis: "Eventually we may well discover that . . . 'idiopathic' mental illness indeed involve[s] subtle [physiological] abnormalities that have so far eluded us . . . ."[14] In view of the relatively unsophisticated state of our understanding of neurophysiology and neuropathology, it is more than likely that there are diseases of the human brain, just as there are diseases of the human immune system, that have not yet been discovered. However, ordinary honesty, not to mention scientific integrity, requires that we distinguish between proven and putative diseases, lest we discover diseases by fantasy and fiat, as we do when we attach disease labels to disapproved behaviors, such as gambling.

Mental Disorder as a Species of Medical Disorder

For a long time, psychiatrists have viewed mental disease on the model of medical disease, which, in turn, meant a somatic lesion (lesion understood both in an anatomical and physiological sense). Implicitly—that is, judging from the character of psychiatric research and the emphasis on drug treatment—they still view it as a somatic lesion. But in their explicit definition of mental illness, psychiatrists have made a fundamental switch which has failed to receive the attention it deserves.

Perhaps because they have been unable to demonstrate a somatic basis for mental illness, or perhaps because they realize that the idea of mental disease is basically unrelated to the idea of the body as a machine, psychiatrists have changed their basic criterion and tactic for defining mental illness: first, they define illness as a genus; then, having created a suitably elastic category of illness, they define mental illness as a member of the genus called *illness.* This is precisely what Robert Spitzer, professor of psychiatry at Columbia University and the moving spirit behind DSM-III, does by offering this definition of mental illness (now called disorder): "A mental disorder is a medical disorder."[15] So much for that.

Having placed mental illness where he wants to find it, Spitzer continues:

> A medical disorder is a relatively distinct condition resulting from an organismic dysfunction which in its fully developed or extreme form is directly and intrinsically associated with distress, disability, or certain other types of disadvantage. The disadvantage may be of a physical, perceptual, sexual, or interpersonal nature. Implicitly there is a call for action on the part of the person who has the condition, the medical or its allied professions, and society.[16]

It is unlikely that any dermatologist, surgeon, or pathologist would take this definition seriously; or, for that matter, that anyone could, or would want to, defend it on intellectual or scientific grounds. However, this definition is clearly defensible as useful—indeed, perhaps now as necessary—for legitimizing the feverish medicalization of modern life, an endeavor whose value psychiatrists seem not to question. "To the man who wants to use a hammer badly," observed Mark Twain, "a lot of things look like nails that need hammering."[17] To doctors, politicians, and the public today, a lot of things look like diseases that need treatment. Some of these things Spitzer classifies as mental diseases (excuse me, disorders). "A mental disorder," he writes, "is a medical disorder whose manifestations are primarily signs or symptoms of a psychological (behavioral) nature, or if physical, can be understood only using psychological concepts."[18]

Donald F. Klein, a colleague of Spitzer's at Columbia, hammers home this tautology with the finesse of a piledriver. "By mental illness," he declares, "we mean a subset of all illnesses . . . ."[19] This certainly makes it easy for the psychiatrist to prove that mental illness is an illness, and that the psychiatrist is a medical specialist: it is all accomplished by fiat. (See Figure 3.1.)

Mental Illness as a Treatable Condition

Psychiatrists now often claim that a particular form of behavior is a mental illness because, as they put it, "it responds to psychiatric treatment." This perspective, too, implies a radical change in criterion—from lesion to intervention, from a medical to a criminological model of illness.

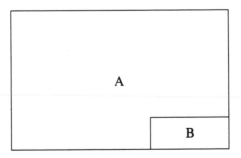

Figure 3.1. Mental illness as literal disease. A = Illness (any condition called and officially recognized as a disease). B = Mental illness (any condition called and officially recognized as a mental disease).

Actually, it is not unreasonable to define crime from such a cart-before-the-horse point of view—that is, as what legislators prohibit and judges and juries punish. Psychiatrists now propose the same perspective for mental illness: A mental disorder is what psychiatrists so identify and use drugs to treat. For example, Morris Lipton, a professor of psychiatry at the University of North Carolina, states: "There is good reason to believe that neurotransmitters and their receptors are involved in mental illness because pharmacological manipulations of these are our most powerful methods for . . . treating the illness."[20]

There is, of course, method in the madness of defining disease in terms of what doctors do to *it:* In the process, psychiatrists conceal the traditionally coercive-paternalistic perspective on treatment characteristic of psychiatry. In other words, this definition doubles as a disguised defense of a policy of psychiatrists treating diseases, rather than patients and of consent to psychiatric treatment being either irrelevant or more easily obtained from sane surrogates than insane patients. The following example, from a Nader Group report on the "homeless mentally ill" in Washington, D.C. is illustrative:

> It is important to stress that schizophrenia is a treatable disease in the majority of cases. It is therefore remarkable that a situation is tolerated in which most of the approximately 1,200 persons with a treatable disease live untreated on the streets and in shelters; imagine the outcry if 1,200 untreated diabetics were living on the streets and in shelters.[21]

This is a characteristically selective use of the disease analogy. Because schizophrenia is a disease like diabetes, schizophrenics, we are admonished, should not go untreated. What the authors neglect to mention is that most diabetics are not children; they are adults responsible for securing their own treatment for their own illness. (Only exceptionally is a diabetic treated without his consent, and virtually never is he treated against his will.) If one were to develop the analogy between diabetes and schizophrenia fully and fairly, one would have to say, and say just as indignantly: "Imagine the outcry if 1200 untreated diabetics were incarcerated in asylums for diabetics and subjected to involuntary treatment!"

It must be noted, finally, that not only is treatability not a legitimate criterion of illness, but that psychiatrists and their acolytes use the idea in a thoroughly debauched way: they simply ascribe what they call *treatability* to any form of behavior they want to coercively control. One typical current example should suffice.

Is taking illegal drugs an illness? Of course, says Torrey Brown, medical consultant to the National Basketball Association. Why does

Brown believe this? Because, "It's something that needs treatment, is treatable, and you can recover from it."[22] Perhaps the time has come to expunge the names of Ignaz Semmelweis, Paul Ehrlich, and Robert Koch from the annals of the history of medicine: for if the criterion of what constitutes disease is what Torrey Brown and all those who agree with him say it is, then what the pioneers of modern medicine studied, and the diseases and treatments they discovered, had nothing to do with what we now regard as some of our most important and serious diseases.

Actually, the idea of treatability as a criterion of illness represents a perversely ironic inversion of what, until recently, characterized most serious diseases, and still characterizes many: namely, untreatability. It would be folly to forget that the scientific concept of illness, developed in the nineteenth century and still accepted as its literal meaning, has nothing whatever to do with treatability. Bacterial endocarditis was untreatable when I was a medical student and is treatable today: it was a disease then and is a disease now. The psychiatrists' current emphasis on treatability is especially perverse. "Schizophrenia," Jung reminds us in his autobiography, "was considered incurable [in the early decades of this century]. If one did achieve some improvement with a case of schizophrenia the answer was that it had not been real schizophrenia."[23] Jung was an honest man and he rejected psychiatry as a dishonest enterprise. Today, psychiatry is an even more dishonest enterprise than it was then. The contemporary psychiatric definition of mental illness as a *treatable condition* reeks of a foul combination of arrogance and stupidity.

Distress, Disability, Disadvantage

These "three D's," as Spitzer calls them, are the cardinal criteria of mental illness underlying DSM-III. All three must be present for a condition officially to qualify as a mental illness. As we shall see, it is easy to juggle them so that one or more are present or absent, as the classifier desires.

Consider, first, distress, defined thus: "This means that either the subject complains about the distress that he experiences or distress is inferred from his manifest behavior."[24] Regrettably, the word *inferred* here means, as the history of psychiatry shows, that the psychiatrist can *attribute* distress to anything and everything he wants to: for example, he may infer distress from smoking and not being able to stop, or from being able to stop but wishing to smoke. Nor must we forget, in this connection, that most odious of psychiatric inferences, namely, interpreting the affect of a person who brags about being Jesus, or who feels high for whatever reason, as distress.

The second criterion, disability, is equally elastic and meaningless: by disability Spitzer "means that there is impairment in more than one area of functioning."[25] To illustrate this criterion, Spitzer offers the following example:

> As a consequence of the requirement of generalized impairment, it is possible for a condition to be associated with impairment in a single function and not be classified as a disorder, providing that the condition does not result in any of the other two D's (distress, disadvantage). Thus, homosexuality per se, which represents an impairment in functioning in the area of heterosexual relationships, is not considered a mental disorder because the area of impairment is often limited, and this condition does not qualify for either of the other D's, as we have defined them.[26]

The third D, disadvantage, must, according to Spitzer, be a disadvantage "not resulting from the above [two D's]."[27] Surely, this is all so absurd that no one would pay attention to it were it not for the powers inherent in, and the social consequences of, the APA's official nomenclature of mental diseases.

Normality, Suffering, Unhappiness

As satire, the idea that everyone is mentally ill occurs already in nineteenth century belles lettres.* It remained for Freud to take this idea seriously. "Thus," states Freud in his *Introductory Lectures on Psychoanalysis,* "a healthy person, too, is virtually a neurotic . . . ."[29] Asserting that health is illness is base rhetoric at its most brazen, which is why, elsewhere, I have characterized Freud as a base rhetorician.[30] Kenneth Minogue, a professor of political science at the London School of Economics, views this intellectual style as characteristic of the "ideologist [who] resembles Sigmund Freud in thinking it is always the pathological that reveals the character of the ordinary."[31] Of course, Freud was following the footsteps of some distinguished ideologists

---

*It should be kept in mind that before the Freudian revolution, the psychiatrist was a physician who worked in a mental hospital, typically, a public insane asylum; and that being categorized as insane meant being treated as a fit subject for psychiatric incarceration. For a marvelously entertaining and instructive spoof of what happens when a psychiatrist begins to view everyone around him as crazy, see the classic short story, "The Psychiatrist" by the nineteenth-century Brazilian physician-writer, Machado de Assis.[28]

and base rhetoricians who had pioneered the tactic of conceptual and moral inversion long before Orwell dreamt of it. Proudhon, for example, is remembered for asserting that "Property is theft," a dictum warmly embraced by socialists and communists. Freud's dictum has similarly been embraced by psychoanalysts. For example, an acolyte in New York writes: "The normal character disorder is a fairly well-recognized disease."[32] One wonders if insurance underwriters have any idea of what lurks in the minds of the soul-doctors.

The universality of mental illness implicit in this line of thinking was given its imprimatur by a study that, in its day, was hailed as the most important post-World War II inquiry into the nature and epidemiology of mental illness. In *Current Concepts of Positive Mental Health*, the book that became the bible of the Community Mental Health Movement, Marie Jahoda writes:

> If it is reasonable to assume that such [human] conflicts are universal, we are all sick in different degrees. Actually, the differences between anyone and a psychotic may lie in the way he handles his conflicts . . . apart from extremes, there is no agreement on the types of behavior which it is reasonable to call "sick."[33]

Karl Menninger agrees. In *The Vital Balance*, he writes:

> . . . we say that all people have mental illness of different degrees at different times, and that sometimes some are much worse, or better. And this is precisely what recent epidemiological studies have demonstrated . . . . Gone forever is the notion that the mentally ill person is an exception. It is now accepted that most people have some degree of mental illness at some time.[34]

Menninger's view that everyone is mentally ill has now made its way into the very heart of the official diagnostic system of American psychiatry. In court testimony, under oath, Jay Katz, a professor of psychiatry at Yale, admitted that "If you look at DSM-III you can classify all of us under one rubric or another of mental disorder."[35] Does this make Katz reject mental illness as a valid medical diagnosis? Of course not. The importance of all-inclusiveness as a characteristic of the criterion of mental illness will become clear when we consider its strategic uses (see Chapter 9).

Since suffering is a universal human experience, the view that everyone has mental illness may be bracketed with the view that suffering is a criterion of mental illness; indeed, according to Menninger, who espouses this view, suffering is a criterion of all illness, not just of mental illness. He writes:

. . . we can define illness as being a certain state of existence which is uncomfortable to someone and for which medical science offers or is believed by the public to offer relief. The suffering may be in the afflicted person or in those around him or both.[36]

Lest this definition be dismissed as that of a crank, it must be remembered that Karl Menninger was the undisputed dean of post-World War II American psychiatry.

Finally, the idea of *unhappiness with one's own lot* as a criterion of illness is now supported not only by psychiatrists but also by members of so-called minority groups with special axes of their own to grind (such as women and homosexuals). For example, is pregnancy a disease? Or homosexuality?

Abstractly, pregnancy is not considered to be a disease; but, concretely, unwanted pregnancy—that is, unwanted by the woman who is pregnant—*is*. Similarly, homosexuality *as such* is not considered to be a mental illness; but *ego-dystonic homosexuality*—that is, homosexuality unwanted by the subject—*is*. Some of these definitions may seem especially compassionate or humane, as they appear to respect the subject's wishes concerning whether or not she or he wishes to be treated as ill. But this is a dangerous illusion. Physicians continue to define disease independently of whether the subject is or is not satisfied with his condition: they regard a person suffering from, say, diabetes or leukemia as ill, regardless of whether or not the patient is satisfied with having diabetes or leukemia (or even recognizes himself as having an illness); similarly, psychiatrists define persons exhibiting what they call schizophrenia or mania as ill, even though such persons typically insist they are not ill and reject psychiatric help. (Psychiatrists say that such patients *deny their illness.*)

Nor have psychiatrists really given up on homosexuality. According to Donald Klein, "If an obligate homosexual becomes unhappy with his lot, tries to perform heterosexually and cannot, he thereby demonstrates operationally an intrinsic involuntary incapacity sufficient to elicit social concern, should be considered ill, and is entitled to the sick role."[37] But suppose the homosexual is happy? Klein is not willing to declare him mentally healthy: "The happy homosexual may be suspected of underlying disease, but currently the issue is moot."[38] Is there anyone who may not be "suspected of underlying disease," especially by psychiatrists?

Mental Illness as Committability

Precisely because there is no objectively verifiable criterion—like a blood test or biopsy—for ascertaining whether or not a person is mentally ill, the presence of this illness is often, and characteristically, inferred from the fact that the supposedly mentally ill person occupies the role of mental patient. This is the reason why persons who assume the role of mental patient (by asserting that they are mentally ill or seeking admission to a mental hospital), as well as those to whom the role is ascribed against their will (by commitment to a mental hospital), are all viewed as mentally ill. This is also the reason why many official forms—such as applications for employment, driver's license, license to carry a gun—ask whether the applicant has ever been a patient in a mental hospital. If the person answers yes, there is no way he can ever prove that he was not mentally ill. Moreover, an affirmative answer creates the presumption that he is still mentally ill, a presumption the subject might find difficult to overcome.

The fact that the presence of mental illness is typically inferred from the suspected subject's occupancy of the role of mental patient gives rise not only to circular definitions of the condition but also to purely dispositional definitions of it (masquerading as descriptions). For example, in 1954, the Group for the Advancement of Psychiatry (GAP), an organization of leading American psychiatrists, proposed the following definition of mental illness: "Mental illness shall mean an illness which so lessens the capacity of a person to use (maintain) his judgment . . . as to warrant his commitment to a mental institution."[39]

This idea may now seem antiquated, because, according to the present rules of forensic psychiatry, a person cannot be committed for mental illness alone: he must *also* be dangerous to himself or others. This is another reminder of the fact that it is quite impossible to understand mental illness without knowing a good deal about its history, that is, about the changing fashions in psychiatric rhetoric and mental health policy.

Committability as a criterion of mental illness illustrates most dramatically the dissimilarities between bodily illness and mental illness, and the similarities between crime and mental illness—the latter two being identified, in part, by their consequences: incarceration in prison in case of felony, in a mental hospital in case of folly.

The semantics of psychiatry also points to, and reveals, an intimate connection between insanity and incarceration. For about two centuries, from 1700 until 1900, the only persons regarded as suffering from a bona fide mental illness were patients legally classified as mad, usually called "certified lunatics." Although the adjective *certifiable* as applied to mental patients has an increasingly old-fashioned ring to it, laymen, reporters, and even legal writers sometimes still use terms such as *certifiable madman* or *certifiably insane*. We must remember, too, that during the eighteenth and nineteenth centuries the institution in which mental patients were housed were called *lunatic asylums*, not mental hospitals; the persons who did the confining were called *alienists* or *mad-doctors*, not psychiatrists; and the persons confined were *committed* to the asylums by law, like criminals to prison. Thus, before about 1900, the term *voluntary mental patient* would have been an oxymoron, just as the term *voluntary convict* would be now. In other words, the idea of mental illness (as a condition) is inextricably tied to the idea of being a mental patient (as a social role); further, the social role of mental patient, in turn derives from, and rests on, a legal definition or imposition of a particular social status.

Mental Illness as Nonintentionality

The belief that the mentally ill person cannot form intent—that his behavior is unintended, like a reflex—plays an important part in the idea of mental illness, especially in its legal applications. The belief that the mentally ill person is a passive victim of compulsions, irresistible impulses, or unconscious forces, is a closely related notion.

The image of the insane person as someone *not really himself*—that is, as someone who engages in behavior he does not really intend—is very old. Building on it, Freud claimed that there are two kinds of mental states and behaviors, conscious and unconscious; and that mental symptoms are unconsciously motivated or determined. This combined psychiatric-psychoanalytic imagery sustains the present view that the behavior of mentally ill persons is (or may be) unintended and that nonintentionality is one of the criteria of mental illness. The following scenario, taken from a newspaper story, illustrates this use of the idea of nonintentionality in psychiatry.

Steven Smith (fictitious name), a hospital technician, complains of being unable to walk or see and is diagnosed as suffering from multiple sclerosis. Confined to a wheelchair for $4\frac{1}{2}$ years, he receives more than $40,000 in Social Security Disability Benefits. During church service one day, he gets out of his wheelchair and declares: "It's not a miracle that I'm standing here." Smith tells the astonished audience that he had been faking his symptoms, adding, "I could have claimed a miraculous recovery, and everything would have been fine. But that wouldn't have helped my problem." The minister, the Reverend T. Jones (fictitious name), hastens to explain to the congregation that "he [Smith] *did not do this intentionally.* He said he [Smith] was planning to seek psychological care to find out why he did it" (emphasis added).[40] By viewing Smith's malingering—sustained over a period of more than 4 years—as nonintentional, Smith himself, the minister of his church, and the congregation could all conclude that Smith was mentally ill and that his behavior was the result of mental illness. Had Smith's behavior been viewed as deliberately contrived, his minister and the congregation would have had to conclude that Smith was a sinner rather than a sick person.

Indeed, so basic is the idea of nonintentionality to the legal concept of insanity that it is often listed as its indispensable, pathognomonic characteristic. For example, Benjamin Greshin, an attorney, states: "The lunatic is . . . by *definition* . . . subject to a disease that creates *forces beyond his control* . . . . The lunatic is regarded as unable to form intent" (emphasis added).[41] As I shall show later, this is patently untrue (see Chapter 7). However, it is precisely because this contention is false that it is so useful as a legal and scientific fiction.

Consider, in this connection, the current view of alcoholism as a disease and the curious role of intentionality in it. The now-fashionable psychiatric-popular view of alcoholism exhibits a revealing double-think and double-talk. Asserting that alcoholism is a disease like diabetes, the advocates of this view add that blaming the alcoholic for his alcoholism is therefore just as mistaken and mischievous as would be blaming the diabetic for his diabetes, and that intentionality or will-power has nothing to do with getting well; working the analogy for all it's worth, the propagandists assert that the alcoholic can no more intend or will to get over his disease than can the diabetic. On the other hand, the proponents of this view contend that, in order to get over his disease, the alcoholic must abstain from drinking alcohol. But not drinking is an act of abstinence that only the alcoholic can intend or perform. This double-think is nicely conveyed in the following letter written to "Dear Abby," which she brings to us with her enthusiastic agreement:

> The American Medical Association does classify alcoholism as a disease. There is documented research showing that alcoholics have a different physiological makeup than non-alcoholics; their enzymes, genes, hormones, and brain chemistry work together to create their abnormal reaction to alcohol. And yes, it is a genetic disease.[42]

It must be wonderful to know all this without having had to go to medical school. The writer and "Dear Abby" also know how to treat this disease: "The alcoholic is never 'cured,' but by abstaining from alcohol one day at a time, he can escape the hell of compulsive drinking."[43] So, after telling us that alcoholism is a disease, the writer suddenly says it is hell. Perhaps he and "Dear Abby" and a few other people are a little mixed up about what is a bodily disease, what is a mental disease, and what is hell. Are these three different things? Or are they only three different names for the same thing?

Mental Illness as Irrationality

The view that the insane person is irrational, and vice versa, is as old as the idea of mental illness itself. Often, the two terms are used synonymously. Nowadays, psychiatrists like to emphasize that the mentally ill person is sick, whereas lawyers like to emphasize that he is irrational. Thus, there is an interesting difference between them with respect to where, in the anatomy of madness, each locates the lesion: Psychiatrists (typically) say that mental illness is a disease because it is a proven or putative brain disease, manifested by mental symptoms; whereas lawyers (often) say that mental illness is a disease because it is irrationality, manifested by mental symptoms.

This legal perspective on mental illness is most forcefully articulated by Herbert Fingarette, a professor of philosophy at the University of California in Santa Barbara. "Insanity, mental illness, mental disease—these are not medical concepts," he asserts.[44] While that may sound as if Fingarette were zeroing in on the metaphorical character of the idea of mental illness, nothing could be further from the truth. Fingarette wants to legitimize, not delegitimize, the psychiatrist's authority based on the idea of insanity, as the following excerpt shows:

> Who are the insane? . . . The insane are madmen, crazy persons bereft of reason. They are persons whose conduct is irrational because they themselves are irrational persons. To those who have observed an insane person, it is evident . . . .[45]

But, surely, we can observe an insane person only when we know he is insane. And how do we know that? Fingarette's voluminous writings on the subject leave no doubt that he regards the psychiatrist as the proper expert to tell us. Since Fingarette wants to legitimize the notion of insanity, he fills it with the content that would do so most convincingly for philosophers and other devotees of pure reason—namely, irrationality:

> There is a notion which lies at the heart of the idea of insanity—it is irrationality. . . . having seized upon the notion of irrationality, we have grasped what is the most distinctive element in insanity. . . . Mental health and mental illness are thus categories rooted in the spiritual: both the mentally healthy and the mentally ill suffer; but the suffering of the mentally ill is rooted in irrationality. . . . The mind that is ill is the mind that is irrational.[46]

Clearly, Fingarette uses the term *mental illness* as an analogue to bodily illness; since he maintains that the mentally ill person is not responsible for his criminal acts and should be incarcerated by psychiat/ equally clear that he uses the term *mental illness* as a literalized _ to serve the traditional purposes of institutional psychiatry.

"Rationality is mental health," concludes Fingarette.[47] Why not piety, or obedience to authority, or social adjustment? Yet, Fingarette's interpretation is by no means idiosyncratic. For example, Michael S. Moore, a professor of law at the University of Southern California, carries the idea of insanity as irrationality even further, reaching the most astonishing conclusions about the humanity of the human beings he calls *mentally ill:*

> We predicate "mentally ill" of a person whenever we find his past behavior unintelligible in some fundamental way . . . . When is there this fundamental failure of understanding of a fellow human being? The answer lies in those attributes that allow us to see another member of the human species as a person, that is, having the attributes of autonomy and rationality. . . . it is the lack of rationality that prevents us from understanding mentally ill human beings to the same extent that we understand more normal persons. . . . Being mentally ill means being incapacitated from acting rationally in this fundamental sense.[48]

The difficulties this definition poses are obvious. In the first place, it puts a premium on the observer's inability to understand another person. What Moore neglects to mention, moreover, is that it is not enough for A to be unable to understand B's behavior in order to be able to declare B irrational and insane. A must also have more power than B (specifically, A must have the power to place B in a legal and social category in which B does not want to be). Actually, if this definition were taken seriously, whenever A does not understand B, A could conclude that B is irrational. And who would be judging A's rationality?

The parochial nature of this perspective is obvious. After all, we know that there are several categories of human beings whose behavior normal adults often find difficult, or impossible, to understand, for example, small children and foreigners. Are they to be judged irrational and insane? (The ancient Greeks believed that anyone who did not speak Greek was a barbarian, and misogynic men now believe that all women are crazy.)

It is wonderfully revealing of the nature of psychiatry that whereas in natural science there is a premium on the expert observer's *ability to understand* what he observes (and to understand it better than the object he observes, which is typically inanimate), in psychiatry there is a premium on the expert's *inability to understand* what he observes (and to understand it less well than the object he observes, which is typically another person eager to proffer his own understanding of his own behavior).* The psychological advantages of not understanding human behavior is, of course, a subject amply illuminated by both writers and psychologists. Its strategic—economic, political, and social—advantages are explored in detail in the present volume.

Mental Illness as Irresponsibility

The connections between insanity and irresponsibility, and between insanity and irrationality, are similar. Historically, insanity was synonomous with irresponsibility. Juries, Moore observes, have always "perceived that madness itself precludes responsibility."[49] Of course, since that is the way madness is defined. Moore also alludes to mankind's "intuitive judgment that mentally ill human beings are not responsible."[50] Of course, if paternalism is accepted as the natural state of human affairs. Indeed, the time-honored prejudice about the nonresponsibility of the insane is enshrined in the various formulations of the insanity defense. The once famous and now infamous Durham Rule puts it this way: ". . . an accused is not criminally responsible if his unlawful act was the product of mental disease . . ."[51] (For further discussion see especially Chapter 8.)

Mental Illness as Deviance and Crime

The commission of certain sensational crimes has long been equated with insanity. This equation is asserted more strongly today than ever before in history, and more strongly in the United States than anywhere else in the world. For example, if a mother murders her young children, or if a street person pushes a waiting passenger to his death under a subway train, there is an automatic assumption that the murderer is mentally ill. When such a case comes to trial, the prosecutor rarely objects to the psychiatric exculpation of the criminal's conduct and is satisfied if the culprit is committed to a mental hospital.

Curiously, this conflating of the ideas of illegality, immorality, and insanity is now considered to be scientific. For example, according to James Marshall, a legal scholar: "A history of unconventional behavior, of deviance from social norms, may indicate mental illness."[52] Jesus,

---

*This observation is consistent with, and may in part explain, the seemingly perverse fact that American state mental hospitals have long been, and continue to be, staffed mainly by foreign physicians whose ability to understand, interpret, and speak English, especially idiomatic English, is slight or nonexistent.

Luther, the Founding Fathers, Lenin, Hitler, and Martin Luther King, to mention only a few historical figures, have all violated social norms and engaged in unconventional behavior. Did they all have a mental illness? The positivistic-psychiatric understanding of mental illness as social deviance stands condemned by its utter insensitivity to ethical and political issues.

Other Miscellaneous Criteria and Concepts of Mental Illness

Although the criteria and concepts that lead psychiatrists (and others) to conclude that a particular behavior counts as a mental illness already listed are long enough, by no means do they encompass all of the odd suggestions that have been advanced in the psychiatric quest for the holy grail of defining this elusive condition. For example, in an essay purportedly presenting a philosophical analysis of the idea of mental illness, Marshal Edelson, a professor of psychiatry at Yale, defines mental illness as "the morbid process—and the effects of attempts to recover from it—initiated by some degree and duration of frustration of a wish to attain a symbolized desirable state of affairs that remains unmitigated by adaptive mastery of external reality, substitution, or sublimation."[53]

Insofar as Edelson's statement makes sense at all, it offers an astonishingly silly criterion for mental illness: for what has a process initiated by a frustrated wish got to do with illness? The word *process*, a vacuous abstraction, functions here simply as a semantic prop, enabling the author to attach to it the adjective *morbid*, thus creating a disease by word-magic, pure and simple. The idea that a frustrated wish causes a *morbid process* which in turn constitutes a mental illness is preposterous, philosophically as well as practically. On the basis of this criterion there is no human action that could not be interpreted as a mental illness. For example, suppose that a poor person, despairing over his prospects of ever earning a sizable amount of money, robs a bank. This action is motivated, in part at least, by a frustrated wish, therefore it is a (symptom of a) mental illness. That way, surely, lies madness, but we now call it psychiatry.*

---

*Compare the definitions reviewed in this chapter with Hobbes' description of madness in 1651:

> The passion, whose violence, or continuance, maketh madness, is either great vainglory; which is commonly called *pride*, and *self-conceit*; or great *dejection* of mind. . . . In sum, all passions that produce strange and unusual behavior, are called by the general name of madness.[54]

It is folly to think that modern psychiatric definitions of mental illness are improvements on Hobbes' view of madness.

Although in a contest for psychiatric obscurantism it would be diffi-cult to decide who deserves first prize, this pellucid pronouncement by Judd Marmor, emeritus professor of psychiatry at the University of Southern California, must, like Edelson's, be counted as a formidable entrant: "An awareness of the pluralistic, multifactorial origins of psy-chopathology broadens our understanding and increases our therapeu-tic potential. The psychiatrist who thinks in systemic terms is a true generalist in medicine . . . ."[55] Most psychiatric propagandists are sat-isfied with claiming that mental illness is a bona fide illness and that the psychiatrist is therefore a bona fide medical specialist. Marmor goes one giant step further: He claims that the psychiatrist "is a true general-ist in medicine." But would anyone in his right mind ask a psychiatrist to remove his inflamed appendix—or his ingrown toenail, for that mat-ter. Mental patients have been diagnosed as having delusions of grandeur for less.

Since human beings are known to be creatures of habit, experts intent on inflating the concept of mental illness have also proposed repetitiveness—especially if the repetitive behavior is undesirable—as a criterion of mental illness. "The best clinical evidence of kleptomania or pyromania," pontificates James Marshall, is "the very repetitive char-acter of the deviance."[56] Spitzer, too, likes this criterion:

> Two distinct conditions which have been identified and which will be in-cluded in DSM-III on this basis are kleptomania and pyromania. Certainly, the incomprehensibility of these conditions to the untrained observer is further support for viewing these conditions as evidence of an organismic dysfunction.[57]

The psychiatrist's eagerness to find mental illness wherever he looks is matched only by his reluctance to define mental illness. Thus, while some respected psychiatric authorities insist that at least one-quarter of the American population suffers from identifiable mental illness or that, sometime in their lives, everyone is mentally ill, others tell us that mental illness simply cannot be defined. Lawrence C. Kolb, professor of psychi-atry at Columbia University's College of Physicians and Surgeons and the author of the classic *Noyes' Modern Clinical Psychiatry*, writes:

> Since all behavior is but a reaction to personality and life factors, it is not always easy to define criteria of mental illnesses. An unbroken line of continuity exists from normal behavior to neurotic and psychotic behavior. . . . Perhaps the criteria of mental illness are largely the degree to which behavior becomes undesirably substitutive and symbolic and the extent to which problems are dealt with in a neurotic manner rather than by rational decision.[58]

Since this was written (1968), the term *neurosis* has been eliminated from the official diagnostic vocabulary of psychiatry, but the definition of *mental illness*—a term that has also been purged—has not become any more precise. In DSM-III *mental illness* is replaced by *mental disorder,* which is defined as follows:

> Although this manual provides a classification of mental disorders, there is no satisfactory definition that specifies precise boundaries for the concept "mental disorder" (also true for such concepts as physical disorder and mental and physical health). . . . In DSM-III each of the mental disorders is conceptualized as a clinically significant behavioral or psychological syndrome or pattern that occurs in an individual and that is typically associated with either a painful symptom (distress) or impairment in one or more important areas of functioning (disability).[59]

The authors of DSM-III are, of course, wrong when they assert that there is no satisfactory definition of physical disorder. Most bodily illnesses—for example, arthritis, arteriosclerosis, hypertension, myocardial infarction, tuberculosis, syphilis, mumps, measles, poliomyelitis, malignant melanoma, subdural hematoma, need one go on?—are clearly defined and can be objectively and reliably identified. The assertion that physicians have the same difficulty defining medical diseases as psychiatrists have defining mental diseases is false. The rest of this passage, with its plethora of semantic pretensions—exemplified by the terms *clinically significant, syndrome, distress,* and *disability* that do the work of code words—is reminiscent of Edelson's obscurantism. In short, the authors of DSM-III offer us a definition of *mental disorder* so obscure and all-inclusive as to be meaningless.

Although modern existential or so-called will-psychologists like to emphasize their disagreements with the deterministic philosophy underlying psychiatry and psychoanalysis, they, too, love the ideas of mental health and mental illness, which they define in accordance with their own concepts of virtue and wickedness. Thus, to Colin Wilson "schizophrenia is a disorder in which the robot takes over from the 'I.'"[60] Enamored with Abraham Maslow's idea of "peak experience"—which, I fear, is merely another pretentious way of talking about living life to the fullest—Wilson latches on to the absence of such experiences as a criterion of mental illness. "It would not be inaccurate to say," he writes, "that we are mentally ill all the time we are not having peak experiences."[61] This is going from the medical model of mental illness to what we might dub the *artistic model* of it: everyone who is *not creative* (whatever that might mean) is mentally sick. Under the band-aid of existential rhetoric, there remains the festering old sore of mental illness.

This survey of the current criteria of mental illness would be incomplete without mentioning religiosity as psychopathology. A good deal of the voluminous literature on this subject is devoted to showing that religion is a cause or symptom of mental illness. For example, Eli S. Chesen, a psychiatrist and author of a book revealingly titled *Religion May Be Hazardous To Your Health*, writes:

> Religion is actually a kind of a consumer good that is without question potentially harmful to the user's mental health. . . . I am not espousing atheism or any other religious stance. I am merely setting down a series of conclusions based upon the observations of case histories. . . . There is a common, close association between religion and psychotic disorders. . . . There is absolutely no question in my mind that many ultrafundamentalist preachers are themselves suffering from a schizophrenic psychosis.[62]

Acting on the proposition that a certain kind of religiosity is a mental illness, Richard Yao, a former Wall Street lawyer, has founded an organization he calls Fundamentalists Anonymous. "The best kept secret in America," he contends, is that "fundamentalism could be a serious health hazard to millions." By health hazard, Yao of course means mental health hazard. Fundamentalism, he says, "causes a disease of the mind that should be taken seriously."[63]

But all is not lost. M. Scott Peck—a psychiatrist, an avowed bornagain Christian, and a best-selling author—has discovered that mental illness is due to demonic possession. Describing himself as "the highest-paid shrink in the world," Peck claims to have "twice encountered Satan. . . . [and] predicts that within a decade, demonic possession will be a psychiatric diagnosis."[64] Evidently subscribing to the principle that if a person is going to reinvent the wheel, he might as well go back to the original model, he enjoins us to recombine the concepts of illness, mental illness, and God's will as they used to be united in the good old days. "Mental illness," Peck explains, "occurs when the conscious will of the individual deviates substantially from the will of God."[65]

Finally, I want to mention one more criterion of mental illness, namely, rhetorical power justifying the claim that the psychiatrist is a bona fide physician. The content of this claim changes with changing fashions in medicine and psychiatry, as the following reflections illustrate.

When I was a young psychiatrist, my colleagues rationalized their medical pretensions by claiming that unconscious conflicts in the human mind caused bodily diseases. The "medical value of psychoanalysis" thus lay in discovering and demonstrating the supposedly psychiatric etiology of bodily diseases—such as asthma, peptic ulcer, or ulcerative colitis—and in promising to cure them by means of psychotherapy.[66] Accordingly, the magic phrases justifying the psychiatrist's inclusion in the medical community—in which his role has rightly been that of a perennial pariah—were *psychoanalysis* and *psychosomatic medicine.* Now that I am an old psychiatrist, my colleagues rationalize their medical pretensions by reviving the antique claim that diseases of the brain cause diseases of the mind. Thus, the medical value of psychiatry now lies in discovering and demonstrating the biological etiology of mental diseases—such as depression and schizophrenia—and promising to cure them by means of drugs. Accordingly, the magic phrases justifying the psychiatrist's inclusion in the medical community are *biological psychiatry* and *psychopharmacology. Plus ça change* . . .

CRITICAL OBSERVATIONS CONCERNING THE CRITERIA OF MENTAL ILLNESS

In the previous section I have only scattered some critical comments on the various criteria of mental illness. Now I want to expand on what I consider to be their most serious shortcomings.

Mental Illness as Brain Disease: Psychiatry's Savior or Destroyer?

While the idea that mental diseases are brain diseases is as old as psychiatry, the popularity of this view has waxed and waned during the past two centuries: It was dominant at the beginning of the nineteenth century; was replaced by the concept of moral insanity at mid-century; became dominant again toward the end of the nineteenth century; was eclipsed by the psychoanalytic-psychodynamic perspective during the middle decades of the twentieth century; and is now dominant once more. Thus, in a guest editorial in the influential *American Medical News,* John Hanley, a professor of psychiatry at the University of California at Los Angeles, states:

> Now, it is in the tradition of such experts [medical specialists] that they are masters of a body of knowledge about an organ system. What is the organ system of psychiatrists? If the domain of the cardiologist is the heart and circulatory system, then surely the domain of the psychiatrist is the brain and its system therein. To qualify and survive as physician specialists, we must become better brain scientists.[67]

This definition is at once descriptive and prescriptive: it not only identifies psychiatry as the study of "the brain and its system therein," but also promotes this definition as necessary for the psychiatrist's survival as a physician specialist. It is not clear, however, why the psychiatrist's survival as a physician should concern us or why we should assume, *prima facie*, that it is desirable. Phrenologists and homeopaths failed to survive as medical specialists and few would regard their passing as a loss. In short, except for psychiatrists who place their loyalty to their guild above their loyalty to science, human welfare, or just plain common sense, the demise of psychiatry as a medical specialty is not, ipso facto, a calamity.

To be sure, if psychiatrists are especially knowledgeable about the brain and the diseases that affect it, as Hanley and others claim, then they have a legitimate claim to being regarded as medical specialists. But if "the domain of psychiatry is the brain and its system therein," then the difference between neurology and psychiatry is the same as that between a glass half full and a glass half empty. Maintaining such a distinction-without-a-difference is indefensible both scientifically and economically. Given such a case—and if academic institutions aspire to be scientific and the law rationally enlightened—educators ought to teach either neurology or psychiatry, but not both; the law ought to recognize either neurology or psychiatry, but not both; and the government and insurance companies ought to pay for either neurological or psychiatric illnesses, but not for both. However, I would not advise anyone to hold his breath until that day arrives.

I am pointing to a contradiction in the classic psychiatric claim that, I think, most people, and especially psychiatrists, overlook: namely, that as soon as a disease thought to be mental is proven to be physical, it is removed from the domain of psychiatry and placed in that of medicine, to be treated henceforth by internists, neurologists, or neurosurgeons. This is what happened with paresis, pellagra, epilepsy, and brain tumors. It is an ironic paradox, then, that while definitive proof that mental illnesses are brain diseases would destroy psychiatry's *raison d'être* as a medical specialty distinct and separate from neurology, the claim that mental illness is a brain disease has served, and continues to serve, as the psychiatrist's most effective justification for legitimacy as an independent medical discipline.

Are Mental Illnesses Brain Diseases?

What shall we make of the persistent psychiatric claim that the major psychoses—schizophrenia and manic-depression in particular—are *proven* neurochemical disorders of the brain? For example, Abram Hoffer and Humphry Osmond—two prominent schizophrenia researchers and the originators of megavitamin therapy for mental illnesses—assert that "schizophrenia is a physical *disease*, in the same way that pellagra and diabetes and mental retardation are physical diseases. . . . the schizophrenic is a victim of a metabolic error in the chemistry of his body."[68]

Is this true or false? I am not an expert on the physiology of the central nervous system, I do no neurochemical research, I do not even prescribe drugs in my practice. But I can read. Hence, I know that ever since the earliest days of psychiatry, psychiatrists have *claimed* that mental diseases are brain diseases; *that pathologists have never been able to confirm these claims;* and that, nevertheless, these claims have *sufficed* to establish psychiatry as a medical specialty. Today, aided and abetted by a vast nonmedical mental health industry and many lay mental health groups, psychiatrists have at last succeeded in elevating the claim that mental illness is brain disease to the status of unchallengeable dogma. From the contemporary, conventionally accepted, psychiatric point of view, rejecting the reality of the somatic basis of schizophrenia is just as absurd as rejecting the reality of the somatic basis of diabetes. Still, I believe this crucial psychiatric claim is either a monumental error, or a monumental fraud, or a combination of both. In this book and in many of my previous writings I have assembled certain kinds of evidence in support of my position. Now I want to offer additional evidence of a different sort in support of it—namely, the opinion of experts on diseases of the body, that is, pathologists.

The Testimony of Pathology

Psychiatrists, as we saw, insist that schizophrenia and manic-depressive psychosis are brain diseases. Textbooks of pathology describe and discuss all known bodily diseases, including brain diseases. Accordingly, one way to verify whether schizophrenia and manic-depressive psychosis are brain diseases is to see what the authors of textbooks of pathology say about them. Well, the answer is that they do not say anything at all about these alleged diseases: they do not mention them, as they simply do not recognize mental illnesses as (bodily) diseases. The significance of this much-neglected fact is enhanced by the pathologists' recognition of *mental retardation*—not as a disease, to be sure, but as the manifestation of certain genetic disorders, such as Down's syndrome (formerly known as mongolism). In order to show that the psychiatric claim—now widely shared by lay mental health groups—that the major psychoses are proven brain diseases is completely unsupported by the opinion of pathologists, I have reviewed the principal contemporary textbooks of pathology, with the following result.

Stanley L. Robbins, professor of pathology at Boston University Medical School, is the senior author of what is perhaps the most widely used textbook in the field, *Pathologic Basis of Disease* (3rd ed.).[69] In this work, running to almost 1500 pages, there is no mention of schizophrenia, manic-depression, or any mental illness. Revealingly, the authors, who thus implicitly reject the reality or somatic basis of mental illness, do recognize the reality of the somatic basis of mental retardation: in the chapter on "Genetic Disorders," they describe and discuss Down's syndrome as well as Klinefelter's syndrome (two genetic disorders causing intellectual impairment).

Anderson's Pathology—a two-volume work running to nearly 2000 pages, edited by John M. Kissane, professor of pathology at Washington University in St. Louis—also makes no mention of schizophrenia or manic-depression.[70] Finally, the most comprehensive contemporary text on pathological physiology—*Sodeman's Pathologic Physiology* (7th ed.)— is also completely silent on the subject of schizophrenia and manic-depression.[71] In short, the authors of textbooks on pathological *anatomy, biochemistry,* and *physiology* do not mention the major mental illnesses— treating them either as if they did not exist or were not diseases.*

Viewed against this background, the claims of clinical psychiatrists—who have no special competence in anatomy, biochemistry, or physiology—may seem less convincing. For example, E. Fuller Torrey, a zealous propagandist for the view that schizophrenia is a brain disease (and for the policy of treating it involuntarily), flatly asserts: "In the last decade research evidence has become overwhelming that these [schizophrenia, manic depressive psychosis] are indeed brain diseases, just as multiple sclerosis, Parkinson's disease, and Alzheimer's disease are brain diseases."[72]

Evidently, Torrey's research evidence has not yet overwhelmed pathologists who write textbooks of pathology: as we saw, they recognize multiple sclerosis, Parkinson's disease, and Alzheimer's disease as brain diseases, but they do not so recognize schizophrenia and manic-depressive psychosis. It is perhaps worth mentioning that defenders of the psychiatric faith ceaselessly criticize me for holding that mental diseases are not (proven) brain diseases, but never—absolutely never— address the inconsistency between their views and the pathologists' views on schizophrenia. It seems to me not unreasonable, however, that

---

*I have checked several other related texts—on endocrine and metabolic physiology, the metabolic basis of disease, and immunology—and have not found a single such work that even mentions, much less supports, the various psychiatric claims concerning the somatic basis of the major psychoses.

psychiatrists ought to convince pathologists that schizophrenia is a brain disease before they take it upon themselves to tell the public that it is such a disease or try to silence those who disagree with them on this crucial issue.

The Testimony of Internal Medicine

In contrast to the way textbooks on pathology treat mental illnesses, textbooks of medicine, with chapters on schizophrenia and mood disorders written by psychiatrists, now present the major psychoses as proven brain diseases. For example, the reader of the Ninth Edition of the prestigious *Harrison's Principles of Internal Medicine* (1980)—the leading American textbook in the field—is authoritatively informed, as if it were a fact, that schizophrenia is "a hereditary life-long disease of the nervous system."[73] Only three years later, in the Tenth Edition (1983), the reader is told a quite different story:

> The dopamine hypothesis currently offers the most popular explanation for a biochemical mechanism of schizophrenia. . . . The clinical potency of anti-psychotic medications has been correlated with their ability to compete with dopamine at stereospecific dopamine binding sites. Furthermore, there is evidence that the schizophrenic-like psychosis produced by amphetamines is evoked either by a release of dopamine or by a heightened sensitivity in the dopamine receptors in the brain.[74]

Note that the explanation of schizophrenia offered here is advanced because it is *the most popular,* not because it is supported by the best evidence. The view that mental illness is brain disease, has of course, always been popular, and the writers of textbooks of medicine are evidently not above pandering to the craven desire of wanting to be on the winning side of a popularity contest. Indeed, *Harrison's* presents the affective psychoses in the same matter-of-fact way as proven brain diseases:

> Good evidence exists for the presence of genetic predisposition toward mood disorders. . . . Recent work suggests that HLA-linked genes on chromosome 6 influence suspectibility to depressive disorders. . . . Less work has been done on the neurochemical basis of mania, but it is believed to be due to an excess of norepinephrine, just as depressions are thought to be caused by a dearth of this neurotransmitter.[75]

These claims conflict with the views of experts on pathological anatomy and pathological physiology, who, as we saw, make no mention of such genetic and chemical lesions in their textbooks.

The second major medical text, *Cecil's Textbook of Medicine* (17th ed., 1985), offers the reader the same unverified psychiatric claims as if they were well-established facts. Written by Paul R. McHugh, a professor of psychiatry at the University of Oregon, the material on schizophrenia and manic-depression is placed in a chapter titled "Neurologic and Behavioral Diseases"—making it appear that behavioral diseases are diseases of the nervous system. Here is how this prestigious textbook of medicine misinforms its readers:

> The genetic constitution has been decisively demonstrated to be one of the "causes" of schizophrenia. . . . As with schizophrenia, an important genetic contribution to the etiology of the manic-depressive disorder seems certain. . . . A pharmacologically induced disorder has enhanced confidence that . . . the mechanism for affective disorders is a neural one.[76]

How are we to account for this diametrically different handling, by the authors of textbooks of pathology and medicine, of the psychiatrist's claims concerning the somatic basis of the major mental illnesses? Why do pathologists ignore and implicitly (or even explicitly) reject the psychiatrists' claims about the somatic basis of schizophrenia and manic-depression, and why do specialists in internal medicine accept these claims so eagerly and uncritically? I believe the reasons are, again, practical. In his daily work, the pathologist has no need whatsoever for the psychiatrist. Moreover, since the psychiatrist's claims about somatic pathology concern the pathologist's own expertise, the pathologist has no more reason to accept the fantastic and unsupported claims of psychiatrists than, say, an astronomer has to accept the fantastic and unsupported claims of astrologers. Accordingly, pathologists ignore, as unworthy of attention, the claims of psychiatrists concerning the somatic bases of mental illnesses.

The situation of the specialist in internal medicine is quite different. Unlike the pathologist, who deals with organs, tissues, and cells, the practicing physician deals with patients; unlike the pathologist who examines cadavers or specimens of tissues or body fluids, the physician examines living persons. Persons behave and misbehave, and when they misbehave, the physician needs the psychiatrist to relieve him of the difficult patient. This, in my opinion, is why authors of medical textbooks treat psychiatric claims so differently than do the authors of textbooks of pathology. Because he needs the psychiatrist, the practicing physician cooperates with him and is often corrupted by him: the result is that the specialist in internal medicine shows his respect for psychiatry by accepting and legitimizing the psychiatrist's classic claim that mental illness is like any other illness.

Schizophrenia Reconsidered

As we have seen, there is vexing ambiguity inherent in the very idea of mental illness: Does it, or does it not, refer to a brain disease? Instead of confronting this ambiguity and trying to resolve it, psychiatrists have engaged in double-talk, characterizing the same mental illnesses alternately as functional and organic—and even if functional, as organic. This posture is exemplified by the way psychiatrists treat the paradigmatic mental illness, schizophrenia. Typically, most psychiatrists now assert that while schizophrenia seems to be a functional illness, its organic basis will soon be discovered—a claim that suffers from all of the problems of definition, verification, and naming discussed earlier. Let me try once more to clarify the contemporary psychiatric claim— advanced with increasing vigor in recent years—that schizophrenia is a brain disease. What can we learn from this claim?

Since contemplating the possibility that schizophrenia is not a disease is taboo to psychiatrists, they make no effort to clarify how the term *schizophrenia* is defined. Instead, they dramatize with horrifying examples what a terrible disease it is, and how terrible I am for "denying" its existence. For example, Heinz Lehman, a professor of psychiatry at McGill University in Montreal, refers to my views on schizophrenia as follows: "In fact, some psychiatrists call schizophrenia a myth and a metaphor (Szasz, 1961) . . . *denying* it the status of a disease" (emphasis added).[77] Similar language is used by Guze, who begins an article on "Mental disease classification" by raising the "seemingly fatuous question of whether there is actually such a thing as mental disease."[78] After observing that "most doctors would answer 'Of course,'" Guze notes that there are some dissenters. "And since the *denial* of mental disease may crop up among patients or their relatives," he writes, "such a view merits a brief discussion" (emphasis added). However, instead of discussing my views, Guze dismisses them by disparaging "the *attitudes* of people who *deny* the very existence of mental disease. . . ." (emphasis added).[79]

In a sense, psychiatrists like Lehman and Guze are right in using the word *denial* to characterize my position concerning mental illness. However, I deny the miraculous transformation of malicious behavior into medical disease only because psychiatrists assert it, and I am accused of denying it only by those who believe in it—just as Jews deny the divinity of Jesus only because Christians assert it, and are accused of denying it only by those who believe in it. However, such assertions and denials mislead us from the nature of the controversy: The contention is about deeds, not words; about economic and political power, not theological or psychiatric abstractions.

Before considering the content of the claim that schizophrenia is a brain disease, it is essential that we take notice of who are the persons who advance this claim most aggressively: they are psychiatrists and the relatives of schizophrenics. (Nonpsychiatric physicians and schizophrenic patients are notably unenthusiastic about this claim or expressly oppose it.) For example, following the publication of a series of articles in *The New York Times* (in March 1986) on schizophrenia as a brain disease, Ira Rose, the President of People Acting Together with Hope, wrote to thank the *Times:*

> We, as a parent support group, are extremely grateful for your series on schizophrenia. . . . Recognition has long been overdue that this terrible brain disease is the fault neither of the victims nor their families, but is of neurobiological or genetic origin. . . . We need the understanding and help of all society to see this disease as it truly is—a disabling brain disease.[80]

Although the information conveyed in such newspaper reports on schizophrenia may be untrue, the reports are very useful for answering the *cui bono* question (Chapters 9–12). Moreover, if scientists, journalists, and educated people shut their eyes to the fact that the contention that schizophrenia is a brain disease pleases those who do *not suffer* from this alleged brain disease much more than those who supposedly *do,* then this observation itself ought to be considered an important element in what we mean by the term *schizophrenia.* I might add here, too, that the claim that schizophrenia is a brain disease does not prevent psychiatrists from also claiming that "long-term psychotherapy [is] useful in treating schizophrenia."[81] Long-term psychotherapy is not notably useful in treating other brain diseases, such as neurosyphilis or subdural hematoma.

In their attempt to prove that schizophrenia is a disease, psychiatrists have gone to desperate lengths. For example, the late Silvano Arieti, recognized as one of the foremost modern authorities on schizophrenia, offered this nonsense to support his claim:

> When we consider the impact of schizophrenia on the present generation (there are about 40 million schizophrenics in the world), we conclude that no war in history has produced so many victims, wounded so many people. No earthquake has exacted so high a toll; no condition that we know of has deprived so many young people of the promise of life.[82]

After a lifetime of studying schizophrenia, Arieti seems to have forgotten that life can be a threat as well as a promise, and not only for young people. How does Arieti establish that schizophrenia is a disease?

By asserting that *it* causes much suffering; by claiming that *it* is a disease characterized by "an alteration . . . in the way some cells function";[83] and by the fact that some critics of psychiatry deny that schizophrenia is an illness:

> Some people—unfortunately among them even a few professionals—insist that schizophrenia does not exist, that it is a myth, and they succeed in getting considerable attention from the public and from the press because of the sensational nature of their statements . . . . If we scratch the surface and search for the *unconscious reasons* for *denying the existence of what is obvious* and greatly disturbing, we eventually come to recognize that this *denial* is founded on a common and ancient prejudice toward mental illness . . . . The fear of mental illness . . . leads to its *denial*. The belief that, we, too, . . . may be wrongly labeled as schizophrenics, leads to its *denial*. The apprehension that we may be secretly suffering from this disorder, leads to its *denial* (emphasis added).[84]

Arieti was sincere about the literal reality of psychiatry's sacred symbol, and was duly rewarded for his faith by the keepers of the psychiatric keys. But sincerity is not necessarily a virtue. Assuredly, it is not a virtue when what the writer is sincere about is his firm belief that anyone who disagrees with him on a fundamental tenet of the psychiatric faith can be doing so only because he is insane. Many modern thinkers have faulted psychiatry and psychoanalysis for this debauchment of the rules of intellectual debate, but perhaps none severely enough. Isaiah Berlin, for example, although much troubled by this tactic, leans over backwards to excuse Freud for his role in promoting it and giving it a semblance of intellectual integrity. "Freud, too," writes Berlin, "contributed to this; not in his work of genius . . . but as the originator, however innocent, of the misapplication of rational psychological and social methods by muddle-headed men of good will and quacks and false prophets of every hue."[85] After thus making the obligatory gestures of deference to Freud, the mythic hero, Berlin articulates elegantly the ugliness exemplified by Arieti's previously quoted statement:

> It was left to the twentieth century to do something more drastic than this. For the first time it was now conceived that the most effective way of dealing with questions, particularly those recurrent issues which had perplexed and often tormented original and honest minds in every generation, was not by employing the tools of reason . . . but by obliterating the questions themselves . . . . Questions for whose solution no ready-made technique could easily be produced are all too easily classified as obsessions from which the patient must be cured.[86]

Like Arieti, most psychiatrists now believe that schizophrenia is a brain disease. Moreover, most of them now say this because they believe that scientists have *recently discovered* that what had been thought to be a functional illness is, in fact, an organic illness. This claim, too, is false. When we say that a person has an organic illness, what we mean is that there is something demonstrably wrong with his body: for example, when we say that a person is blind because of cataracts, we mean there is something wrong with his eyes; whereas when we say that a person is blind because of hysteria, we mean that there is nothing wrong with his eyes. The ambiguity in such statements is due to the fact that the term *blindness* may be used to describe complaints as well as the effects of somatic lesions. Because the term *schizophrenia* may also be used to describe strange behaviors as well as the (proven or putative) effects of somatic lesions, it is similarly ambiguous. Hence, asserting that "schizophrenia is a brain disease" is *choosing a particular definition for the term, not necessarily discovering a hitherto undetected brain lesion.*

To be sure, it is possible to discover hitherto unidentified brain lesions. But that can be done only on the brains of specific patients. If certain never-before-seen lesions were identified in the brains of mental patients and considered to be lesions specifically identifying schizophrenia, then, given the way schizophrenia is in fact diagnosed, it is certain that many schizophrenics would not have such lesions, and that many nonschizophrenics would. Would schizophrenics without schizophrenic lesions still be considered to be schizophrenic or psychotic or ill? Or, would they be considered to be suffering from another, still unidentified, mental illness? Or would they be considered to be mentally healthy?*

MAKING AND UNMAKING MENTAL ILLNESS

To understand what mental illness is, and also what it is not, it is necessary to ask, and to examine three closely interrelated questions: (1) How do psychiatrists arrive at, or generate, psychiatric diagnostic categories? (2) Why do they pay so much attention to classifying mental diseases? and (3) *Cui bono?* Who benefits (and who is harmed) by psychiatric classification and the idea of mental illness itself? I shall

---

*In this connection, note that a standard American text for primary care physicians emphasizes that one of the criteria *necessary* for diagnosing schizophrenia is the *"absence of signs of organic brain disease"* (emphasis in the original).[87] The cacophony of voices among establishment psychiatrists about the very subject matter of their discipline is an obvious symptom of the disorder whose anatomy I lay bare in this book.

address all three questions at length in the following chapters. Here I limit myself to a few observations about the APA's current role in psychiatric classification.

In November 1985, Robert Spitzer and his colleagues, charged with revising DSM-III, held the first of several meetings to consider three new mental diseases as possible additions to the existing list. The most important thing about these proceedings, a report in *Time* magazine cogently noted, "is that DSM-III is of crucial importance to the profession [because] . . . its diagnoses are generally recognized by the courts, hospitals, and insurance companies."[88]

Although the social consequences of psychiatric diagnoses have always been important, the situation regarding psychiatric taxonomy was quite different a century ago. Then, a single diagnosis was sufficient: a person was either insane, in which case he was incarcerated in a madhouse, or he was not, in which case he was left alone. The idea of insurance companies or government agencies paying privately practicing physicians to *give* psychotherapy to seemingly normal individuals would have been unthinkable—and not because what we now *call psychotherapy* did not exist.

Another feature that characterizes the way psychiatric diagnoses are now made and that differs from the way they were made a hundred years ago is equally revealing. Before identifying this difference, I want to anticipate what might occur to anyone reading this—namely, that because of great technological advances during the past century, all physicians use different methods for making diagnoses now than they did then. Of course! But psychiatrists had no technical methods for identifying *mental* diseases a century ago, and have none today. The change in their technique for generating new psychiatric categories is not technological, but political. A century ago—especially in German-speaking countries, from whence all of our major nineteenth century psychiatric diagnostic categories come—new psychiatric discoveries were made by *individuals*. For example, Ewald Hecker invented/discovered hebephrenia; Emil Kraepelin, dementia praecox; Eugen Bleuler, schizophrenia. No individual American today would dare to do such a thing: it would be unseemly to be so individualistic, so autocratic, so undemocratic. Ours is the age of psychiatric group-think: group therapy has long been a popular method of mental healing; now group invention/discovery, defined as diagnosis, has been added to it. The APA now has *task forces* and *consensus groups* to make and unmake psychiatric diagnostic categories. This is how, in 1973—under pressure from gay rights groups—homosexuality was deleted from the roster of mental illnesses.

No doubt anticipating problems with newly discovered mental

diseases like "paraphilic rapism" and "premenstrual syndrome," the psychiatrists invited several feminists and psychologists to their 1985 meeting. The proposal that rape is a disease so upset feminists—fearing that the diagnosis would provide an instant insanity defense for men who sexually assault women—that they threatened to sue.* So Spitzer backed down: "We probably will withdraw the diagnosis of rapism . . . ," he told *The New York Times.*[90] It would be laboring the obvious to dwell on the fact that Spitzer and his colleagues are acting like legislators introducing new bills in Congress and supporting or withdrawing them, depending on how the political winds blow. This is not the way real doctors act: Medical research on AIDS has provoked violent responses of outrage from African authorities who feel their countries are stigmatized by the high incidence of the disease among their people; but these protests have not prompted western AIDS researchers to withdraw their findings.

Moreover, according to the report in *Time* magazine, when the feminists threatened to sue over the invention/discovery of "masochism"—mainly afflicting women who stay in abusive marriages—the psychiatrists changed its name to "self-defeating personality disorder." This surprised the feminists, who did not expect the meeting to descend "into the usual picturesque result of successful lobbying: a bit of old-fashioned horse-trading."[91]

Psychiatrists have, indeed, come a long way from the autocratic-Teutonic days of Kraepelin and Bleuler, when solitary, male, psychiatric investigators staked their reputations on claiming to have discovered new diseases. Now we have psychiatric democracy or mobocracy—that is, psychopathology by a consensus of charlatans, with women meticulously included among the mischief-makers, with a stake in expanding the business. One of the invited psychologists—naively expecting something scientific to happen—complained: "The low level of intellectual effort was shocking. Diagnoses were developed by majority vote on the level we would use to choose a restaurant. You feel like Italian, I feel like Chinese, so let's go to a cafeteria. Then it's typed into a computer."[92] However, it does not seem to matter how openly political—

---

*In December 1985, the APA's Board of Trustees approved, by vote, Paraphilic Coercive Disorder as a new mental illness.[89] With this diagnosis, the APA has taken another giant step toward psychiatrizing crime, since Paraphilic Coercive Disorder is, in fact, the Association's term for rape and other violent crimes that males commit against females. But, crime is crime, whether the motive is economic, political, religious, or sexual. There is no distinction in law between committing murder to make money or to eliminate a sexual rival; I believe that there need be, and should be, no distinction between committing assault to gain revenge or to gain sexual gratification.

how obviously nonmedical and unscientific—are the ways and means by which psychiatrists create categories of mental illness: the medical and scientific community, as well as the lay public, continue to view psychiatry as a bona fide medical specialty and mental illness as bona fide illness. Carol Nadelson, the president of the APA (for 1985–1986), smugly asserts:

> Thanks to the use of DSM-III, the diagnosis of mental disorders is now generally as reliable as the diagnosis of physical ills. . . . Psychiatry has emerged as a mature medical specialty whose methods of diagnosis and treatment are guided by a rational scientific approach. Psychiatry has proved itself in the laboratory.[93]

Is that so?

Some Hidden Agendas of Classifying Mental Illnesses as Diseases

As we have seen, psychiatrists love to talk and write about *how* they classify mental diseases, but are considerably less eager to discuss *why* they do so—usually dismissing the latter question with some uplifting references to research and treatment. But the questions remain: Why do psychiatrists dwell so insistently on classification? Why do they periodically issue official documents—reminiscent of papal bulls—concerning formally recognized mental diseases? And why do they sometimes decide that previously recognized mental diseases are no longer diseases? No other medical specialists act this way. Only by observing these gross features of the psychiatric landscape—from an airplane flying overhead, as it were—will we be able to see the forest as a whole. Otherwise—if we enter the forest by foot—we will soon get lost, lurching from tree to tree, each stump demanding our complete attention with its heartrending tale of woe.

Why do we place persons, animals, and things in definitional categories or boxes? One important reason is to enable us to act. The division of foods into those that are edible or inedible—or, more precisely, into those God permits us to eat and prohibits us from eating—is a case in point. Here is a contemporary American example: Who is an American? There are at least three different answers to this question. One is: native-born citizens of the United States—since only they qualify for the office of the Presidency. Another—disregarding the exclusion specified in the Constitution as unimportant for most people—is: anyone who legally qualifies for citizenship—that is, native-born as well as naturalized citizens. Finally, in the opinion of some people—for example, clergymen demanding unrestricted immigration from Central and South America—the answer is: anyone who resides in, or wants to come to, the United States.

The question of which phenomena we should admit to citizenship in the land of medicine—that is, which phenomena we should recognize as bona fide diseases—poses a similar problem. The issue is not only or even primarily scientific, but practical and political. As some would benefit and others suffer from unrestricted immigration into the United States, so some people benefit and others suffer from elasticizing the definition of disease. To make matters more complicated, the people who benefit and suffer may be the same persons. It is important that we clearly understand this process as it applies both to disease and mental disease.

Let us call the box into which we place all officially recognized diseases DX (for diagnosis). Who profits from enlarging the number of items we put in this box? The persons who profit—not only economically but also existentially—are those who treat diseases and care for persons who have diseases. This is why physicians, especially psychiatrists, evangelize for the supposed benefits of viewing everything under the sun, from personal unhappiness to mass poverty, as a disease. Such persons act as if this perspective could yield only benefits through the compassionate treatment of victims by health care professionals and the generation of discoveries by research scientists.

But that is not true. There are some glaringly obvious costs associated with the medical-therapeutic perspective on life: one is economic, the other existential-political. I shall briefly describe each.

The Economic Consequences of Enlarging the Category DX

The economic consequences of what we place in category DX depend on the economic organization of society. In a purely individualistic-capitalistic society, it makes little difference what professional or governmental organizations classify as a disease. Since health care and medical research are paid for by private persons, the judgments of those economically uninvolved in these affairs are relatively unimportant. Private persons decide for what diseases (of their own, or of others) to seek treatment and at what cost, and what medical research they choose to support. Obviously we do not now live—nor have people ever lived—in this kind of society. I do not mention it because I believe that, medically, it would be the best of all possible societies (although it might be). I mention it only to set the stage for clarifying the implications of disease definitions in the kind of society in which we do live.

Today, regardless of where we live, we live in a society in which medical services—unlike liquor, cigarettes, or tickets to rock concerts— are not paid for by individuals out of their own pockets. In the United States, most of the money for health care comes from the government (federal and state) and from insurance companies (whose services are monitored by the government), and from a complex intermingling of these two sources. The definition of *disease*—as well as of *physician, patient, hospital,* and so forth—thus becomes a paramount factor in the calculations of third parties who hold the money bag: they are likely to pay for diseases that are in box DX, and will certainly not pay for those that are not in it.

As a result, nearly everyone is both helped and harmed. For example, physicians and other health care professionals—insofar as they are the beneficiaries of a mammoth medical-industrial complex—are helped; at the same time—insofar as they become the employees, slaves, or even scapegoats of the system—they are also harmed. Similarly, people in general—insofar as they are the beneficiaries of a system of health care free of direct cost to them—are helped; at the same time, people— insofar as they lose control over the definitions of disease and treatment and the terms of their relationship with their physicians—are also harmed. (In the end, the harm will far outweigh the help; but it will be too late to go back. Perhaps a new beginning will still be possible.)

The Existential Consequences of Enlarging the Category DX

As everyone now realizes, changes in health care policies in the United States during the past several decades have resulted in many physicians making economic gains but suffering existential losses. Insofar as the issue before us is the existential consequences of enlarging or constricting the category called *disease,* the following observations are relevant.

Inasmuch as pathologists study cells, tissues, and organs, they would lose much and gain nothing if they accepted conditions such as agoraphobia or kleptomania—not to mention masochism or terrorism—as bona fide diseases. Since they could never hope to find the cellular basis of these diseases, accepting them as bona fide diseases would only disfigure their own discipline. Similar considerations hold for all medical specialties, except psychiatry: No hematologist would claim diabetes as a blood disorder; no neurologist would claim prostatic hypertrophy as a neurological disease; no dermatologist would claim multiple sclerosis as a skin disease; and so on. But there is no disease— already known or not yet discovered—that psychiatrists do not claim as their own—that is, as a mental illness; or, if it is not a mental illness, then as a disease that is nevertheless relevant to psychiatry—because its *etiology* might be mental or emotional, or because it might respond favorably to *psychotherapy,* or because it might exhibit a significant *psychiatric overlay.* All this makes the relationship between various medical specialties and psychiatry absurdly lopsided—the psychiatrist cast simultaneously in the roles of grandiose therapist and impotent charlatan. A few examples, familiar to anyone acquainted with the contemporary medical scene, will illustrate what I mean.

There is no disease—acute or chronic, minor or major—into which psychiatrists do not now feel entitled to meddle; no patient—voluntary or involuntary—for whom they do not now claim to feel responsible. Here are some of the typical psychiatric rationalizations and justifications that make this possible: the patient with an acute life-threatening illness, like myocardial infarction, *denies* his illness; the patient with a chronic, debilitating illness, like lupus, is *depressed* by it; the patient with a minor illness, like basal cell carcinoma of the skin, *overreacts* to it; the patient with a major illness, like severe hypertension, *underreacts* to it; and so forth. No matter how a person—especially if he is already considered to be a patient—reacts, the psychiatrist can—and often does—interpret his behavior as a manifestation of mental illness, requiring the salvific interventions of the specialist in mental healing. In contrast, the dermatologist, hematologist, immunologist, oncologist, and other medical specialist does not view every mental illness—from agoraphobia to schizophrenia—as an opportunity for meddling or proving his importance.

The grandiosity of psychiatric claims reaches its climax in modern psychosomatic fantasies of the mental causes and cures of various bodily diseases. These claims are, of course, merely the recycling, in secularized garb, of age-old religious fantasies attributing the cause of bodily illness to misbehaviors, and its cure to miracles. Psychiatric research demonstrating that depression causes cancer illustrates the former type of claim; while the amazing anecdotes of Norman Cousins and other peddlers of bodily-health-through-mental-health illustrate the latter. These remarks should not be interpreted as meaning that I deny the influence of our personal life style and social circumstances on acquiring or overcoming certain diseases. On the contrary, I regard such a connection as self-evident: countless epidemiological and sociological studies illustrate its ubiquity. One of my favorite examples is the study reported in an article titled "Is an educated wife hazardous to your health?" The investigators answer their question with a resounding yes:

A significant risk of all-cause and ischemic heart disease death was seen in men whose wives were more educated than they, compared with men whose wives were less educated. The risk was the highest for the least educated men with the most educated wives. . . . These data support a causal role for status incongruity and fatal ischemic heart disease.[94]

To psychiatric imperialists, this proves the ubiquity of mental illness and the all-importance of psychiatry. To me it proves only that since psychiatry deals with life, and since disease and death are a part of life, psychiatrists, not surprisingly, address themselves to disease and death in all their diversity.

Actually, crisis intervention, liaison psychiatry, family therapy, suicide prevention, drug abuse counseling, grief therapy, and all the other variations on this tired theme add up to a rather ridiculous conclusion, namely, that under the psychiatrist's microscope, every speck of dirt looks like a pathogenic microorganism—with a sinister-sounding name to prove its dire disposition. It is a comic performance that is, however, no longer funny. The following witticism, said in jest about psychoanalysis in the 1930s, is now misinterpreted with absurd earnestness by psychiatrists and the public alike. The joke is this: If the patient arrives early for his appointment, he is anxious; if he arrives late, he is hostile; and if he is on time, he is compulsive. Mental illness *über Alles.*

This, then, is why—absurdly—the subclass called *mental illness* actually comprises more members than does the class called *disease,* of which it is itself supposed to be a member. The category called *mental illness* includes everything from Alzheimer's disease and brain injury to racism and terrorism, whereas the category called *disease* includes only somatic pathology. (See Figures 3.1 and 3.2.) This paradox is due neither to accident nor to error; instead, it is due to the elasticity of the category called *mental illness* (comprising fictitious diseases) and to the nonelasticity of the category called bodily illness (comprising hematologic, metabolic, infectious, and other diseases). Our capacity for describing phenomena is *limited* by our powers of observation; whereas our greed for practical advantage and a sense of control over others is *unlimited.* Barrows Dunham was not referring to psychiatric classification when he wrote the following, but he might just as well have been:

When you want to organize knowledge, therefore, you will be careful to base the classifications upon essential qualities. You will thus derive classes in which the members have the greatest amount of resemblance to one another and the greatest amount of difference from the members of other classes. But suppose that, instead of organizing knowledge, you set out to organize ignorance and prejudice. You will then do precisely the opposite. . . . You will keep the classification vague and flexible, so that it can be made to include just whatever individuals you choose.[95]

Finally, I want to reemphasize that since the legitimation of the patient role—that is, the official acceptance of a person as a patient with a bona fide disease—has similarly far-reaching practical consequences, the boundaries of category DX will also depend on what kinds of persons the official definers of disease want to credit or discredit as patients.* The legal consequences of occupying the mental patient role are, of course, especially important.

This brief overview of the economic and existential consequences of expanding the category of DX should make it clear that it is absurd to debate what is or is not a mental illness in medical or scientific terms. Science—in the sense of disinterested taxonomic description—has virtually nothing to do with the matter. In practice, the question is basically a consequential one: People agitate for or against enlarging the category of mental illness—for example, for or against counting masturbation, homosexuality, smoking, or rape as mental diseases—because they desire or detest the consequences.

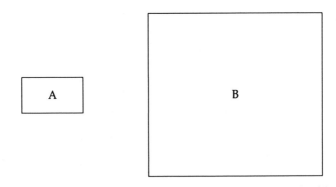

Figure 3.2. Mental illness as metaphoric disease. A = Illness (bodily disease). B = Mental illness (nondiseases called diseases and treated as if they were diseases).

---

*It is worth noting in this connection that American psychiatrists smugly dismiss, as pseudodiagnoses, certain mental illnesses popular among Soviet psychiatrists, such as *creeping schizophrenia*[96]—but feel deeply offended when similar skepticism is shown toward the products of American psychiatric manufactories, such as *oppositional disorder.*

MENTAL ILLNESS AND THE MEDICAL MODEL

In recent decades, the term *medical model,* ostensibly denoting a *medical* approach to *mental illness,* has gained wide currency. I consider this usage misleading, mainly because if mental illness is defined and accepted as an "illness like any other," it makes no more sense to adopt a nonmedical approach to it than it would to any other illness; on the other hand, if there is no such thing as mental illness—that is, if the phenomena so named are *not diseases*—then it makes no sense to adopt a medical approach to it. A reconsideration of paresis as the model of mental illness will help to clarify my argument.

The Paradigm of Paresis

The classic psychiatric model of mental illness has always been, and still is, general paresis (syphilis of the brain). This disease often first manifests itself by means of mental symptoms, such as depression, excitement, and paranoid thinking. Untreated, the disease progresses rapidly to mental deterioration, dementia, and death. In addition to mental symptoms, the patient also exhibits objective neurological signs, for example, an abnormal pupillary reflex. It is important to keep in mind that before 1909, when organic arsenic compounds were discovered to be moderately useful against syphilis, there was no treatment for the disease; and that the effective treatment of the syphilitic infection, and hence the prevention of paresis, did not become a reality until the discovery of penicillin. In the nineteenth century—indeed, prior to the First World War—paresis was characterized by a rapidly downhill course, usually ending in death, within a year or two.

When Bleuler invented/discovered schizophrenia, his model for it was paresis, and he said so:

> It is not yet clear just what sort of entity the concept of dementia praecox [schizophrenia] actually represents. It probably includes one or very few diseases, in the narrower sense, which constitute the major portion of cases, in the same way as general paresis embraces the majority of all cases of the *dementia paralytica* of the previous century.[97]

However, there is a curious paradox about paresis as the paradigm of the psychoses. The patient with *dementia paralytica*—which is what paresis was called in Kraepelin's day—exhibited objective neurological signs; the illness was characterized by a rapidly downhill course with an invariably fatal outcome; and at autopsy, the patient's brain showed easily identifiable morphological (structural) abnormalities. In contrast, the patient with dementia praecox—which is the name Kraepelin gave to what we call schizophrenia—exhibits no neurological signs; the illness is not characterized by a rapidly downhill course and is never fatal; and at autopsy, the patient's brain shows no identifiable morphological abnormalities. Some analogy.[98]

Ignoring these differences between paresis and schizophrenia, the early psychiatrists concentrated instead on two things: one was that both classes of patients acted crazy ("demented") or were called crazy by others; the other was their own so-called "clinical method," in reality only a euphemism for the psychiatrists' description of the behavior of persons locked up in insane asylums. By accepting such biased accounts as the manifestations of brain diseases—putative at the moment, proven as science progresses—psychiatry, as Mark Sedler writes, "rather suddenly found itself to be a bona fide medical science."[99] I shall summarize how this happened.

The first psychiatrist to describe what is now called "schizophrenia, disorganized type," was Ewald Hecker (1843–1909). Like all the early psychiatrists, Hecker "believed that the etiologies of the major psychoses were to be discovered through neuropathological investigations."[100] Psychiatrists, and now lay persons too, still believe this. But to believe something does not mean that it is true. Indeed, doubt about this belief must have arisen because of the important differences between paresis and the other psychoses which I just mentioned. The suspicion that such doubt arose is supported by Hecker's following remarks in his original paper on hebephrenia written in 1871:

> The final proof that hebephrenia is a unified form of mental illness in its own right can, of course, be established *only on anatomico-pathological grounds.* But, because of the still provisional character of our knowledge of brain anatomy, *we must renounce this proof,* possibly for a long time to come. This is all the more likely given that our patients generally *live to a ripe old age* (emphasis added).[101]

I submit that a brain disease so severe as to cause a rapidly progressive and virtually complete "dementia" (as the early psychiatrists saw it), but nevertheless compatible with a long and physically healthy life, is, *prima facie,* highly improbable, if not impossible. This, too, must have occurred to nineteenth century psychiatrists, for Hecker remarks that "hebephrenic patients are often accused of malingering," an accusation he dismisses as absurd.

It seems clear that the discipline of psychiatry was made possible by the general acceptance of the proposition that it is not necessary to demonstrate that a patient has a brain disease in order to gain credence for the claim of having discovered one; it is enough to postulate it, and to claim that the "clinical method" enables the specialist in mental diseases to diagnose it. What is this clinical method? It is, according to Hecker, "the necessary conjunction of a phenomenological method, a longitudinal perspective, and a commitment to the project of identifying discrete disease forms."[102] And here, once more, is Sedler eulogizing Hecker for this achievement:

> Hecker's concept of hebephrenia . . . constituted a reliable and highly specific *nosological instrument* that enabled subsequent investigators to focus their medical perceptions on a clinically homogeneous population with a characteristic symptom complex and a predictable course. . . . Taking *general paresis* as the standard example of a separate and distinct entity, he argued that hebephrenia is similarly unique . . . [partly] in consequence of its early onset and deteriorating course (emphasis added).[103]

Again, we witness the psychiatric observer leaving the well-trodden path of proving brain disease and instead spinning metaphors: *nosological instrument, focusing, symptom complex, deteriorating course* — metaphors all, each substituting psychiatric prejudice for critical thinking and scientific investigation. (For a discussion of metaphors, see Chapter 5.)

The Neurology of Mental Illness: A Case Study

Although the authors of DSM-III reject pathoanatomical or pathophysiological lesion as the cardinal criterion of mental illness, psychiatric researchers continue to concentrate their efforts on attempts to discover the somatic basis of psychiatric disorders. Typical of such studies is a report by E. D. Ross and A. J. Rush on "the neurology of depression."

According to these authors, "A major problem confronting both neurology and psychiatry is to define the neuroanatomical basis of psychiatric disorders."[104] But if the neuroanatomical basis of psychiatric disorders is as irrelevant to the definition of mental illness as psychiatrists now claim, why is its discovery so important? In order to establish depression as a disease of the brain rather than of the mind, Ross and Rush detach the experience (symptom) of feeling depressed from the putative underlying disease. Brain-damaged patients with depression, they tell us, "actually may deny being depressed or dysphoric."[105] In other words, even though these persons are not depressed and do not seem depressed to those around them, they nevertheless *are* depressed. But this is not the way psychiatrists interpret the therapeutic effects of lobotomy on intractable pain: When the patient ceases to complain of pain after such a procedure, the physicians do not say that he still has pain but denies it; on the contrary, they say that the patient has been relieved of his pain. The linguistic and logical tour de force implicit in asserting that persons who are *not depressed* suffer from *depression* thus deserves a brief comment.

Depression is the name we give to a particular affective experience, our own or someone else's. Consider, then, the case of a person who does not feel depressed and whom, because he does not seem or act depressed, no one else considers to be depressed. Comes now the modern psychiatrist who says: "You are wrong, this man is depressed. I know because I have found that he *has* the clinicopathological correlates of depression." Without examining the validity or the invalidity of this claim, it seems to me reasonable to ask: When a psychiatrist who writes this way uses the word *depression*, does he mean the same thing people ordinarily mean when they say, for example, about someone who has just suffered a personal loss, that *he is depressed?* I think not. I submit that, once again, instead of discovering an illness—as do the medical researchers who describe the pathology of AIDS and discover the virus that causes it—psychiatric researchers merely continue to announce a program intended to demonstrate "that depression is primarily a disorder of the brain." To be sure, if psychiatric researchers find something wrong with a particular person's brain, then they have demonstrated that the person has a brain disease; but if the person in question is not depressed, then the researchers have, in my opinion, not discovered depression without symptoms of depression—or, as they claim, asymptomatic depression as a discrete brain disease—but have only changed the meaning we usually attach to the word *depression*.

If the history of psychiatry were a film played continuously in a movie theater, we might now say, "This is where we came in," and get up and leave. Almost 200 years have passed since psychiatrists have seriously begun to advance the claim that mental diseases are brain diseases. And that is exactly what they are still doing. "The article," Ross and Rush conclude, "presents an initial inquiry into the neurology of depression utilizing the technique of the clinicopathological correlations . . . . This in turn should establish firmly that depression is primarily a disorder of the brain and not simply a dysfunction of the 'mind'".[106] Surely, this is a grandiose conclusion from the evidence at hand. However, because people want to believe this, the claim seems credible. Thus, although psychiatrists still give us only a program for proving that mental illness is a brain disease—instead of proof—the scientific community and the public accept the program as proof more eagerly than ever before.

The Somatic Model of Mental Illness: Medical or Pediatric?

When a speaker or writer on psychiatric matters uses the phrase *medical model*, he usually means or implies two things: first, that mental illness *is* an illness; second, that we *ought to* treat it *as if* it were an illness. Neither proposition is novel. Why, then, did the fresh phrase *medical model* become so fashionable? And why do I say that it is misleading? Here, briefly, are the reasons why.

Supporters of the medical model—typically psychiatrists—act as if they believed that if they could convince mental patients, their families, and, above all, politicians, that persons called *mental patients* are truly sick, then they could treat them for their illness, regardless of whether or not the patients want to be treated. But such psychiatrists act not like internists but like pediatricians, who must convince parents that their child is sick before they can treat the child—and having convinced the parents, can treat the child regardless of whether or not the child wants to be treated.

Similarly, the opponents of the medical model—typically antipsychiatrists—act as if they believed that if they could convince mental patients, their families, and above all, politicians, that the persons called *mental patients* are not really sick, then they could prevent psychiatrists from treating them, regardless of whether or not the patients want to be treated. In short, they, too, act like pediatricians, who, if they can convince parents that their child is not sick, can prevent the child from being treated, whether or not the child wants to be treated.

These observations illustrate that both psychiatry and antipsychiatry rest on a coercive pediatric model characterized by relations of domination and subjection, rather than on a noncoercive medical model of respect for persons characterized by relations of mutual cooperation and contract.

MENTAL ILLNESS AS A CLAIM

Before concluding this survey of what counts as mental illness, I want to offer some brief remarks on one of the most interesting differences between bodily illness and mental illness, namely, that while the former may be asymptomatic, the latter cannot be. The notion of an asymptomatic mental illness is a self-contradiction.

Symptoms, Signs, Illness

Physicians as well as sophisticated lay people distinguish between two basically different kinds of manifestations of, or clues to, illness: subjective symptoms, such as fatigue or pain; and objective signs, such as elevated blood pressure or cellular abnormality in a biopsy or blood smear. This distinction corresponds to the distinction physicians make between bodily illness and mental illness: The former diagnosis (strictly interpreted) requires the presence of abnormal signs; the latter does not. Indeed, when confronted with a difficult diagnostic problem, physicians follow a procedure revealingly called "ruling out organic disease": if no bodily disease can be demonstrated, a diagnosis of mental disease is usually made.

With the distinction between symptom and sign—or complaint and lesion—firmly in mind, let us look at the similarities and differences between bodily illnesses and mental illnesses. It is obvious that bodily illnesses may, and often do, cause discomfort, pain, and suffering. It is equally obvious, however, that bodily illnesses may not cause any symptoms at all: they may, in other words, be asymptomatic. How do we know that a person has an asymptomatic disease? By the signs the disease produces. Especially in their early or latent stages, many diseases are, or may be, completely asymptomatic, for example, diabetes, leukemia, hypertension, malaria, malignant melanoma, syphilis. In short, an illness may manifest itself in two ways, by symptoms and signs, and may accordingly be identified in two ways, from symptoms and signs. (Since in medical discourse symptoms point to signs, or lesions, diagnoses of bodily diseases ultimately rest on the identification of signs or lesions.)

The situation with respect to mental illness is radically different. Why? Quite simply because mental diseases manifest themselves in only one way, by symptoms, and can accordingly be identified in only one way, from symptoms. It is important to note, in this connection, that the authors of DSM-III are either confused about, or want to obliterate, the crucial distinction between sign and symptom, as their following statement shows. After emphasizing that their approach to classifying mental disorders is "descriptive in that the definitions of the disorders generally consist of descriptions of the clinical features of the disorders," they add that "the characteristic features [of the disorders] consist of easily identifiable behavioral *signs or symptoms*, such as disorientation, mood disturbance, or psychomotor agitation" (emphasis added).[107] There is, however, no such thing as a "behavioral sign": the items the authors so designate are simply behaviors described in psychiatric jargon rather than in plain English.

To put the matter simply and succinctly, there are, and can be, only symptomatic mental illnesses; an asymptomatic mental illness is an oxymoron. How could a person who does not gamble suffer from pathological gambling? Or a person who does not drink alcohol suffer from alcoholism? Or a person who is never manic suffer from mania? Ironically, this fundamental conceptual identity between mental illness and mental symptom is tacitly acknowledged by the authors of DSM-III in their characterization of what counts (for them) as a mental disorder: "In DSM-III each of the mental disorders is conceptualized as a clinically significant behavioral and psychological syndrome or pattern that occurs in an individual and that is typically associated with either a painful symptom (distress) or impairment in one or more important areas of functioning (disability)."[108] Judged by these criteria, there can, in the absence of distress or disability, be no mental illness. Since it is obvious that this is not true for bodily illness—diseases such as asymptomatic and undiagnosed hypertension or coronary atherosclerosis immediately spring to mind—it is difficult to see how psychiatrists can, in good faith, maintain that mental illness is like any other illness.

By treating symptoms and signs as two independent variables, I have summarized in Table 3.2 the four combinations to which they give rise, namely: symptomatic and asymptomatic bodily illness, symptomatic mental illness, and no illness. Asymptomatic mental illness does not appear in this table for the simple reason that such a disease would have to be either a bodily disease (for example, schizophrenia defined as a chemical abnormality of brain function*), or a mental disease whose diagnosis is based on past symptoms or behavioral abnormalities (for example, a history of drinking or of depressed behavior). What I say here is not intended to minimize the practical importance of past behaviors. After all, if a person spoke French fluently a week ago, it is likely that he may do so again; the same is obviously true for the behaviors we call alcoholism, depression, or pathological gambling. Repetitive behavior is, however, still just behavior, notwithstanding the efforts of psychiatrists to interpret it as a sign of somatic pathology.

---

*If the claim that schizophrenia is a brain disease, exhibiting chemically demonstratable abnormalities, is true, then, in that sense, schizophrenia is a brain disease; such a disease could, of course, be latent. The postulated analogy between paresis and schizophrenia would then be fulfilled.

TABLE 3.2. **Bodily Illness and Mental Illness: Signs and Symptoms**

Sign	Symptom	Condition
+	+	Symptomatic bodily illness
+	–	Asymptomatic bodily illness
–	+	Symptomatic mental illness (May be mistaken for undetected and possibly as yet undetectable bodily illness and vice versa)
–	–	No (detectable) illness

In their zeal to imitate physicians, psychiatrists have, of course, constructed asymptomatic mental illnesses: the most characteristic member of this class is—or, better, was—*latent* homosexuality. We must say *was* because even overt homosexuality is now no longer considered to be a mental illness.* Revealingly, it was Freud and the psychoanalysts who created this doubly metaphoric mental illness—that is, an illness that consists not merely of disapproved desire or behavior, but of desire or behavior assiduously resisted or avoided by the subject who supposedly suffers from it.

Symptoms: Literal and Metaphorical

Our efforts to understand bodily illness and mental illness are hampered—indeed paralyzed—by a fundamental misunderstanding of the nature of symptoms and signs: they are not two similar manifestations of disease, as commonly believed; instead, they are two radically different phenomena. Symptoms are verbal communications or claims; signs are objective measurements of bodily structures or functions, or publicly verifiable observations about the body (not about how a person feels about his body). This is the reason why bodily illness is typically diagnosed when—and because—a person exhibits a physical-chemical abnormality in the structure of his body: for example, bleeding, jaundice, a fractured bone (visible to the naked eye or by x-ray), fever, high blood pressure. Mental illness, on the other hand, is typically diagnosed when—and because—a person makes certain claims about the behavior of a person (himself or others) considered to be a *designated patient.* (A person's nonverbal behavior may of course also be evidence for or against mental illness: for example, a person who kills a group of

---

*In 1973, the APA abolished homosexuality as a mental illness, unless the subject wants to assume the patient role, in which case *it,* again, becomes an illness.[109]

people he does not know is now likely to be characterized, on the basis of his behavior alone, as mentally ill. I shall say more about this presently.)

Since the act of lodging a claim is intrinsic to the origin and nature of the phenomena we call mental illnesses, but is irrelevant to the origin and nature of the phenomena we call bodily illnesses, it is remarkable that this distinction has been so neglected not only by psychiatrists but also by philosophers (who often make reference to mental illness). To put it simply, bodily disease can be, but mental illness can never be, discovered and diagnosed without any claims of illness being lodged either by or about the patient. For example, a person undergoing a routine medical examination for admission to college or entrance into the armed forces may be discovered, on the basis of blood or urine tests, to have diabetes or leukemia. Before the testing, neither the subject nor anyone else claims that he is ill. Yet it is discovered that he is ill. Clearly, it is not possible to discover mental illness in a similar way. Why not? The answer to this question further highlights the linguistic problems hidden behind the phenomena we now call mental illnesses.

The reasons for the distinctions between bodily illness and mental illness lie in part in the different ways we use and interpret the word *symptom* in medicine (in reference to bodily illness) and in psychiatry (in reference to mental illness). An example will clarify what I have in mind. Suppose a middle-aged man complains of precordial pain. That is a symptom. What does it mean? To the patient it might mean that he has coronary artery disease. But it does not mean that to a good doctor. To the physician, the patient's precordial pain is a clue pointing to something unknown: it might be coronary artery disease, or gall bladder disease, or arthritis, or the fear of heart disease, or none of the above. The word *symptom* here is used literally: it means that it may be the manifestation of some pathological process in the body (disease).

In psychiatry, not only is the word *illness* used metaphorically and interpreted literally, but so also is the word *symptom*. This is crystal clear from the way we use what we call the two *classic symptoms of psychosis*, namely *hallucinations* and *delusions*. For example, unlike precordial pain, which may or may not point to coronary insufficiency, hallucinations and delusions *do not point* to psychosis; they *are* (the same as) psychosis. If a psychiatrist acknowledges or recognizes that Jones is having hallucinations and delusions, he has no choice but to conclude that Jones is psychotic. The reason for this lies in the *prejudgments* that words such as *hallucination* and *delusion* carry with them.

Consider some simple examples. When a lonely, deinstitutionalized ex-mental patient populates his world with imaginary persons who talk to him, we say that "he is hearing nonexistent voices" and is "hallucinating." But when Beethoven hears melodious sounds in his head, we do not say that "he is hearing (nonexistent) music" and is "hallucinating."* Similar considerations apply to the false ideas of religious leaders, which we do not call *delusions* (unless we want to delegitimize them and those who hold them); but we do call the false ideas of mental patients *delusions.*

Here is another, less abstract example illustrating the role of language and power in determining what is a mental symptom/mental illness. Johnny, a high school student, acts distracted, neglects his studies, and makes it otherwise clear by word and deed that he is quite smitten by his girlfriend. The father reassures his wife: "Don't worry, Johnny is just showing symptoms of being in love." Everyone treats the word *symptom* in this sentence as a metaphor (even persons who do not know what a metaphor is). However, with only a slight change in the scenario, the situation might be very different. Johnny, now in college, gets poor grades, drops out of school, comes home, mopes around the house, acts taciturn and withdrawn, refuses to look for a job or help around the house, and perhaps makes some veiled threats about killing himself. The mother tells her husband: "I am worried about Johnny showing symptoms of schizophrenia." Everyone treats the word *symptom* in this sentence as if it were a literal use of the term—that is, as if it pointed, possibly or probably, to the existence of a real disease. Suppose, further, that—more or less against his will—Johnny is carted off to a psychiatrist. The psychiatrist examines him, obstensibly to determine whether or not he is mentally ill. Insofar as the psychiatrist's examination is directed to answering this question, it is bound to be a charade. How can any psychiatrist worth his salt conclude that Johnny, exhibiting such behaviors, is not mentally ill? Clearly, unless the report about Johnny's behavior is false, the psychiatrist has no choice but to find mental illness: his options are limited to finding one or another mental illness, a relatively benign one or a very malignant one. The reason for this is that, in psychiatry, mental symptom equals mental illness, an equation quite undisguised in so-called extreme cases.

For another example, suppose that, in a rural area, neighbors summon the police to complain about offensive odors emanating from a

---

*"You may ask me where I obtain my ideas," wrote Beethoven. "I cannot answer this with any certainty: they come unevoked . . . turn . . . into tones . . . which resound, roar, and rage until at last they stand before me in the form of notes."[110]

ramshackle house inhibited by a recluse and his old mother. The police go to investigate. They find a middle-aged man in tatters, malnourished, with a multitude of cats and dogs in a filthy house and with the man's aged mother dead in bed. When asked what happened, the man tells the police he had to strangle his mother because she complained of being in pain and God told him he must help her. Who would doubt that the man is mentally ill? What are the symptoms of his illness? The very behavior I have described. Whether the problem is this hypothetical man's behavior, or the behavior of any other person committing a bizarre crime—John Hinckley, Jr. is a good example—the mere idea of asking for an explanation of what happened makes the ordinary person impatient. He already *knows* what happened: "Only a crazy person would do such a crazy thing." Crazy act equals mental symptom; mental symptom equals mental illness. Mental symptom *does not point* to a possible illness; *it is* (the same as) a mental illness.*

Mental Illness as Religious Symbol

In this chapter I have begun to sketch the outlines of the idea of mental illness. By the time the reader comes to the end of the book, I hope I will have succeeded in painting a life-sized portrait of it. One important feature of this concept is, however, already clear, namely, that mental illness is an idea without boundaries: it blends into everything around it. First and foremost, mental illness blends into medicine. Then it blends into history, politics, education, law, criminology, sociology, art criticism, literature, mythology, religion—everything except the hard sciences. And therein lies an observation I want to offer before ending this chapter.

I have long argued that there are important parallels between religion and psychiatry, a theme I do not want to belabor here.[111] However, the absence of a clear boundary between mental illness and everyday life warrants a brief restatement of my core argument—namely, that the ideas of mental health and mental illness have replaced the idea of God and the Devil, and that the institutionally legitimized explanations, justifications, and interventions of psychiatry have replaced those of organized religion. "During the Middle

---

*It may be objected that certain symptoms suggestive of bodily illness may also be pathognomonic, for example, the classic symptoms of angina pectoris: in such cases objective tests may still confirm or disconfirm the diagnosis. However, in the cases characterized by the syllogism "Only a crazy person would do such a crazy thing," there is nothing to confirm or disconfirm: the conclusion is self-evident and is felt not to require further proof.

Ages," James Turner observes, "no clear lines separated the religious from the secular. . . . The church and the world blended."[112] Today, no clear lines separate the psychiatric from the nonpsychiatric: the explanations, justifications, and interventions of psychiatry permeate the world and blend with it.*

---

*Despite the dramatic growth of (nonpsychiatric) medicine in our age, there is a clear boundary between it and the world: hematology and the world do not blend; oncology and the world do not blend; neurology and the world do not blend. Only psychiatry and the world blend.

4

BEING A MENTAL PATIENT

Admission to hospital often takes place against the will of the patient and therefore the psychiatrist finds himself in a different relationship to his patient than other doctors. He tries to make the difference as negligible as possible by deliberately emphasizing his purely medical approach to the patient . . . .

—*Karl Jaspers*[1]

Who are mental patients? How is this class of persons defined and identified? How does a person become a mental patient and how do such patients differ, if at all, from other, nonpsychiatric, patients? These questions, and the answers usually given to them, will be my subject in this chapter.

I should like to begin by anticipating an objection that might be raised at this point against my argument. "If you do not believe in mental illness," the reader might want to say to me, "how can you speak of mental patients? Shouldn't you also disbelieve in the existence of mental patients? Aren't you contradicting yourself?" The answer is no,. and it is important that we clearly see why.

Atheists do not believe in God. Such disbelief in the existence of a deity does not mean that atheists do not recognize the existence of priests and worshippers. Clearly, the existence of God is not a fact in the sense that the existence of persons preaching about or praying to

God is a fact. Similarly, my disbelief in mental illness does not mean that I do not recognize the existence of psychiatrists and mental patients. It is precisely because supernatural beings and mental diseases are abstract or imaginary constructs, without material existence, that their existence is claimed or inferred, in a circular fashion, from the existence and belief of priests and worshippers, of psychiatrists and mental patients.

However, it would be a mistake to believe that the existence of St. Peter's Cathedral in Rome proves that Jesus is the Son of God, or that the existence of the National Institute of Mental Health in Bethesda proves that mental illness exists—although this has, more than once, been seriously suggested to me by people listening to me lecture on the myth of mental illness. In short, although mental illness may not exist, mental patients do. Who, then, are they? What is wrong with them? Why are they considered to be *ill* and why *mentally?*

BECOMING A MENTAL PATIENT

Psychiatrists rarely consider the question of how a person becomes a mental patient, and when they do, their answers are likely to be wrong. For example, Jack Ewalt and Dana Farnsworth, both professors of psychiatry at Harvard, write:

> A person thus becomes a patient when his capacity to compensate for all the unfavorable factors in his emotional environment breaks down, and he is unwillingly or unknowingly impelled to indulge in behavior which is unacceptable to himself or those with whom he is associated or comes in contact.[2]

It is not true, however, that a person becomes a patient *when* there is a change in his capacity to cope, or *because* he unwillingly or unknowingly misbehaves. The truth is that a person becomes a patient when he defines himself, or when others define him, as a patient, and when that definition is formally or officially supported as legitimate or valid. Specifically, for a person to become a psychiatric patient, two circumstances must come together: (1) an individual must make certain claims about himself or others must make certain claims about him—that is, he must designate himself or be designated by others as mentally ill; (2) a psychiatrist or judge must concur with this claim—that is, he must diagnose or validate the designated person as mentally ill. When this process has run its course, the product is the social phenomenon called a *mental patient* or, more accurately, a *designated mental patient.*

The Mental Patient: Voluntary or Involuntary?

Persons assume, or are assigned to, the role of mental patient in several ways. Some come from among persons identified in Table 2.1, Row 3. Typically such an individual seeks out a physician with what he, the patient, believes or claims to be the symptoms of a medical disease; the physician examines him but can find nothing wrong. If the patient persists in making demands on his doctor, and if the doctor grows tired of his demands, then the doctor is likely to refer the patient to a psychiatrist. It is estimated that 60, 70, or even 80 percent of patients seen by general practitioners and family physicians have no demonstrable bodily illness. Many of these persons are recruited into, and join the ranks of, mental patients.

Another group of mental patients is comprised of persons who seek out psychiatrists on their own initiative for the help they hope to obtain from them. Although these patients are physically healthy—or, if not, their diseases are considered to be unrelated to their complaints—they want some sort of psychiatric help and willingly cooperate with a variety of so-called psychiatric treatments, psychological as well as physical. Insofar as a person assumes the role of mental patient voluntarily, his situation resembles that of any other client seeking professional help. The clients of architects, attorneys, accountants, and physicians differ in terms of the sorts of service each seeks, but are similar in that each is free to initiate and terminate his relationship with the expert who, as the saying goes, is on tap, not on top. However, it is precisely with respect to the ability or power to control the expert-client relationship that the situation of the mental patient typically differs from that of the medical patient. To understand this difference we have to consider the history of psychiatry as well as the connection among the ideas of insanity, incompetence, and irresponsibility.

Medicine, Psychiatry, and Self-Ownership

With the exception of psychiatry, the practice of modern Western medicine is premised on the principle of the self-ownership of adults. Typically, doctors and patients are free to reject each other: in other words, each must *consent* to the relationship—the doctor to providing medical care, the patient to receiving it. Diagnostic and therapeutic interventions are *medically legitimate* because they are scientifically prudent, and *legally legitimate* because the patient consents to them. (See Table 4.1.)

This fundamental political principle of self-ownership—which undergirds not only medical but also economic and legal relations in free societies—was nearly fully articulated by Aristotle. According to it, a

TABLE 4.1. Illness and Consent: The Politics of Medical Intervention

(Bodily) Disease	(Patient) Consent	Nature and Name of Medical Intervention
+	+	Medical intervention in the presence of disease with the sane subject's consent: conventional treatment of injuries, infections, tumors, etc.; literal treatment.
+	−	Medical intervention in the presence of disease without the sane subject's consent; medically: treatment without consent; legally: assault and battery.
−	+	Medical or psychiatric intervention in the absence of disease with the sane subject's consent: abortion, voluntary psychiatric interventions, etc.; metaphoric treatment (not treatment; "help").
−	−	Medical intervention in the absence of disease without the subject's consent: involuntary psychiatric interventions; (not treatment: social control; punishment; torture).

person owns himself, body and soul, and has the right to use himself as he deems fit, so long as he does not injure others. (Aristotle's only reservations to this principle were with respect to suicide and slavery: he considered suicide to be a violation of man's obligations to the State and slavery to be the "natural condition" of the slave.) Defining a *voluntary agent* as "one who knows both the person he is affecting by his action and the instrument he is using," Aristotle concluded that "it is not possible to treat oneself unjustly. . . . no one can commit adultery with his own wife or housebreaking on his own house or theft on his own property."[3]

It is this principle that has led to the adoption of the legal rule that no one—*except infants, idiots, and the insane*—ought to be medically diagnosed or treated without his consent. (I am stating this in the classic idiom of English law dating from a time when a man was regarded as insane only if he was like a *wild beast*.)[4] There are two ways in which major departures from this principle may be rationalized and justified.

One way is to expand the class constituting exceptions to the rule, typically by treating certain persons—for example, women, criminals, blacks, mental patients—*as if* they were children. This, of course, is called *paternalism*, and I shall say more about it presently.

The other way out of the political constraints of self-ownership is to reject the principle altogether—or to qualify it with strong claims of co-ownership, as it were—in favor of possession by other parties, such as God or the State. For example, if God owns the body and wishes it to be inviolate to human prying, then dissection will be considered a crime. This perspective is by no means extinct today; those who do not share it, call it *religious fundamentalism*. Similarly, if the State owns the body, then the drugs legislators condone will be considered licit and therapeutic, whereas those they condemn will be considered illicit and pathogenic, and suicide will be illegal not because it is an affront against the Rules of God but because it is an affront against the Rules of Health. Many years ago I proposed the term *Therapeutic State* for the political system generated by and embodying this principle.[5]

Ironically, many of our contemporary medical and psychiatric dilemmas arise from the fact that the more physicians are recognized as experts on health, the more power they are given to determine the social behavior of sick persons. Chemists know how to distinguish gold from other elements better than ordinary people, but the State gives them no power over the conduct of persons possessing gold. However, supposedly because psychiatrists know how to distinguish sick minds from healthy minds better than ordinary people, the State gives them power over the conduct of persons allegedly possessing sick minds. The following statement by Norman Fowler, British Secretary of State for Social Services, is sadly revealing. "I think that schizophrenia is a medical illness," Fowler told *The Times* (London), "and patients should have whatever treatment *the doctors think necessary*" (emphasis added).[6] Well, arthritis and atherosclerosis are also medical diseases. Does Fowler propose that patients no longer be permitted to reject being treated for these diseases? If this is how the second-highest ranking British politician in charge of health policies thinks and talks, can we expect anything else but a further strengthening of the powers of a centralized-medicalized Therapeutic State?

Like marriage, the relationship between psychiatrist and patient involves two persons. Accordingly, it is the combination of the former's penchant for paternalism with the latter's desire for dependency that creates the relationship that ultimately develops between them. The truth is that not only are many psychiatrists not interested in a reciprocal type of relationship with their patients, but many mental patients are not interested in such a relationship either. Whether we like to or not, what characterizes many psychiatric patients and situations is precisely that they are coercive: schizophrenic self-disregard, agitated depression, threats of injury to self or others are intensely coercive communications. Indeed, in the interview in *The Times* from which I just quoted, a typical problem presented by schizophrenic patients was seen as this: "Have you [the interviewer asks Fowler] any other ways you can help for example widowed mothers living in terror of being attacked physically by very strong sons . . ?" Some *illness.* "I have no blanket solution for that," replies Fowler.[7] Thomas Hobbes would have had a solution for it. When Britain was the cradle of Western liberties, its leaders knew that crime was not a disease, and that disease was not a crime.

Obviously, anyone who interacts with a violent person—especially if he chooses to do so, and if the violent person is called a *mental patient* or a *schizophrenic*—finds himself in a situation where he is expected to *do something.* The superior person—family member, psychiatrist, policeman—placed in such a position has essentially three options: (1) He can countercoerce, for example, by committing the patient as psychotic; (2) he can allow himself to be coerced, for example, by catering to the demands of the patient; or, (3) he can escape from the field, for example, by severing the relationship with the coercing person (or he can take care and not enter the field in the first place).

Medicine and Psychiatry: Becoming a Patient and Becoming a Mental Patient

Medicine originates from the facts of injury and illness, the discomfort and disability they cause, and the search for relief they generate. Persons become medical patients because they suffer, seek relief from their suffering, and turn for relief to experts whom they endow, rightly or wrongly, with the power of healing. In short, medical practice originates from below, from the patient—and medicine is as old as mankind. Moreover, the feature of voluntariness is crucial to being a medical patient: Indeed, it is so basic that we take it for granted. Unless unconscious, a person typically enters a hospital by checking in, much as he enters a hotel; and he can, of course, check out whenever he wishes. There is no legal mechanism for forcing a person to enter a hospital, or remain there, against his will. (Unconscious persons are regarded as having given tacit consent to being patients.)

Unlike medicine, psychiatry originates from the facts of deviant and disturbing behavior (sometimes caused by brain disease), the discomfort and distress such behavior causes others, and the search for the control of the disturbing behaviors and persons by those disturbed. Persons thus become psychiatric patients because they make others suffer, because those they make suffer seek relief from their discomfort, and because these sufferers turn for relief to experts whom they endow, rightly or wrongly, with the power to restrain and treat the offending person who is designated as mentally ill. In short, psychiatric practice originates from above, from those having power over the patient—and psychiatry is only as old as is this particular social arrangement for controlling those who burden or offend others.

Historically, psychiatry is synonymous with involuntary and institutional psychiatry: originally all mental patients were *involuntary patients incarcerated in mental institutions*. This arrangement prevailed from the first invention of madhouses in the seventeenth century, until the early part of the twentieth century. As recently as the early 1940s, when I was a medical student in Cincinnati, a person could not be a voluntary patient in an Ohio state mental hospital. That arrangement was consistent with the view that madness or insanity—now called severe mental illness or psychosis—is a condition characterized by a loss of competence or rationality. "It is the nature of psychiatry," write Albert Jonsen and Burr Eichelman, two medical ethicists, "to work with patients who suffer from impaired perceptions of themselves and the world. It is an impairment of the 'consenting organ' itself which is being treated."[8] The authors go on to observe that:

> Of course, this has always been the condition of psychiatry: its patients have always been the troubled, the confused, the deranged. . . . [As a result, psychiatric treatments] such as commitment, the shock therapies, and psychosurgery . . . were often imposed on the supposedly incompetent . . . .[9]

It is important to reemphasize that the medical patient has typically been presumed to be competent, whereas the mental patient has typically been presumed to be incompetent. Competence is one of those troublesome concepts that combines an observer's subjective judgment with an objective condition supposedly exhibited by the subject. In actual use, such concepts are bound to be corrupted by the self-interests and prejudices of the judging parties. For centuries it was taken for granted, and it is still widely believed, that an insane person is irrational and legally incompetent. The range of this incompetence varies, but typically includes such things as looking after one's own best interests, executing binding contracts, being responsible for the crimes one commits, and standing trial. These remarks—on which I shall expand later (see Chapters 8–11)—are intended to remind the reader that although incompetence and insanity are not purely medical concepts, or perhaps are not medical concepts at all, modern societies use physicians, and physicians use these concepts, to implement mental health laws. Thus, while experts on forensic psychiatry often disclaim insanity and mental disease as medical concepts, legislators deputize doctors to enforce laws based on these very concepts. For example, Herbert Fingarette, who writes frequently on forensic psychiatry, states:

> In our earlier examination of the notion of mental disease, we saw that it is not a medical concept. That is, it is in fact not defined by current medical doctrine, could not even in theory have any systematic role within purely medical doctrine, and moreover is now increasingly recognized by the courts as a legal rather than a medical concept.[10]

Notwithstanding many similar assertions in the legal literature, physicians are legally authorized to commit a person to a mental hospital, detain him there as a patient, and treat him for his mental disease against his will. Thus, under the 1959 British Mental Health Act, "any qualified medical practicner . . . can sign an emergency order. No expertise in psychiatry is required."[11] Perhaps because insanity has, in fact, no medical meaning, many mental health laws require that not one but two doctors sign the commitment papers—presumably in order that one could act as a corrective to the other, but actually to strengthen the medical legitimacy of the procedure.

Today, the importance of involuntariness in the role of mental patient is as great as it ever was, perhaps greater. This fact is concealed, however, both by private psychiatric practice and by what is, ostensibly, voluntary mental hospitalization. I say ostensibly, because no person can properly be said to be a voluntary mental patient so long as he can be intimidated by the threat of involuntary incarceration. Indeed, because of the overt and covert threat of involuntary mental hospitalization, it is impossible to say how many persons now enter or stay willingly in mental hospitals. Moreover, even the person who enters a mental hospital voluntarily cannot leave at will: his status is easily converted from voluntary to involuntary. Finally, there is a large and important class of mental patients comprised of persons who become patients by breaking the law and are then diverted from the criminal justice system to the mental health system. Such persons are, in effect, sentenced to incarceration in a mental hospital instead of a prison; it is now also possible to sentence such persons to involuntary patienthood in psychiatric outpatient facilities.

Let me now summarize the similarities and differences between the conventional uses of the terms *patient* and *mental patient*. The term *patient* is reserved for persons who *assume* the sick role by asserting that they are ill or by having some type of identifiable relationship with a physician or hospital. Persons complaining of being ill, regardless of where they may be, and persons situated in hospitals, nursing homes, clinics, and physicians' offices are thus all called *patients*. On the other hand, if a person does not seek medical help and has no identifiable (formal) relationship with a medical personage or institution, he is not—even if he has a demonstrable bodily illness—considered to be a patient. For example, it would be wrong to call a Christian Scientist suffering from cancer but refusing medical help a *patient*.

Insofar as a person voluntarily assumes the role of mental patient—either by asserting that he is mentally ill or by establishing an identifiable relationship with a mental health professional—the roles of patient and mental patient are similar. The two roles differ, however, in all those ways in which it is possible to *ascribe* the role of mental patient—but not of (medical) patient—to a person against his will. For example, virtually anyone in conflict with the law may be declared mentally ill; such persons are then typically called *mental patients*, especially if their involuntary psychiatric scrutiny is legally legitimized—for example, as part of a court-imposed plea of insanity or ruling of incompetence to stand trial. This is why we are often told not only that there are millions of mentally ill persons in this country who do not receive the psychiatric care they need, but also that there are millions of *mental patients* who do not receive such care. By contrast, there are millions of poor people suffering from leprosy or malaria in underdeveloped countries who are never called *patients*. In short, anyone *called* mentally ill is, ipso facto, also considered to be a mental patient, and vice versa. I view this conflation of the alleged condition called *mental illness* and the social role of *mental patient* as further support for my contention that mental illness is a nonexistent or fictitious condition: Because there is no way of objectively establishing that a person suffers or does not suffer from mental illness, the condition is inferred from the social role, and vice versa.

BEING A MENTAL PATIENT AND HAVING A MENTAL ILLNESS: IS THERE A DIFFERENCE?

As I have shown, having an *illness* and being a *patient* are concepts that vary independently: It is possible to have an illness and not be a patient, or to be a patient and not have an illness. This is not true for the relationship between having a *mental illness* and being a *mental patient* (especially if the role is ascribed rather than assumed): It is not possible to be a properly certified mental patient and not have—that is, not be considered to have—a mental illness. For example, even if a person is regarded as having been improperly hospitalized, he is still considered to have been a patient. A single illustration should suffice. Between 1980 and 1984—a period during which psychiatrists have continued to trumpet the triumphs of the pharmacological treatment of mental illnesses making hospitalization largely unnecessary—*adolescent admissions to private psychiatric hospitals* increased more than 350 percent, from 10,765 to 48,375. According to a report in *Newsweek,* "In many cases young people are being hospitalized . . . [for] *afflictions* such as 'conduct disorder' and 'adolescent adjustment disorder' . . ." (emphasis added).[12] Nowhere do the reporters for *Newsweek* question that these youngsters have *bona fide mental diseases* or *are bona fide patients.*

My contention that psychiatrists have succeeded in combining and equating mental illness as a condition and the mental patient role is also exemplified by the psychiatric approach to malingering, now called *factitious disorder:*

> The unique aspect of these "factitious" disorders is that the sole objective is to assume the role of a patient. Without an acute emotional crisis or a recognizable motive . . . indeed, without a need for treatment, many of these patients make hospitalization itself a primary objective and often a way of life.[13]

Here a person is defined as a patient solely because he *wants* to be a patient, and as mentally ill solely because he *is* a patient. Revealingly, psychiatrists do not consider such alleged maladies to be metaphoric: "As in all forms of factitious illness," assert the authors, "the production of the illness is factitious, but these patients are *truly ill* . . ." (emphasis added).[14] The authors seem to relish the internal contradictions inherent in their image of this non-illness-that-is-really-an-illness: after emphasizing that persons suffering from factitious disorders assume the patient role even though they are "without a need for treatment," they explain that "the introduction of these disorders into the official psychiatric nomenclature is expected to . . . stimulate research in the area of treatment . . . ."[15]

When the Mental Patient Is Not a Patient

Since classifying persons as patients serves the purposes of the classifier, some people will try to enlarge the category called *patients,* and others will try to constrict it. I have cited some examples of the effort to expand this category, and now want to cite some examples of the effort to constrict it—specifically, of defining persons conventionally regarded as mental patients as *not patients.*

I have always believed that people appreciate a service in proportion to what they pay for it, and vice versa. This principle is certainly supported by the fact that companies selling health insurance have traditionally rebelled against the idea that mental illness is like any other illness. During the past several decades, however, they have increasingly been forced, by psychiatric lobbyists and their supporters in the various state legislatures, to accept this absurd proposition. The coverage of alcoholism, chemical dependency, and other autogenous diseases has, of course, contributed its share to the burgeoning cost of health insurance. "You may be startled to read," observes financial columnist Sylvia Porter, "that a large percentage of the total health-care bill employers pay goes to mental health care—often as high as 20 percent." As a result, she continues, "psychiatric care will be *separated* from other medical expenses in employee assistance programs. For *funding purposes,* such programs are treated apart from group health benefits" (emphasis added).[16]

A specific effort to constrict the category called *mental patient* is reflected in certain health insurance policies. Many insurance companies offer policies paying benefits in case of illness; some reimburse hospital and related medical expenses, while others pay cash benefits directly to the policyholder for being in a hospital. How do policies of the latter type define whether a person should be counted as a patient and hence a proper recipient of benefits? They do so by reference to whether or not he resides—as a *patient*—in an institution called a *hospital.* This makes the criteria for determining whether an institution qualifies as a hospital crucial, since it is the definition of a hospital that will determine whether the insured person is or is not a bona fide patient. The typical health insurance policy providing direct cash payments in case of confinement in a hospital defines *hospital* as follows:

> Hospital means an institution which diagnoses and treats *injured* and *sick persons* . . . . "Hospital" does not mean a . . . *mental institution* or a place for the care and treatment of *drug addicts or alcoholics* (emphasis added).[17]

If the insurance industry insisted that mental hospitals are not hospitals, period, there would perhaps be less confusion about the differences between bodily illness and mental illness. Instead, the industry has chosen to legitimize mental illness as a bona fide illness, underwriting special coverage for it, thus creating one of the most lucrative business enterprises of our day, the private mental hospital corporation.

The Most Frequently Encountered Mental Patient

My foregoing analysis is supported by the account American psychiatric authorities give of the most commonly encountered mental patient, namely, the person suffering from a *personality disorder*. Here is what the authors of *The Comprehensive Textbook of Psychiatry/III* tell us about him:

> Those with personality disorders crowd the rosters of clinic dropouts, treatment failures, and referrals to other agencies; for the very persons whom psychiatry labels with the term "personality disorders" are the same persons called bad or deviant, sinning or loathsome. Doctors hate hypochondriacs; attempted suicide is still a felony on many statute books; and the righteous and intolerant single out paranoiacs for special disdain. . . . Those with personality disorders make up a large percentage of people in jails, on welfare rolls, and in the general practitioner's waiting rooms.[18]

The mind boggles: Hypochondriacs, paranoiacs, individuals who attempt suicide, "bad persons" are all sick, suffering from the dreaded disease called *personality disorder.* I want to emphasize that the authors of this prestigious text do not claim that persons suffering from personality disorders exhibit demonstrable brain diseases (as do persons with organic mental disorders); or that they suffer from the manifestations of probable brain disorders (as, according to them, do persons with schizophrenia); or that they want to assume the role of mental patient (as, they say, do persons with neuroses). In short, although persons with personality disorders exhibit none of the criteria of mental illness used in the other chapters of this textbook—that is, proven brain disease, putative brain disease, or assuming the role of mental patient— they are nevertheless classified as suffering from a mental illness. Why? Because they are "functionally disabled."

Concerning the social functioning—or, rather, nonfunctioning—of persons with personality disorders, we learn that "Although until recently psychiatrists were reluctant to acknowledge it, those with personality disorders are functionally more disabled than the neurotics psychiatrists prefer to treat."[19] The contradictions multiply. First we are told that people with personality disorders have no bodily disease and do not want to be mental patients, but, nevertheless, are mentally ill and psychiatric patients. Now we learn that psychiatrists do not like to treat persons suffering from personality disorders, yet these patients are more commonly encountered in psychiatric practice than any others. Moreover many nonpatients also suffer from this malady: "Personality disorders account for the most irrational elements among the leaders of society."[20] Then, even before finishing the "Introduction," the authors offer us the following remarkable passage, completely contradicting claims advanced elsewhere in the book where they assert that the neuroses are diseases:

Those with personality problems are not easy to understand. The neurotic is often a self-diagnosed sinner who willingly begs for psychiatric help, confesses his problems, and often thereby cures himself. . . . In marked contrast, someone with a personality disorder is far more likely to refuse psychiatric help, point out the psychiatrist's problems, and, by persisting in his annoying behavior, cause colleagues in other disciplines to scoff at psychiatrists' competence.[21]

Virtually all of the issues I have discussed earlier are wonderfully illustrated in these lines. Note, for example, the authors' disdain for the neurotic: he is a *sinner* who *begs* for help and *confesses* his problems. It would seem, then, that the neurotic's problems are existential or moral, rather than medical or psychiatric. Nevertheless, psychiatrists eagerly embrace him as a *sick patient*. Note further the authors' explicit acknowledgment that persons sick with personality disorders *refuse psychiatric help*. It is not surprising that the authors find them *not easy to understand*: they do not want to understand such persons; they want to define them as mentally ill and coerce them into becoming psychiatric patients. Finally, the fact that the person afflicted with a personality disorder wants to stay away from psychiatrists is interpreted as follows: "Because those with personality disorders do not routinely acknowledge pain from what society perceives as their symptoms, the person is often regarded as unmotivated for treatment . . . ."[22] This is an absurd assertion. The persons the authors here describe are not *regarded* as unmotivated for treatment, they *are* unmotivated for it—because they simply do not want it.

Despite these seeming obstacles to therapeutic cooperation, the authors proceed to a "Clinical Overview" of the disease. After having read their "Introduction," one wonders how they will identify this disease and what rationale they will offer for claiming it as a disease. Personality disorder, they state, is a mental disease with four characteristics:

The first characteristic is an inflexible and maladaptive response to stress. The second characteristic is a disability in working and loving that is generally more serious and always more pervasive than that found in neurosis. The third characteristic is that personality disorders almost always occur in response to a social context. And the fourth characteristic is a peculiar capacity to get under the skin of others.[23]

A remarkable list indeed. The authors' suggestion for therapy is even more remarkable:

Reliable diagnosis depends on what the psychiatrist can observe with certainty. However, the successful management of patients who insist that nothing is the matter must be based on what he can infer.[24]

The authors simply ignore the vexing question of what entitles psychiatrists to regard a person as a patient if he insists that "nothing is the matter," and what entitles them to treat such a person against his will.

BEING INCARCERATED: THE MENTAL HOSPITAL PATIENT AND THE PRISON INMATE

Long before I became a psychiatrist, I was impressed by the fact that in modern societies many individuals are incarcerated like prisoners in institutions—but are called *patients*. No doubt, others have been impressed by this also. I assume they have dismissed it, however, as a social arrangement justified by medical considerations. I could never believe this.

Because of my attention to the role of coercion in psychiatry, my critics have consistently accused me of overemphasizing its importance. I, for my part, feel that psychiatrists underestimate its importance, and for an obvious reason. The social role of the mental hospital patient resembles the role of the prison inmate much more than it resembles the role of the medical patient. Karl Jaspers, who abandoned a successful psychiatric career to become a philosopher, recognized this embarrassing similarity but chose not to pursue it:

> Admission to hospital [he wrote] often takes place against the will of the patient and therefore the psychiatrist finds himself in a different relationship to his patient than other doctors. *He tries to make the difference as negligible as possible by deliberately emphasizing his purely medical approach to the patient,* but the latter in many cases is quite convinced that he is well and resists these medical efforts (emphasis added).[25]

Psychiatrists, politicians, and others concerned with mental health policy systematically reject this insight, a denial that immediately derails their efforts to help the persons they insist on calling mentally ill. Moreover, this hypocritical equation of the situation of the mental patient with that of the medical patient obstructs the more relevant and fruitful comparison of the situation of the mental hospital patient with that of the prison inmate: like criminal behavior, mentally ill behavior is a deviation from psychosocial—that is, conventional, ethical, legal—norms of conduct; like conviction for crime, commitment for mental illness cannot come into being without someone's lodging a complaint about the offender/patient, and without that complaint being legitimized by appropriate social authorities.

The Social Anatomy of Crime (with and without Victims)

Lawbreaking is a phenomenon; *law* and *crime* are social constructs. For a crime to exist, there must be a triangular relationship, such as the following: *Smith steals* Jones' car and wallet in New York, drives to Boston, and lives it up using Jones' credit cards. *Jones complains* to the police about the theft. *The police arrest* Smith (and a *judge sends* him to jail). In short, there is an offender, a victim, and a social authority with legitimacy to validate or invalidate the complaint and with power to coerce the offender. Although people sometimes naively believe that crime consists simply of lawbreaking, that is not so: a crime can be said to exist only when a person lodges a complaint against another person and when his complaint is formally legitimized as valid.

Suppose that Jones does not complain to the police about the loss of his car (perhaps because it contains evidence of his own criminal activity). How would the police know that a crime had been committed? They couldn't. My point here is similar to that of the classic question about a tree falling in a deserted forest: Does it make a sound? The answer is no: It generates sound waves, but not sound, since the term *sound* refers to "that which is heard" (*Webster's*). A similar distinction obtains between lawbreaking as an event, and crime as a legal concept. This is not hairsplitting. On the contrary, it is a distinction with supremely important practical consequences. As I noted, if a robbery is not reported, there can be no prosecution because there is no suspect. Suppose, however, that the police catch the culprit by accident and charge him with the crime. There may still be no crime unless the victim is willing to testify against the offender. In the practical administration of the criminal law, it is the plainest common sense that even if an accused is in fact guilty, the police may have no case against him if the victim refuses to cooperate with the prosecution. If pressed to testify, all an unwilling witness has to do is say in court: "I don't remember . . ." (if that is the man who robbed me, or whatever), and the case against the accused collapses. This is one of the reasons why many gangland crimes committed by professional criminals against each other are impossible to prosecute.

Typically, then, (ordinary) crime presupposes two conflicting parties—one asserting that he has been victimized, the other (usually) denying that he is at fault. This is why the concept of so-called victimless crime is inconsistent with Anglo-American legal principles and practices. Suppose, for example, that Jones buys marijuana from Smith. Jones is not, literally, a victim; he has no more grievance against Smith than if Smith were selling him newspapers or candy. Nor has Smith a complaint against Jones. In short, crimes *with victims* are literal crimes, whereas crimes *without victims* are metaphorical crimes. Of course, once people literalize their metaphors—religious, legal, or psychiatric—it becomes difficult or impossible for them to see this distinction. Yet the distinction remains and continues to bedevil those who try to treat victimless crimes like ordinary crimes. It must suffice here to indicate a few of the consequences of the literalization of this particular metaphor.

Because a metaphorical crime produces no literal victim, a victim is created by legal fiat: it is (said to be) society. This allows agents of society to create and lodge complaints of such lawbreaking. But how do they know that a law has been broken? By themselves engaging in an unlawful act: for example, an undercover policeman *impersonates* a john or a drug user and entraps a prostitute or drug seller. Since there is no literally aggrieved party in such a transaction, the policeman lodges the complaint—unless he succumbs to the temptation of extorting a bribe from the prostitute or becoming a drug dealer. The rest is modern American history: organized crime, police corruption, disrespect for law, unprotected streets and homes.

The Social Anatomy of (Serious) Mental Illness

As we distinguish between lawbreaking and crime, so we must also distinguish between peculiar behavior and psychosis. A formal diagnosis of psychosis requires the same sort of triangular relationship as does a formal finding of crime. Here is an example. Mr. Jones persecutes his wife with complaints that she is poisoning his food and making him impotent. As long as Mrs. Jones remains silent or perhaps mentions this only to her timid elderly mother, we cannot properly speak of Mr. Jones as being psychotic. However, once Mrs. Jones goes to the local mental health center and complains about her husband's *delusions,* she sets in motion a social process that normally ends in Mr. Jones being formally diagnosed and perhaps committed to a mental hospital. Of course before that happens, there is likely to be a confrontation between Mr. Jones and Mrs. Jones, with certain representatives of social authority— social workers, psychiatrists, judges—entering the fray and adjudicating the conflicting claims. How do they do that? On the basis of the evidence presented to them. For example, Mrs. Jones may, in the last minute, withdraw her complaint and volunteer that she has made it up to punish Mr. Jones for his past infidelities; and Mr. Jones may behave in a socially appropriate manner in front of those formally judging his mental state—in which case, he would not be committed to a mental hospital. Conversely, Mrs. Jones may stick to her accusations, called *giving a history of Mr. Jones's illness;* and Mr. Jones may insist that not only is his wife poisoning him but that she is also a secret KGB agent, and that God has told him he must kill her—in which case he will surely be committed to a mental hospital.

The parallels between crime and mental illness could thus hardly be more perfect. In each case: (1) claimants advance conflicting claims concerning each other and themselves; (2) representatives of social authority judge the validity of the conflicting claims and decide in favor of one or another party; (3) the person adjudicated as properly accused (of crime or mental illness) is detained for further investigation (trial, mental examination); (4) if the accused is confirmed in the suspected role (guilty, psychotic), he is incarcerated (in prison or mental hospital). As a rule, the person imprisoned or hospitalized in a mental institution is the individual accused of crime or mental illness. In exceptional cases, however, the accusation can backfire and result in the accuser's becoming the accused and ending up incarcerated. This is what happened to Alger Hiss, who was convicted of perjury, not of espionage. And this is what happens in James Thurber's "A unicorn in the garden," where the nasty but normal wife who tries to commit her harmlessly eccentric husband ends up incarcerated in the "booby-hatch."[26]

In short, a person cannot become a criminal unless and until he is accused of a crime, nor can a person become a (committed) mental patient unless and until he is accused of mental illness. In both cases the accusation may be lodged by: (1) an aggrieved party (victim or relative); (2) an unaggrieved agent of the State (entrapment by policeman, recommendation by psychiatrist); or (3) the subject himself (criminal seeking conviction confesses to crimes; self-identified mental patient seeking mental hospitalization volunteers psychotic symptoms).

However, the situation of the prison inmate and mental hospital inmate differ in the ways in which complaints against them are perceived and adjudicated. Briefly put, Americans see merit in the principle that a person accused of crime should be considered innocent until proven guilty and that it is better to let a thousand guilty persons go free than incarcerate a single innocent person. In the case of the person accused of mental illness, Americans see merit in exactly the opposite principle: namely, that such a person should be considered mentally sick until proven otherwise, and that it is better to hospitalize a thousand persons who do not need treatment than to deprive a single person of the treatment he needs for his mental illness. This is why lawyers who help a person accused of a crime to rebut the charges against him are not considered to be the enemies of the social order, whereas psychiatrists who help a person accused of mental illness to rebut the charges against him are considered to be such enemies—as the following example illustrates.

Ann Landers, a staunch advocate of mental health, systematically misidentifies treatment for mental illness as identical to treatment for medical illness. The following is her reply to a letter from a woman who complained about the difficulties facing parents trying to get their mentally sick child to accept psychiatric help:

> You've honed in on one of the most frustrating aspects of helping a psychotic. It is getting that person to accept treatment. Often a parent must file a *complaint* to enable the *police* to *force the patient* to go to a psychiatric hospital for evaluation (emphasis added).[27]

In the case of crime, Miss Landers no doubt distinguishes between a complaint filed with the police and the guilt of the accused, and supports the Anglo-American legal principle that the accused and his agents are entitled to a defense against the accusation. In the case of mental illness, however, her attitude is just the opposite. "Well-meaning civil libertarians," she writes, "in an effort to protect the rights of the mentally ill, have in some instances prevented such action."[28] In short, Miss Landers views the effort to prevent a person's imprisonment in a mental hospital as unjustified. Her mindless endorsement of psychiatric deception and coercion is dramatically illustrated in the closing lines of her reply:

> Medication [for psychotics unwilling to go to mental hospitals] has been a godsend. In the old days, it was a major hassle every four hours to get a mental patient to take his medicine. Today, one shot of Prolixin can keep a psychotic under control for approximately two weeks. Enormous progress has been made, and it's the drugs that have produced miracles.[29]

Medication, miracle drugs, godsend: clearly, there is no justification here for obstacles to the transformation of American citizens from persons into mental patients. Such is the logic of the psychiatric ideas and interventions endorsed by Miss Landers and, no doubt, eagerly accepted by most of her readers.

Since at this point the reader might wonder just what is wrong with Miss Landers' recommendations for therapy, her endorsement of the "enormous progress [that] has been made" in psychiatry—and, in general, with the way so-called psychiatric problems are now managed in our society—I shall briefly restate my objections to the use of legally recognized excuses, incriminations, and incarcerations based on psychiatric criteria. Simply put, my objections rest on the classic philosophy of individual liberty according to which it is just to punish a man for what he has *done,* but it is unjust to do so for what he *is* or *thinks:* this is all we mean, and can mean, by *freedom under law:*

> To punish a man [wrote Thomas Macaulay] because he has committed a crime, or because he is believed, though unjustly, to have committed a crime, is not persecution. To punish a man, because we infer from the nature of some doctrine which he holds . . . that he will commit a crime, is persecution, and is, in every case, foolish and wicked.[30]

I submit that what we now call *psychosis* is either crime or doctrine: That is, it is either an act we should call *crime* and treat accordingly, or it is what Macaulay called *doctrine* and we should treat it accordingly. The modern, psychiatrically enlightened intellectual believes our moral duty is to do exactly the opposite: If a dangerous psychotic commits a crime, we must not punish him, because it would be unjust to do so; whereas if he is merely dangerous, we must restrain him, because he is ill and it would be uncaring not to do so. This tendency of falling into therapeutic despotism and paternalism must have been apparent to classical liberals. "Man," warned Macaulay, "is so inconsistent a creature that it is impossible to reason from his belief to his conduct, or from one part of his belief to another."[31] From this flows the principle that we must punish overt acts, not inward mental states. Obviously, once the incarceration of certain classes of persons is accepted as not a loss of liberty but a gain of treatment, the whole classical liberal argument for individual liberty and responsibility becomes meaningless.

But let us return, for a final observation, to our comparison of the criminal and the mental patient. The differences between crime and mental illness are actually the greatest when the subject and the object of a criminal or psychiatric complaint is the same person, the agent himself. When a person lodges a criminal complaint against himself, it is investigated the same way as if someone else had lodged it. For example, when a grisly, unsolved crime is reported by the press and the police look for the person who did it, innocent people often come forward and confess to the crime. Such a confession is never accepted on its face value as true; on the contrary, it is treated with the utmost skepticism. On the other hand, when a person lodges a psychiatric complaint against himself, it is not investigated at all. When, for example, a man says that the FBI is sending messages to him through his gold teeth, the patient's assertion is accepted on its face value as true; indeed, psychiatrists view it as a *symptom of mental illness* when, in fact, it is merely a *claim*. These considerations explain why pseudoscientific experiments with so-called pseudo-mental-patients excite so much interest and why such experiments are worthless. (See Chapter 6.)

Classifying the Rule Violator

Persons do not become patients but may become mental patients, by breaking the law, being arrested, and then being coerced into the sick role. While this is not the way people discover that they have a duodenal ulcer or leukemia, it is the way they often discover they have schizophrenia or an antisocial personality disorder. The psychiatric diagnoses then obscure why these persons are called patients and why they are confined involuntarily in buildings called hospitals.

"Mental patient taken to movie, escapes," reads a typical newspaper headline.[32] Arrested and charged with 16 crimes—including kidnapping, threatening to murder, assault and battery with a deadly weapon, and forcible rape of a child—this offender, instead of being imprisoned to await trial, was sent to a mental hospital for psychiatric examination to determine his competence to stand trial. Automatically, such a person is called a *patient*. This linguistic habit, reflected in countless similar reports, makes me conclude that American doctors, lawyers, newspapermen—and the American people in general—are now perfectly comfortable with the idea that a person such as this malefactor *is a mental patient*, and that the building in which he is forcibly—but, evidently, not forcibly enough—confined *is a hospital*. In other words, they are comfortable with the practice called *diverting offenders from the criminal justice system to the mental health system*. The result is that the conditions *in* mental hospitals and prisons, as well as the conditions *of* the persons incarcerated in them, tend to be similar. This is so familiar that documenting it is like beating the proverbial dead horse. But I will beat it once more, if only for a moment.

In June 1985, a Senate committee headed by Senator Lowell P. Weicker (R.-Conn.) released the results of its six-month-long investigation of state mental hospitals. The committee—whose findings included "numerous injuries among patients and staff, severe understaffing, physical abuse of patients, lack of treatment programs"—came close to noting that many mental patients are in fact criminals guilty of violence against others, but stopped short of doing so: "Now that dangerousness is the only criterion for involuntary hospitalization, and now that new barriers exist to treating patients, hospitals are filling up with dangerous patients who are merely being housed."[33] I maintain, however, that the term *dangerous patient*, is a dangerously misleading way of describing individuals who violate other people's rights to life, liberty, and property.

Actually, one of the most important functions of the mental patient role—and of the idea of mental illness itself—is to obscure certain crimes and the psychiatric methods of dealing, or failing to deal, with them. The upshot is that people now repress the obvious criminality of violent mental patients in much the same way as, in Victorian times, they repressed the obvious sexuality of women. However, as Freud warned, the repressed inexorably returns—and when it does, hardly anyone recognizes it for what it really is. The following newspaper story is illustrative:

"Psychiatric centers fail to report patient crimes, State panel says," reads the headline.[34] But what do the authorities expect? They keep telling people that mental hospital inmates are mad, not bad. How, then, can they be criminals? Easily, as the rest of the report demonstrates:

> Albany, Dec. 21 (1985), (AP)—Directors of state psychiatric centers are breaking the law by failing to report possible crimes among patients to the police, a state commission has concluded. . . . At three centers in April, there were 136 incidences of suspected assault on patients, 16 of which resulted in major injuries . . . . In one incident withheld from the police, a patient was beaten into semiconsciousness by another patient. . . . there is a perception among facility directors that the police do not vigorously investigate such crimes . . . .[35]

The latter observation is a gross understatement. Psychiatrists would have to be crazy to report crimes committed by patients to the police; and they would have to be even crazier to report crimes they themselves commit.

Ironically, after insisting that criminals are sick, and after forcibly evicting mental patients from mental hospitals, psychiatrists now criticize the handling of persons they call mental patients by complaining about the "criminalization of mentally disordered behavior." Characteristically, psychiatrists who address this subject pretend that the clients served by the criminal and institutional-psychiatric systems are the incarcerated inmates rather than those who incarcerate them. From that perspective, they see the situation this way:

> The finding that substance abuse and antisocial personality disorder are most often ascribed to psychiatrically ill incarcerated offenders supports the assertion that individuals are selectively *unable to gain access to treatment.* If the "forfeited" patients continue to be socially disruptive and continue to be excluded from psychiatric facilities, they will readily be *accepted* by the criminal justice system. . . . The fact that the criminalization of the mentally ill is taking place can be considered a comment on the failure of psychiatry in its association with government (emphasis added).[36]

Is it true, however, that what we are witnessing is the *criminalization of the mentally ill,* as many psychiatrists now contend? Or is it, instead, merely an occasional reversal in the centuries-old process of the *psychiatrization of the criminal?* As I have tried to show, individuals do not exist in nature labelled as criminals or mentally ill; what do exist are persons who violate social norms and who are then categorized in various ways. When masses of men, especially the pillars of society, automatically prejudge rule violators as heretics, witches, or mental patients, then we witness one of the most fundamental social mechanisms by means of which groups secure the cohesion of their members— namely, scapegoating.[37]

THE ROLE OF THE PSYCHIATRIST

Since the roles of mental patient and psychiatrist are complementary, there remains for us to see if we can throw more light on the former by illuminating the latter. As we have had occasion to observe already, the psychiatrist's relationship with his patient is not only often paternalistic, like the physician's, but also coercive, quite unlike the physician's.

Paternalism: Medical and Psychiatric*

There is a large, and largely inadequate, body of literature on paternalism in medicine and psychiatry.[38] I am critical of this literature because it is long on self-congratulatory abstractions and short on candid analyses of, and clear stands on, concrete medico-ethical issues. Sometimes the very definition of paternalism used by writers on medical ethics is unsatisfactory, for example, when it is defined as "interfering with the decision of the patient for the sake of benefitting the patient."[39] By omitting the adjective *ostensibly* before "for the sake of . . . ," these writers reveal their deep-seated bias in favor of "medical paternalism," which they then proceed to defend as follows:

> When this [medical paternalism] occurs with competent patients, so-called strong paternalism occurs. Such paternalism is taken to be unjustified on most accounts in the literature. . . . On this basis, almost all medical care turns out, we believe, to be strongly paternalistic and thus unjustified. However, if this is so, why do patients so readily accept such care? . . . But if all of medicine is unjustifiably paternalistic, then in a strong sense none of it is.[40]

---

*I use the term *paternalism* to characterize the relationship between an adult, typically a professional person, and another adult, called *client* or *patient*, where the former treats the latter as if he were a child or like a child; and the term *coercion*, to refer to the use of force, or threat of force, by one person to secure the compliance of another person.

This meditation ignores the simple fact that many people, especially when they are ill, want to be treated paternalistically. The crucial question before us is not whether medical paternalism is, abstractly, justified or unjustified, but whether, in any particular case, it is what both doctor and patient want: If one party wants it and the other does not, there is a conflict between them that often generates another question, namely: Is either party resorting to deception or coercion to press his partner into the role-performance he wants? Psychiatrists do this formally, by legally committing patients and treating them against their will. Patients do it informally, by producing emergencies such as suicide attempts. In my opinion, the paramount issue is whether the relationship is *consensual* or *coercive;* whether it is *paternalistic-dependent* or *reciprocally respectful* is a secondary consideration.

Apparently, there is no limit to the arrogant foolishness to which doctors, especially after they take up medical ethics as a hobby, will not go. For example, Edmund Pellegrino and David Thomasma, two prominent medical ethicists, declare that the ethical aim of medicine is to "assure and facilitate the patient's moral agency."[41] Medical paternalism—especially the coercive paternalism characteristic of psychiatry—may serve many ends, but "assuring and facilitating the patient's moral agency" is surely not among them.

Daniel X. Freedman, professor of psychiatry at the University of California in Los Angeles and a former president of the APA, goes even further. In his 1982 presidential address to the APA he declares: "Clearly, all physicians attempt to enhance the individual's wishes for optimal self-regulation of functions—both physiologic and psychologic."[42] If that were true, physicians would be angels in a libertarian heaven. But it is not true. It is the very opposite of the truth. For example, Philip Bean, a British social scientist, offers this account of mental hospitalization in England:

> A GP might call, apparently routinely, but as it turned out usually as a result of a family member making a secretive visit, and a consultant [psychiatrist] would subsequently visit. Sometimes the GP would say he is calling in "a specialist," rarely did he say it would be a psychiatrist. The psychiatrists occasionally colluded with this, for they seldom explained to the patient their specialism.[43]

Ironically, psychiatrists in Britain pride themselves on the fact that a much lower percentage of mental patients are hospitalized involuntarily in their country than in the United States. (The difference may be due to Americans being less submissive to bureaucratic and professional authorities than Britons, or to their being more naive in believing they can effectively resist psychiatric coercion.)

Why do medical ethicists, psychiatrists, and other physicians distort the nature of the medical and psychiatric enterprise so outrageously? Is it possible that they do so precisely because they, too, feel disturbed by the power thrust upon physicians by the State? But the remedy for having too much power lies in renouncing and rejecting it, not in deluding oneself (and others) that one uses power solely to make others independent and self-reliant.* When has power ever been so used by human beings?

The Psychiatrist's Love Affair with Coercion

The modern physician, especially the psychiatrist, is, as I have observed earlier, in love with coercion. Illustrative is the headline in *American Medical News:* "Team MDs call for mandatory drug tests." The coercers explain: "The players' unions are making a big mistake in treating drug rehabilitation not as a treatable medical problem . . . but as a 'bargaining chip' . . ."[45] But what business do doctors have coercing professional athletes to submit to drug testing? Why don't these malicious meddlers propose coercing their fellow physicians to submit to such testing? Or their congressmen and senators?

As if it wasn't bad enough to use medical rationalizations to justify depriving persons of the right to decide what substances they may ingest, such rationalizations are now also used to justify depriving persons of the right to reject ingesting substances they do not want. Moreover, as if it wasn't bad enough to subject committed mental patients to such infantilization and mistreatment, psychiatrists now also insist that psychiatric outpatients be compelled to submit to involuntary treatment. Since the 1960s, the legislatures and courts of at least 29 states have approved a policy called *outpatient commitment,* authorizing psychiatrists to exercise the powers of quasi-therapeutic parole officers—compelling legally competent, unincarcerated persons to submit to psychiatric drugging. "Outpatient commitment," explains a report in *Psychiatric News,* "is aimed

---

*The psychiatrists' self-delusions are aided and abetted by the self-flattering gibberish their leaders speak and write. Here is a typical passage from Freedman's above-mentioned presidential address:

> Lithium in a decade saved $4 billion in costs, while both maximizing productivity and reducing suffering and limitation. Recall that clinical experience and science do incrementally define the selective use of innovations, while policy reflexly greets innovation with prophecies of fiscal doom. In retrospect, the actual gains for health might render such poor prophets a loss! Where policy seeks formulas for determining choice and guiding treatment, science understands the fundamental basis for variability in disease and response and the method for sequentially approximating precision in the clinical process.[44]

at chronic mentally ill patients who respond well to medication while in the hospital but stop taking it once they leave."[46] However, I view this phenomenon as evidence that psychiatrists and patients have different criteria for what constitutes *responding well* to antipsychotic drugs—a heretical interpretation in the eyes of psychiatrists. Moreover, the outpatient commitment process itself is described as being "less formal than that for inpatient commitment, patients [being] ordered to outpatient *treatment*" (emphasis added). I emphasize the word *treatment* because later in the report we learn that judges are committing "patients to outpatient treatment without clinical advice or even against the judgment of the hospital or CMHC [Community Mental Health Center] staff."[47] Are psychiatrists who refuse to treat such patients in contempt of court? Need more be said?

Perhaps nothing demonstrates the depth of the disjunction between rhetoric and reality in psychiatry as clearly as the fact that, while no group of professionals in the United States today protests its paternalistic commitment to being compassionate and wanting to help more loudly than psychiatrists, no group is more reviled by the ostensible beneficiaries of its ministrations. Of course, involuntarily confined mental patients have always complained about the loss of liberty inflicted on them by psychiatrists. However, their traditional protest—that they had been *falsely* committed—only served to reinforce the legitimacy of psychiatric incarceration. Their complaint implied that they accepted the standard psychiatric justification for coercion: in other words, as everyone agreed that persons guilty of murder were rightly imprisoned, so everyone, including former mental patients, agreed that persons correctly diagnosed as insane were rightly committed. The fact that former mental patients insisted that they had been incorrectly diagnosed as insane only proved the accuracy of the diagnosis.

In the early 1970s, after the publication of *The Myth of Mental Illness* and *The Manufacture of Madness*—in which, on epistemological, moral, and political grounds I rejected the legitimacy of civil commitment and the insanity defense—the protest tactics of former mental hospital patients changed radically. Having overcome their belief in the mythology of mental illness, they began, first of all, to call themselves psychiatric *inmates* or *victims*, instead of *patients*. Moreover, freed of the invalidating identity imposed on them by their adversaries (relatives as well as psychiatrists), they were able to relinquish their defensive identification with their oppressors and with it the counterproductive claim of "I have been railroaded"; instead, by assuming their rightful identities as responsible moral agents, former mental hospital patients were able to respect themselves and their fellow victims, combine forces with one another, and, like the members of any other special interest group in a free society, assert their right to speak for themselves. The result was that they began to demonstrate regularly against psychiatrists at their professional meetings. A mimeographed leaflet distributed at the 1983 convention of the APA in New York City included this invitation:

> Come and join us in a day of peaceful protest against the American Psychiatric Association. Each year hundreds of thousands of Americans are deprived of their human rights by psychiatry. . . . STOP PSYCHIATRY BEFORE IT STOPS YOU![48]

I consider this to be a momentous advance in the struggle to return the so-called mental patient to his full stature as a human being: restored to liberty by being protected from psychiatric imprisonment and torture—and, hopefully, restored to responsibility by being deprived of the excuse of the insanity defense.

Nothing like the demonstration of former psychiatric inmates against psychiatrists happens to other medical specialists. The only similar situations that come to mind are the demonstrations against abortion clinics. However, the antiabortion demonstrators claim to represent the fetus whose interest in living undeniably conflicts with the pregnant woman's interest in not wanting to give it birth. Most people, regardless of where they stand on this issue, are able to see merit in the claims of both parties. However, when former mental patients demonstrate against involuntary mental hospitalization and treatment, most people are unable or unwilling to see merit in the contentions of those opposed to psychiatric coercions.

What Psychiatrists Do

Bridging the gap between rhetoric and reality in psychiatry would require greater self-disclosure by psychiatrists concerning what they believe and do, and greater candor by nonpsychiatrists—especially by members of the media—concerning the performance of all the actors who play a role in the human tragedies we now call mental diseases and psychiatric treatment. For starters, I offer the following classification—not of mental patients, but of psychiatrists. My criterion for classifying them, I might add, is based not on what they may say, but on what they do.

A. Psychiatrists in the housing and prison business
  1. Psychiatrists in public mental hospitals: operators of cheap hotels and wardens to the poor and unimportant and their unwanted relatives.

2. Psychiatrists in private mental hospitals: operators of better hotels and wardens to the rich and important and their unwanted relatives.

3. Antipsychiatrists in counterinstitutions: operators of flophouses for the poor and unimportant.

B. Psychiatrists in the business of drugging

1. Neuropharmacological psychiatrists: dealers in psychopharmacologicals.

2. General psychiatrists: dealers in a combination of psychopharmacologicals and advice regarding life-management.

C. Psychiatrists in the business of producing brain damage

1. The lobotomists: dealers in amputating the frontal lobes.

2. The electroshockers: dealers in delivering artificial epilepsy.

3. The insulin-coma producers: dealers in insulin overdosage.

D. Psychiatrists in the business of conversation and moral guidance

1. Psychoanalysts: dealers in the cult of Freudianism.

2. Dynamic psychotherapists: dealers in adjustment to the dominant ethic.

3. Psychotherapists of other persuasions: dealers in the principles and practices of various ethical systems.

The Fallacy of Criticizing the Harmfulness of Certain Psychiatric Treatments

Psychiatrists have always imposed their currently fashionable interventions on their patients without the patient's consent or against his will; and mental patients—not all of them, but many—have always maintained that what the psychiatrists did was not treatment but torture. In view of this history, it is hardly surprising that some former mental patients—and some psychiatrists who feel guilty about having participated in the somatic treatment of involuntary patients—now wage campaigns against certain specific modern psychiatric interventions, especially ECT.* Although, in my opinion, the contention that lobotomy, ECT, and the

---

*For example, R.D. Laing writes: "As a young psychiatrist . . . I administered locked wards and ordered drugs, injections, padded cells and straitjackets, electric shock, deep insulin comas, and the rest."[49] Peter Breggin writes: "As I look back on my career as a psychiatrist, one shame seems unforgivable—my involvement with electroshock treatment. As a resident in psychiatry, I prescribed electroshock, I supervised a ward on which patients were given the treatment, and for a time I personally administered it. Why, then, did I do it even when I knew it was wrong?"[50]

major antipsychotic drugs cause brain damage is valid—indeed, it seems to me, self-evident—pushing this opinion on the public is dangerously misleading and clearly counterproductive. The reason for this is that the claim that a particular psychiatric treatment, say ECT, is bad implies, first, that it is a bona fide treatment, and hence that there is a condition justifiably regarded as mental illness (which it is intended to ameliorate or cure); second, that although this particular treatment may be bad, some other treatment might not be. All this is grist for the mill of conventional psychiatry. Obviously, psychiatrists can generate evidence for the beneficial effects of, say, ECT much faster than the ostensible critics of psychiatry can generate evidence for its detrimental effects. Moreover, this line of argument makes it easy for psychiatrists to abandon the criticized intervention in favor of a newer method, and then claim further advances in their therapeutic powers—as they have done, for example, by substituting antidepressant drugs for ECT. Worst of all, the argument about the ineffectiveness or dangerousness of one or another psychiatric treatment distracts attention from, and indeed undermines, what I consider to be the two most valid objections against contemporary psychiatric interventions: first, that in the absence of literal illness, there can be no literal treatment (in other words, there is, and can be, no such thing as a mental or psychiatric treatment); and second, that without informed and uncoerced consent by the patient, no medical or psychiatric intervention is justified, while with consent every such intervention is justified, even if there is no illness and even if the intervention is considered to be harmful by its critics (provided that the procedure does not injure innocent third parties).

In short, by dwelling on the deleteriousness of ECT or neuroleptic drugs, the ostensible critics of psychiatry try to beat psychiatrists at their own game and on their own grounds. In the process, the critics neglect to use their strongest weapon, namely, insisting that the controversy is not about the effectiveness or ineffectiveness of any particular psychiatric intervention but about consent versus coercion: in other words, that, as I have indicated, with consent even ineffective or worthless treatments ought to be permitted, whereas without it, even treatments officially deemed effective ought not to be.* Unfortunately, in their zeal to combat

---

*Although Hobbes could not even have dreamed of such a thing as compulsory treatment, his principles of political philosophy clearly imply an endorsement of the right to reject such treatment:

> Subjects have liberty to defend their own bodies, even against them that lawfully invade them . . . [and] are not bound to hurt themselves. If the sovereign command a man, though justly condemned, to kill, wound, or maim himself; or not to resist those that assault him; or to abstain from the use of food, air, medicine, or any other thing, without which he cannot live; yet hath that man the liberty to disobey (emphasis in the original).[51]

psychiatry and especially certain brutal interventions, many would-be critics of psychiatry espouse the same intolerance and coerciveness toward those who disagree with them as do their psychiatric adversaries.

Finally, I want to reemphasize the obvious, namely, that people are both similar to, and different from, one another. It is human diversity—or perversity—that accounts for two stubborn facts, one upsetting to psychiatrists, the other to the critics of somatic treatments. The first is that, regardless of how beneficial certain interventions might be according to psychiatrists, some mental patients will consider them to be harmful and reject them: this upsets the psychiatrists who want to force the patients to submit to their care and cure. The other is that, regardless of how harmful and brain-damaging certain somatic treatments might be according to their critics, some persons will eagerly seek out such treatments and willingly submit to them: this upsets the critics who want to coerce both psychiatrists and patients to refrain from engaging in certain consensual treatment relationships. Respect for the liberty and responsibility of mental patients and psychiatrists requires that we eschew both of these postures and look to a mechanism such as the psychiatric will to enhance the autonomy of all the agents participating in this drama. However, so long as most people—including psychiatrists, antipsychiatrists, and psychiatric patients—prefer coercive to contractual relations, there is no reason to expect such a peaceful resolution of the problem.

PATERNALISM AND COERCION RECONSIDERED

The relationship between patient and physician is typically cooperative: the patient wants to *get* treatment, and the physician wants to *give* it. By contrast, the relationship between the mental patient and the psychiatrist is typically antagonistic: the patient wants to *engage* in certain kinds of behavior, and the psychiatrist wants to *prevent* him from doing so. Lest this seem an exaggeration, let me say only that my construction follows inexorably from taking commitment statutes seriously: with monotonous regularity, such statutes focus—and have always focused—on the patient's alleged *dangerousness* to himself and/or others. Clearly, then, the (seriously) ill mental patient is a person who is, or is considered to be, dangerous, and the institutional psychiatrist is a person who tries to cure or control the patient's dangerousness.

Thus, one of the most obvious differences between the medical and psychiatric situations is that the physician controls diseases, not persons; whereas the psychiatrist controls persons, not diseases. This, of course, is an aphorism, not an assertion. And an aphorism, as the Austrian aphorist Karl Kraus noted, is either a half-truth or a truth-and-a-half—which one the reader must decide.[52] Let me add only that so far as the physician's role is concerned, he cannot, strictly speaking, ever treat a disease without taking cognizance of the person who has it: However, in a medical situation that is at once ideally cooperative and technicalized, by treating the patient's disease, the physician also treats the patient. In contrast, since there is no mental disease, the psychiatrist can never treat the patient's disease; however, in a psychiatrist-mental patient situation that is at once ideally coercive and technicalized, by pretending to treat the patient's fictitious disease, the psychiatrist also controls the patient.

But let us return to the medical situation. As everyone knows, until the post World War I years, the typical American physician was a privately practicing professional, whereas the typical American psychiatrist was a state-employed bureaucrat. After the Second World War, physicians began to enter into a progressively more intimate alliance with the State, gradually exchanging their roles as healers for those of employees of medical bureaucracies or agencies of the State.

As a result, doctors now seem completely blind to the fundamental distinction between constructing a scientifically defined and justified criterion of health and coercing a person to adopt a lifestyle that promotes his health. The analogy between health and gold may again help to make this point clear. Let us assume, as scientifically proven, that smoking cigarettes and a diet high in cholesterol are conducive to atherosclerosis: those are then facts, just as the atomic weight or chemical properties of gold are facts. Whether a person in possession of such information *accepts* or *rejects* a medically healthy life style, and whether physicians and the State play a role in directly or indirectly *forcing* a person to adhere to such a life style are, however, matters not of science but of ethics or politics. Obviously, the State could employ and empower chemists to force people to adopt one or another kind of economic attitude toward gold; and, given sufficient monetary of political rewards, there would be no shortage of chemists willing and eager to play such a role. But no chemist *today* would think that such a hypothetical chemist coercing his fellow citizens would be anything other than an agent of the State. Nevertheless, physicians think of themselves as scientists and want to be so regarded by the public.

Actually, aided and abetted by a health-obsessed society, physicians now act as if knowing what health is and what impairs it would give them a special right to interfere with people's right or free will to choose to be unhealthy—a situation illustrating that, regardless of how scientific his medical methods may be, the modern physician has virtually no sense of, and does not value, the ethics of science as truth-finding and truth-telling. I am not saying here that science is better, or worse, than religion or politics. That is not the point: the point is that they are different, and that insofar as the scientist uses his knowledge to justify, and indeed to engage in, coercion, he becomes—conceptually and morally—indistinguishable from the inquisitor or dictator.

After all, not so long ago, the priest, having defined heaven and hell, knew all about them. Accordingly, the priest believed, and people agreed, that he was entitled to coerce individuals to live so that they maximized their chances of going to heaven and minimized their chances of going to hell. Regrettably, the lofty goal called *heaven* sometimes required killing people, a clerical measure warmly endorsed by the theologians. Today, doctors threaten and coerce people so as to make them healthy and live as long as possible. Since many people refuse to cooperate with the doctor's health rules, the physician feels justified, and the people agree, that he is entitled to spoil their pleasures by intimidating and torturing them. Regrettably, the lofty goal called *health* often requires making people mentally sick, a clinical measure warmly endorsed by physicians. (By this I mean inventing mental illness terms and attaching them to certain patterns of unwanted behaviors; see Chapter 3.)

Doctors and patients have come a long way since the nineteenth century, but we had better think twice before we conclude it has all been progress. It is of more than passing interest to note, in this connection, one of the definitions of the word *profession* in the *Oxford English Dictionary.* "A profession in our country," wrote a British gentleman named Maurice in 1829, "is expressly that kind of business which deals primarily with men as men, and is thus distinguished from a Trade, which provides for the external wants or occasions of men." Until recently, this criterion applied particularly to the practice of medicine and law, the relations between practitioners and their clients being based on mutual respect and trust and, of course, the studied avoidance of coercion. Since psychiatrists do not deal with men as men but, on the contrary, deal with men as madmen, psychiatry fails, by this criterion, to qualify as a profession. Although Maurice's definition of a profession may now strike us as quaint and old-fashioned, it should serve as a reminder of how radically the meaning of the word *profession* has changed since the nineteenth century: Formerly, the professional was a person who had a *personal* relationship with his clients based on mutual respect and reciprocity; today, the professional is a person who has an *impersonal* relationship with his clients based on his superior, and their inferior, competence in a specialized area of knowledge or skill.

The Psychiatrist and the Mental Patient as Adversaries

An important feature of legitimate power is that its very existence induces people to submit to it voluntarily—that is, because they believe that the behavior prescribed is right or because they fear punishment for deviating from it. Thus, most people subject to taxation or traffic laws willingly pay their taxes and obey the rules of the road. Similarly, most people subject to mental health laws voluntarily consent to mental hospitalization. This is why the standard psychiatric argument that since only a minority of the persons in mental hospitals is detained involuntarily, involuntary mental hospitalization is not an important issue, is specious and unpersuasive. Actually, so long as incarceration in a mental hospital is a legally legitimate and socially approved procedure, we cannot meaningfully speak of anyone entering or remaining in a mental hospital voluntarily. We must keep this always in mind when we consider the controversy concerning commitment and other coerced psychiatric interventions.

Although official psychiatric rhetoric conceals the frequently antagonistic relationship between psychiatrist and mental patient, informal p^ychiatric publications—the so-called throw-away journals—allow us to see things as they are. The following excerpt, entitled "Types of problem patients on a locked unit," comes from such a source:

> Presumably, if the patient were cooperative, he would not have been admitted or transferred to the locked units to begin with. . . . The most frequent problem encountered is the patient who refuses to do whatever it is we think he should do. Some patients start right out refusing to talk, a rather perplexing problem for a new intern who just finished a course in history-taking and sits expectantly, pen in hand, only to be greeted by a stony silence. Other refusals, not necessarily in order of either importance or frequency, include refusal of medication, refusal to sign consent for electroconvulsive therapy, refusal to go for electroconvulsive therapy after signing the consent, refusal to attend activities and ultimately, refusal to accept discharge plans.[53]

Why do psychiatrists systematically impose themselves on persons who want to have nothing to do with them? I believe they do so because, like most people, psychiatrists love power and exult in pushing others around. "We must take a stand," declares H. Richard Lamb, a professor of psychiatry at the University of Southern California, "for involuntary treatment, both acute and ongoing. Such interventions should not be limited to those who can be proven to be dangerous."[54] Similar statements abound in the psychiatric literature.

Yet, when they are criticized for using coercive methods, psychiatrists often defend themselves by claiming that they dislike treating patients against their will and do it only out of a deep sense of civic and moral duty. However, that is patently untrue, as the whole history of psychiatry proves. Nor, in this connection, must we overlook the fact that the role of psychiatrist, unlike that of mental patient, is entirely voluntary. No one in the United States is forced to become a physician; no physician is forced to become trained as a psychiatrist; no one so trained is forced to practice conventional psychiatry. Accordingly, if a psychiatrist engages in the manufacture of involuntary mental patients either through the mechanism of civil commitment or through the mechanism of the insanity defense, then he proves, by his actions, that he enjoys being a coercive paternalist. Indeed, so passionately convinced are psychiatrists about the rightfulness of treating patients against their will that they contemptuously denounce those remaining few who refuse to treat involuntary patients. Such psychiatrists, say the coercers, reject treating the sick, avoid the most difficult cases, and are unworthy of being psychiatrists.

Be that as it may, distinguishing between paternalism and coercion allows us to lay to rest, once and for all, the claim that, because both medical and psychiatric practices tend to be paternalistic, the differences between them are negligible. In addition, it allows us to identify the various combinations of these two elements and thus reaffirm the crucial differences between *caring* (for patients), *coercing* (mental patients), and *confining* (prisoners). The medical situation may be paternalistic or nonpaternalistic, but cannot be coercive. The psychiatric situation may be paternalistic or nonpaternalistic, and, in addition, may be coercive as well. (Coercion without paternalism characterizes the relationship between a decent jailer and his civilized prisoner.) (See Table 4.2.)

TABLE 4.2. Paternalism and Coercion: Treatment, Coercion, Contract

Paternalism	Coercion	Nature and Name of Medical Relationship
+	+	Paternalism with coercion: most medical interventions vis-à-vis children; all involuntary psychiatric interventions; called (involuntary) *treatment.*
+	−	Paternalism without coercion: medical and voluntary psychiatric interventions vis-à-vis consenting clients treated as if they were dependents rather than partners; called (voluntary) *treatment.*
−	+	Coercion without paternalism: civilized penal sanctions; the lawful punishing of lawbreakers without condescension; called *punishment* (fine, probation, prison sentence).
−	−	Neither paternalism, nor coercion: giving and receiving help based on mutual respect between responsible adults; called *contract, help, therapy, treatment.*

Sadly, however, a persistent professional and popular unwillingness to recognize that mental patients are persons first and patients second, coupled with a stubborn refusal to treat them as persons rather than as mental patients, vitiates all current efforts, sincere or otherwise, to help them. We recognize that a person considered to be sick is a person first and a patient second. If such a person chooses not to be a patient, no one says that he rejects treatment "precisely because of his illness." However, if a person considered to be mentally sick wants to reject treatment, that is exactly what most people say. Politicians are no exception. Witness New York City Mayor Ed Koch's comment that "A person who [is] mentally ill often resist[s] treatment precisely because of his illness."[55]

This image is completely out of focus. Mayor Koch's remark reflects the distortion built into our picture of psychiatry. Like his constituency, the Mayor views treatment accorded the involuntary mental patient as a psychiatric or mental health *service.* But the term *service* implies not only that it is something provided for the recipient, but also that the recipient has the option to reject it. Normally, saying that a person is receiving services involuntarily—for example, from an electric utility company— would be a clear case of talking nonsense: in such a context, the term *involuntary service* is an oxymoron. Only in relation to the involuntary mental patient do we speak of his receiving services and accept the locution as legitimate. This, perhaps, is the most important evidence of how mercilessly we infantilize him.

PART THREE

THE CONCEPTUAL DIMENSIONS OF MENTAL ILLNESS

5

MENTAL ILLNESS AS METAPHOR

But the greatest thing by far is to be a master of metaphor. It is the one thing that cannot be learnt from others.

—Aristotle[1]

Although most people assume that educated persons know what a metaphor is, I have learned that this may not be so. Medical students are educated persons. But most of them do not know what a metaphor is.

Medical students often ask me what I mean when I say that mental illness is not a real illness, and I sometimes try to explain it by drawing a distinction between the literal and metaphorical uses of the word *illness*. One day, before beginning my explanation, I asked if anyone in the group—there must have been about 20 students sitting around the table—could define *metaphor*. Half of them raised their hands. I turned to one and asked him to tell us. He said he knew what a metaphor is but could not define it. I suggested he give us an example. He thought for a moment and then said: "My mind is a blank." And not a single student laughed. It was then I realized that they did not know what a metaphor is; and perhaps why so many people do not, or cannot, distinguish literal diseases, such as cancer and heart disease, from metaphorical diseases, such as lovesickness and mental illness.

For almost 30 years I have maintained that mental illness is a metaphor. What does this contention mean? To many psychiatrists it evidently does not mean much. For example, to Seymour Kety, an emeritus professor of psychiatry at Harvard, it means that "if schizophrenia is a myth, then it is a myth with a powerful genetic component"[2]—a quip often quoted by psychiatrists as a rejoinder to my entire critique of psychiatry. While Kety's remark has some merit as a witticism, it has none as a refutation, for it ignores the fact that virtually any word can be used both literally and metaphorically.

When a psychiatrist hears a joke that another psychiatrist calls *sick,* they both know that they are talking about something other than a real disease. However, when a psychiatrist hears another psychiatrist say "John Hinckley, Jr. is sick," he believes—indeed, all psychiatrists and most other people believe—that they are talking about a real disease. After all, that is why Hinckley is in a hospital—or at least in a building called a *hospital*—and not in a prison. Isn't it astonishing that psychiatrists can be so sure that every time a member of their profession asserts that a person is sick, they are confronted with the task of diagnosing a real disease rather than understanding a figure of speech? Unfortunately, if a person does not understand what a metaphor is, then he will think that my assertion that *mental illness is a metaphor* is nothing but a put-down of psychiatrists and an attack on psychiatry. Let me briefly sketch, therefore, the fundamentals of linguistic analysis necessary for understanding the perspective I have tried to bring to bear on mental illness and mental healing.

THE NATURE OF METAPHOR

The characterization of man as the animal that uses language has become so familiar that it has lost its force. It is particularly ironic, then, that the psychiatrist—the physician specializing in the study and treatment of so-called mental illness—should now turn a deaf ear to his patient's words. For, as Justin Martyr (c. 100–165), one of the Fathers of the Church, put it so well: "By examining the patient's tongue, physicians find out the diseases of the body, and philosophers the diseases of the mind."[3] In other words, to discover diseases of the body, the regular physician examines the patient's body and looks for the manifestations of disease. This is not what the psychiatrist does: To discover diseases of the mind, he examines the patient's speech and looks for its meaning.

Actually, all this is self-evident. If a person bleeds profusely from a bodily orifice or is deeply jaundiced, anyone can tell that he is ill. Similarly, if a person says crazy things—if he *hears voices* or *sees things*—then anyone can tell that he is insane. Nevertheless, people—perhaps especially psychiatrists—forget that mental illness is inferred from language rather than from lesions. In their current enthusiasm for viewing mental illness as brain disease, psychiatrists have convinced themselves (and many others) that abnormal ideas are a symptom of abnormal thought processes, that abnormal thought processes are a symptom of abnormal brain processes, and that the remedy for the mental patient's bad life lies in good chemistry. But how do we know what anyone *thinks?* How do we determine what constitutes true (normal) or false (abnormal) thought or belief? The answer is that we know these things only through the intuitive or explicit analysis of language—that is, through the *meaning* we attach to words, sentences, and figures of speech, our own and those of others.

What Is a Metaphor?

A keen analytical understanding of language and meaning characterizes the writings of Greek and Roman philosophers. Indeed, Aristotle's definition of metaphor is still as good as any: "Metaphor consists in giving a thing a name that belongs to something else."[4] The something else to which the name belongs is the original or core referent of the word used in its *literal* sense. Who determines what the literal meaning of a word is? No one does; it is a matter of convention. How convention does this need not concern us here. What is important for us is that if a person does not have a clear understanding of the literal use and meaning of a word, he will be unable to understand its metaphorical use and meaning, and will also be unable to understand what someone means when he says "that is a metaphor." Since language is metaphorical through and through, and since anyone who speaks a language competently knows this intuitively, two simple examples should suffice.

A man dies and his young son is told that he went to heaven. However, when a man dies and goes to heaven, his going is not the same sort of *action* as that entailed in his widow's going to Italy, nor is heaven the same sort of *place* as Rome.

A man comes home and as he walks through the front door calls to his wife: "*Honey,* I am home."

Like jokes, which they so closely resemble, metaphors like these cannot be explained. If one tries to do so, in the process—to use another metaphor—one succeeds only in *killing* them.

We should note further that the use of metaphor, as Colin Murray Turbayne puts it, "involves the pretense that something is the case when it is not."* The pretense may, or may not, be disclosed by the author, depending mainly on whether, in presenting his analogy, he makes use of the qualification *as if.* For example, a person may say: "I shall view man *as if* he were a machine," or he may say: "Man *is* a machine." Typically, the pretense is not revealed by the grammar. Turbayne offers several pairs of terms that display no grammatical difference, the first member of the pair exemplifying the literal, the second the metaphorical, use of a term, such as "The timberwolf is a wolf/Man is a wolf. Muscle fatigue/metal fatigue."[6] Isn't it possible then, that—*at least sometimes*—the same sort of relationship applies to the pair "Bodily disease/Mental disease?" To put it as modestly as possible, isn't it possible that—at least in some cases—when an assertion is made about a person's being mentally ill, the illness asserted is metaphorical?

There are countless other ways of getting at, or explaining, what metaphor is. Samuel Johnson, for example, said that a metaphor "gives you two ideas for one." Turbayne adds that a metaphor also gives "two ideas *as* one."[7] It is illuminating, in this connection, to cite the synonyms and antonyms dictionaries give for the words *literal* and *metaphoric.* The synonyms of literal are: Verbal, veritable, accurate, true, exact, precise, regular, real, actual, undeviating, veracious, undisputed. Among its antonyms we find, in addition to metaphorical, the following: Wrong, erring, misleading, mistaken, false, erroneous, deceiving, untrue, delusive, beguiling, fallacious, unsound, lying, distorted, unreal, allegorical, allusive, colloquial, symbolical, figurative, and mythical.

Actually, as the examples cited illustrate, everyone who speaks uses metaphors, just as everyone uses nouns and verbs and prepositions—even persons who do not explicitly understand the character of these speech elements. Hobbes saw clearly the benefits and risks that thus accrue to us as a language-using species:

> . . . as men abound in copiousness of language so they become more wise, or more mad than ordinary. Nor is it possible without letters for any man to become either excellently wise, or, unless his memory be hurt by disease or ill constitution of organs, excellently foolish. For words are wise men's counters, they do but reckon by them; but they are the money of fools.[8]

---

*From the vast modern literature on metaphor, I have here chosen to follow Turbayne's analysis. His book, *The Myth of Metaphor*, is a good guide to the literature.[5]

Toward the end of *Leviathan,* Hobbes uses the Roman Catholic doctrine of transubstantiation as his example for driving home his point about the *abuse* of literalizing metaphors:

> *This is my body,* are equivalent to these, *this signifies, or represents my body;* and it is an ordinary figure of speech: but to take it literally, is an abuse (emphasis in the original).[9]

Actually, we have no choice in the matter of using metaphors: "We must," said C. S. Lewis, "use metaphors. The feelings and the imagination need that support. The great thing . . . is to keep the intellect free from them: to remember that they are metaphors."[10] Obviously, doing so cannot be easy, or else wise men would not have felt it necessary—in every age and every language—to keep reminding us of the duty of this remembrance.

One more observation about metaphor may be appropriate here, namely, that there is a close and intimate connection between humor and metaphor. This is because what often gives a joke its mental punch—what makes us sit up, take notice, and laugh—is the subtle switching of criteria for classifying things. The following story, supposedly told by a high-ranking Chinese official to a visiting American dignitary (the context is important) is a good example:

> The Chinese official asks his American guest which is the largest country in the world. "Why, the Soviet Union, of course," is the reply. "No, I am afraid you are wrong. It is Cuba." "Cuba?" says the American incredulously, sensing that he is being put on. "Yes, Cuba. May I explain?" continues the Chinese jokester earnestly. "You see Cuba is very large. Its government is in Moscow. Its army is in Africa. And its people are in Florida."

While this will surely kill it as a joke, let me point out that the criterion by which we measure the size of a country is not the location of its government, or army, or people, but the size of its surface area.

I hope these observations will suffice as building blocks for constructing an alternative—metaphorical—view of mental illness. We must, of course, keep two things in mind. One is that there is no such thing as a metaphor per se: what a metaphor *is* depends on convention and context. This is why I emphasize that if there is no literal meaning—or no *agreement* on literal meaning, which comes to the same thing—then there is also no metaphorical meaning. The other thing to keep in mind is that a metaphor need not be, and usually is not, an isolated word or phrase, such as might be suggested by the examples I have offered. Instead, a metaphor—or a set of related metaphors—is often elaborated into an extended and sustained form, called allegory, parable, fable, model, myth—or even science. In my book, *The Myth of Mental Illness,* I have tried to show that psychiatry is a myth built on the metaphor of mental illness and its extensions, such as psychiatric diagnosis, prognosis, hospitalization, treatment, and so forth.

MENTAL ILLNESS: FROM BRAIN DISEASE TO METAPHORIC (NON-)DISEASE

How does the literal meaning of a word become transformed into its metaphorical meaning, which may then be interpreted literally? For example, how did Jesus' thanksgiving over bread and wine become symbols (metaphors) of his body and blood, and how did the symbols become interpreted literally, as in the doctrine of transubstantiation? We know from history how this complex process, stimulated by the Church Fathers, grew and captured the popular imagination, and how the metaphor was demystified (deliteralized, at least for some Protestants) during the Reformation. Since it is not generally accepted that mental illness is a literalized metaphor, there is no accepted account of how it became so. I shall briefly summarize how I think this has happened.

The Changing Social Context of Mental Illness

For about 200 years, from 1700 to 1900, physicians conceived of madness on the model of medical disease: insanity was a brain disease or a manifestation of such a disease. They were basically right. Until well into the twentieth century, the majority of the patients in state mental hospitals suffered from brain diseases—most of them from general paresis (neurosyphilis), and the rest from a variety of toxic-organic psychoses (caused by alcohol, head injury, and various infections of the central nervous system). When the early (nineteenth century) psychiatrists spoke of mental diseases or diseases of the mind, they understood, and often explicitly stated, that these expressions were figures of speech or metaphors.

Freud's work radically altered this situation. Rightly, Freud is praised for introducing meaning into the discourse about madness. But, wrongly, he is not blamed for introducing the imagery that legitimized a conceptually promiscuous and politically odious use of the idea of insanity. How did Freud do this? By abandoning brain disease as his model for insanity and replacing it with the dream: As he put it, dreams are "the prototypes of all psychopathological structures."[11] Freud thus jettisoned the linkage between insanity and somatic illness and substituted for it an analogy or putative identity between insanity and a normal, everyday feature of inner (mental) experience, namely, dreaming. It is not surprising that Freud should have been so enthusiastic about his model: He was not a psychiatrist and was not even interested in being a doctor. What he wanted was to be a religious (or quasi-religious) leader. For this he needed a powerful, preferably literalized, metaphor, and that is what he fashioned out of the idea of insanity—which, until then, was *only* a disease or putative disease, a notion not especially useful for ideological purposes.

The result was two-fold. The first was a universalization of the idea of insanity, exemplified by Freud's "psychopathology of everyday life": instead of madness being methodical, in Shakespeare's sense, and therefore not an illness, Freud's claim was that everyday life was psychopathological and therefore sanity no less than madness was a form of insanity.[12] The second result was the literalization of the metaphor of mental illness, exemplified by Freud's cryptochemical theories of *actual neurosis* (and other mental illnesses) and by the neurochemical fantasies of contemporary psychopharmacologists.

There is an interesting historical parallel between the Protestant Reformers' and the psychoanalytic psychiatrists' responsibility for transforming inspiring metaphors into dogmatic literalized metaphors (that no longer function as metaphors). During the first thousand years of Christianity, the popes and other church leaders did not insist that the consecrated bread and wine of the Eucharist *were* the literal body and blood of the Savior. Only after the Reformation gathered steam did the Council of Trent, in 1552, proclaim the doctrine of transubstantiation, *insisting* on the interpretation of the sacramental bread and wine as literally (and miraculously) the body and blood of Jesus Christ. Similarly, only after the Freudian revolution got under way did psychiatrists begin to insist—as they now typically do—that mental illness, far from being a metaphor, is literally an illness *like any other illness* (that is, always and without a doubt a disease of the brain). Ironically, while the Protestant Reformers were only indirectly responsible for the doctrine of the transubstantiation of bread and wine into the body and blood of Christ, Freud and his followers are directly responsible for the transubstantiation of personal and social problems into medical diseases.*

---

*It is interesting to mention in this connection that Sophie Freud, a professor of social work at Simmons College (and Freud's granddaughter), has emphasized the danger of literalizing the psychoanalytic metaphors. "These [Freud's] metaphors," she writes, "have seduced clinicians into treating mere ideas as facts or things."[13]

Insanity: From Medical Illness to Medicalization of Conflict

From its beginning as asylum care in the seventeenth century until the advent of the modern psychotherapies at the end of the nineteenth century, everyone knew perfectly well that psychiatry was a hybrid—a combination of confinement and care, law and medicine. It was obvious that the insane person, the subject of psychiatry, was an individual in conflict with others, typically members of his family or the authorities and agencies of society. The psychiatrist's task—in his dual role as physician and agent of society with special powers and privileges granted him by the State—was to manage and resolve this conflict.

The complex consequences of this confrontation (and often collusion as well) between madman and mad-doctor on the one hand, and of the collaboration (and often conflict as well) between the psychiatrist and the patient's family and society on the other, need not detain us here. What should concern us is not losing sight of the fact that psychiatry was born out of this complex context of conflict, cooperation, and collusion and that the problems and solutions thus generated remain its backbone. The advent of psychoanalysis and other individual psychotherapies further confused this already complicated situation by introducing the notion that the psychiatrist was an agent of the patient whose job was to provide therapy for him. But what was the psychotherapist expected to do for the patient? Treat his mental illness, of course. And how did the patient know that he was mentally ill? By suffering from conflicts, of course. A man said he wanted to make love to his wife but couldn't because he was impotent. A woman said she wanted to make love to her husband but couldn't because her tightened perineal muscles prevented the act. And so on. Before anyone quite realized what had happened, a new class of diseases was born— diseases said to be the manifestations of, or caused by, *intrapsychic* conflicts. And what is an intrapsychic conflict? Why, a new name for the most elementary fact of human existence, namely, choice.

Actually, in ordinary usage, conflict is a clash or contest between two discrete opponents, typically individuals or groups. We can also speak of conflicting ideas or values. But to say that a person *has* a conflict—for example, between remaining faithful to his wife and making love to his secretary—is another way of saying that he has a *choice* between two alternative courses of conduct.

The existential-legal transformation of choice into conflict and of conflict into sickness is conditioned partly by an extension of the concept of disease from bodily illness to mental illness, and partly by an extension of the concept of conflict from a clash between opposing persons to a clash between opposing desires in the mind of a single individual. Metaphorization of the concept of conflict and the subsequent literalization of the metaphor are the reasons for the seeming paradox that the more freedom of choice people have the more often they suffer from mental illness. The realization that this is not a statistical correlation or an etiological causation, as it is sometimes mistakenly believed to be, but only a tautology, has apparently escaped most people's attention. Obviously, the more choices a person has, the more conflict he can or may have over selecting one course of action over another. Of course, not every choice generates a conflict; but many do. Hence, the more choices a person has, the more conflicts he is likely to have. If we regard every such conflict as a *problem,* and define every such problem as a *mental illness,* then it will follow that giving a person a choice will be almost the same as giving him a conflict which, in turn, will be seen as giving him a mental illness. Could this be the reason why conventional approaches to the etiology, treatment, and prevention of mental illness are not just unproductive but counterproductive if not positively silly?

Actually, the extension of the core meaning of conflict from a clash between contending persons or parties to opposition between incompatible ideas or values, and thence to a metaphorical conflict between *unconscious impulses* or *intrapsychic forces* has had two vastly important consequences. First, this transformation is responsible for launching us down that slippery slope we call psychiatry, psychoanalysis, or behavioral science. At the top of this slope *stand persons making choices;* at the bottom *lie patients suffering from mental diseases.* How one gets from there to here—in other words, how a person jumps, stumbles, or is pushed down a slope so slippery that, once he begins his downward slide he is virtually unable to stop and climb back up again—I try to explain in this book.

Second, this transformation has led to an important redefinition of the ostensible subject matter and scope of psychiatry, changing it from a forensic into an anthropological-psychological discipline, from the study of insanity to the study of interpersonal and intrapersonal relations. The title and subtitle of one of the most prestigious American psychiatric journals, founded in 1938 by Harry Stack Sullivan, is significant and illustrative. It is: *Psychiatry: The Study of Interpersonal Processes.* Interpersonal processes? Surely, that must encompass religion and law, anthropology and politics, economics and psychology, history, philosophy, semantics—in short, virtually every discipline and field of study other than the hardest of hard sciences.

The change in psychiatry's subject matter—from asylum care to interpersonal relations—had several immediate and important consequences. In the first place, psychiatry gained new prestige both as a basic science and as a clinical practice based on scientific principles. The alleged scientific basis of the new dynamic psychiatry was that it rested on the scientific study of human development and unconscious mental life; while the alleged scientific basis of the new psychological therapies, especially psychoanalysis, was that they rested on the rational application of fresh knowledge discovered by the researches of the depth psychologists. That this psychiatric-psychoanalytic science was, in fact, an ideology and a religion—or antireligion—like Marxist dialectical materialism—has remained one of the best-kept secrets of the twentieth century.*

The upshot is that psychiatry has succeeded in shedding its image as an institutional and forensic enterprise—concerned with protecting the civilly insane by means of confinement, and the criminally insane by means of the insanity defense. Instead of psychiatric ideas and interventions remaining restricted to the narrow confines of incarcerating the obviously insane (whether under so-called civil or criminal statutory auspices), psychiatric principles and practices became diffused into every nook and cranny of social relations, from disputes about divorce and child custody to interpretations of international conflict, terrorism, and war.

Moreover, regardless of how far from medicine they have wandered, psychiatrists, psychoanalysts, and psychotherapists never stopped insisting that they were bona fide doctors doing bona fide medical work. Thus, it would be a mistake to believe, as some psychiatric historians and intellectuals do, that the early twentieth-century physician-psychotherapists—whether orthodox or heretical Freudians—did not cherish their medical identity and did not court the approval of the medical profession for their particular brand of therapy. Illustrative is the fact that, in 1926, a group of German-speaking psychotherapists founded the General Medical Society for Psychotherapy, with the support of such seemingly nonmedically oriented therapists as Alfred Adler, Carl Jung, Karen Horney, and Kurt Lewin.[15] Today, Ronald Laing continues in this tradition, displaying the same desire to appear as a real doctor. "I regard psychiatry," he declared in

---

*All this has been anticipated, in his characteristically allusive fashion, by C.S. Lewis. "I have great hopes [he has Screwtape saying] that we shall learn in due time how to emotionalize and mythologise their science. . . . the worship of sex, and some aspects of Psychoanalysis may here prove useful."[14]

1985, "as epitomizing anti-psychiatry. The approach that I have attempted to develop in theory and practice is an approach which I hope and intend to be a genuine practice of mental or psychic healing. . . . The psychiatrists are the anti-psychiatrists, not the attempt to practice *genuine psychiatry*" (emphasis added).[16]

In this connection, I want to mention another effort to rehabilitate psychiatry. It is a sad and silly episode, now largely forgotten, although it enjoyed considerable attention and acclaim only recently.

The story begins in 1933 with the publication, by Alfred Korzybski, of a book titled *Science and Sanity,* which its author "intended to be a textbook showing how in modern scientific methods we can find factors of sanity, to be tested empirically."[17] Observing that crazy people talk crazy, Korzybski declared that "Our sanity is connected with *correct* symbolism. . . . The *abuse* of symbolism is like the abuse of food and drink; it makes people *ill* . . . ." (emphasis added).[18] No doubt about it, the abuse of symbolism does make people ill—but not by giving them cancer of the pancreas. How does it make them ill? By *metaphorically* giving them a *metaphoric* illness which we *conventionally* call insanity.*

It would be charitable to call Korzybski's attitude toward psychiatry deplorable. A Polish nobleman to the core, he uncritically accepted psychiatric slavery and, indeed, proposed to retrain the serfs with his own methods:

> In hospitals for the "mentally" ill two equally large groups of accessible patients exhibiting similar clinical symptoms should be selected and isolated. A physician who himself has undergone $\overline{A}$ training should attempt to retrain the *s.r* of one group. The other group should not be retrained . . . it would be the control group.[20] ($\overline{A}$ is Korzybski's abbreviation for his "Non-aristotelean system.")

I do not know why it never occurred to Korzybski, who claimed to be especially interested in the metaphorical uses of language, that insanity might be an illness like lovesickness rather than like leukemia. Maybe this is just another illustration of the principle that the human mind is an organ for rationalizing rather than thinking. Korzybski wanted to

---

*Hobbes said the same thing:

> There is yet another fault in the discourses of some men; which may also be numbered amongst the sorts of madness; namely that abuse of words, whereof I have spoken before . . . . When men write whole volumes of such stuff, are they not mad, or intend to make others so? And particularly in the question of transubstantiation.[19]

believe that he had made a fresh discovery about the illness called *insanity;* actually, he was applying his positivistic prejudices to what he, like the psychiatrists, regarded as the crazy speech of crazy people. Be that as it may, Korzybski's work generated a movement, called *general semantics.* Although the semanticists ought to have known better, they didn't. Ignoring that the idea of insanity receives its nourishment from roots deeply buried in psychiatry and the law, they simply appropriated the concept and proceeded to give it their own meaning: Insanity was the improper use of language. And thereby hangs a long and interesting tale whose briefest outline must suffice here.

Led by Anatol Rapoport—who began his career as a mathematician and ended it as a lackey of the psychiatrist lobby—the *general semanticists* (many of whom soon became *general system theorists*) were eager to embrace, and be embraced by, the psychiatrists. Their wish was granted and their work was thereby doomed to failure and oblivion: Instead of scrutinizing psychiatry, they saluted it. What is the evidence for this sell-out of the semanticists? It is that, despite their academic sophistication, they chose to authenticate rather than analyze the term *insanity;* and that, despite their civil-libertarian pretensions, they chose to diagnose the discourse of psychotics rather than denounce the despotism of the psychiatrists. In short, the semanticists did nothing to challenge the theoretical premises and social practices of psychiatry; instead, they hitched their wagon to its economic star and used the idea of insanity to aggrandize themselves and legitimize their self-styled science.[21]

How did Rapoport study sanity and insanity? By observing how sane and insane people talked. How did he know who these people were? By assuming that psychiatrists were sane and psychotics insane. The following illustrates how Rapoport presents his own psychiatric-political prejudices as if they were semantic-scientific conclusions:

> At the other extreme is the language of psychotics and people under the spell of superstition and demagogy . . . [whose] linguistic behavior . . . violates semantic principles. . . . Such reactions make possible gigantic sales volumes unrelated to the quality of the product . . . they make wars inevitable.[22]

It is all here: the uncritical acceptance of the psychiatrist's judgment of who is sane and who is insane; the arrogant anticapitalism and hostility to the free market; the resentment against the ordinary man's desire to make his own choices. Finally, notwithstanding a theory of insanity totally unrelated to biological or medical criteria, Rapoport offers a brazenly flattering endorsement of the *science* of psychiatry: "That is why cultural anthropology is so important a science—and so are psychiatry and semantics. . . . These sciences are all in the forward direction toward self-insight."[23] Clearly, Rapoport learned his psychiatry from his paymasters in the Michigan State Hospital system rather than from Mark Twain or Chekhov.

So much for the efforts to relocate lunacy—from brain to mind to language. I maintain that regardless of whether psychiatry wears the mask of medicine, claiming to be concerned with brain diseases and their cures, or the mask of an anthropological-existential science, claiming to be concerned with man's mental life and the resolution of his conflicts, it remains, inexorably, a fundamentally forensic enterprise. Insanity— mental illness, psychopathology, or whatever *it* may be called—is, in fact, a dual fiction, conceptual and tactical, scientific and forensic. (See Chapter 11.)

METAPHORIC DISEASE IS METAPHOR, NOT DISEASE

Actually, the view that mental illnesses are metaphoric diseases—in other words, that the mind can be sick only in the sense in which a joke can be sick—is about as old as psychiatry itself. This should not surprise us. After all, the nineteenth-century psychiatrists could not have been unaware of the fact that they were reclassifying sins as sicknesses. Moreover, educated men that they were, they must have known what Plato had said about what they were doing:

> And to require medicine, said I, not merely for wounds or the incidence of some seasonal maladies, but, because of sloth . . . and compel the ingenious sons of Asclepius to invent for diseases such names as fluxes and flatulences—don't you think that disgraceful? Those surely are, he said, newfangled and monstrous strange names of diseases.[24]

One can only marvel at the clarity with which Plato had already distinguished between real and false, literal and metaphorical, diseases. He also understood that metaphors are the raw materials out of which the philosopher-king must fashion the Noble Lies necessary for his rule:

> It seems likely that our rulers will have to make considerable use of falsehood and deception for the benefit of their subjects. We said, I believe, that the use of that sort of thing was in the category of medicine. . . . And the way all this is brought to pass must be unknown to any but the rulers.[25]

Moreover, even before there was such a thing as psychiatry in Germany, that country's greatest poet and man of letters foresaw the triumph of the medical metaphor in the modern world and trembled at the spectacle:

> I myself must also say I believe it is true that in the end humanitarianism will triumph; only I fear that at the same time the world will be one big hospital and each person will be the other's humane keeper.

> (Auch muss ich selbst sagen, halt' ich es für war, dass die Humanität endlich siegen wird, nur fürcht' ich, dass zu gleicher Zeit die Welt ein grosses Hospital und einer des andern humaner Krankenwärter sein werde.)[26]

Nearly two centuries elapsed before the world caught up with Goethe. As the semanticist Weller Embler observes: ". . . the nineteenth century saw all too clearly the possibility of machines and the world as a vast factory; and the twentieth century sees the possibility of the whole world as a hospital."[27]

Bodily Disease and Mental Disturbance: An Analogy

So far as I have been able to determine, the first psychiatrist to state that mental diseases are metaphoric diseases was the Viennese psychiatrist Ernst von Feuchtersleben (1806–1848). In his book *Lehrbuch der ärtzlichen Seelenkunde* (*Seele* means soul or spirit), published in 1845, Feuchtersleben wrote:

> The maladies of the spirit alone, *in abstracto*, that is, error and sin, can be called diseases of the mind only *per analogiam*. They come not within the jurisdiction of the physician, but that of the teacher or clergyman, who again are called *physicians* of the mind only *per analogiam*.

> (Die Leiden des Geistes allein *in abstracto*, d.i., Irrtum und Sünde, sind nur *per analogiam* Seelenkrankheiten zu nennen; sie gehören nicht vor das Forum des Ärztes, sondern des Lehrers und Priesters, die man denn auch *per analogiam* Seelenärzte nennt.)[28]

Just as psychiatry was beginning to establish itself as a genuine medical specialty, Feuchstersleben was thus calling attention to the purely analogical relations between medical and mental diseases, regular and psychiatric physicians.

Nor was Feuchtersleben alone in recognizing, during the first half of the nineteenth century, the analogical use of the term *illness* that was developing among asylum doctors, and in pointing out that diseases of the soul or spirit are not diseases. In a debate on the question of the appropriateness of the treatment of the insane by nonphysicians, Maximilian Jacobi (1775–1858)—director of the *Irrenanstaldt Siegburg* from 1825 to 1858—objected to the "collective classification of mental illnesses [*Seelenkrankheiten*] [as illnesses] and to the underlying assumption that, in such cases, the mind itself is diseased."[29] Rejecting the postulate advanced by contemporary German "somaticists," that "every madman [*Irre*] suffers from two illnesses, one of the body and one of the mind," he declared: "I confess that I can no more conceive of an illness of the mind analogous to that of the body than I can of any means by which such an illness could be observed."[30] Finally, honing in on what we would now regard as the existential core of the problem, Jacobi attributed mental illness to "a misuse of self-determination" and insisted that such problems "fall outside the realm of illnesses and have, in fact, nothing whatever in common with them."

Interestingly, Emil Kraepelin (1855–1926), the father of modern German psychiatry, also recognized this analogical relationship, but expressed it in a decidedly less firm voice, saying only that "in the strictest terms, we cannot speak of the mind as becoming diseased."[31] These caveats were ignored, of course, by psychiatrists and nonpsychiatrists alike. The idea that mental illness is a real illness, like any other, was simply too important and useful: It was an idea whose time had come, and its march across the pages of history was not going to be stopped by a person here and there noting its metaphorical character.

The next watershed in the literalization of the metaphor of mental illness is marked by Bleuler's invention of schizophrenia. Bleuler realized that he was basing this diagnosis on the fact that the so-called schizophrenic patient uses metaphors, and yet was willing, perhaps eager, to see the patient as literally sick. One of the cases Bleuler describes in his epoch-making work on schizophrenia is that of a woman who claims that she "'possesses' Switzerland; and in the same sense she says 'I am Switzerland.' She may also say, 'I am freedom,' since for her Switzerland meant nothing else than freedom."[32] What makes this woman a schizophrenic rather than a metaphorist? Bleuler explains:

> The difference between the use of such phrases in the healthy and in the schizophrenic rests in the fact that in the former it is a mere metaphor whereas for the patients the dividing line between direct and indirect representation has been obscured. The result is that they frequently think of these metaphors in a literal sense.[33]

As I showed in my book on schizophrenia, Bleuler was fully aware, and deeply impressed, by the metaphors of schizophrenic patients—which, he insisted, they interpreted literally.[34] In a remarkable passage—one of several that could have been written only by a Protestant psychiatrist—Bleuler states: "I would like to call your attention to the manifold significance of Catholic symbolism. . . . Homo Dei in the image of mortals could just as well have been the brainchild of a modern schizophrenic."[35]

This seems to me bitterly ironic: When the psychiatrist calls physically healthy persons who do not want to be patients *patients,* and the building in which he imprisons them *hospitals,* the psychiatrist insists that he is not using metaphors at all; but when a person who is unhappy and perhaps makes others unhappy uses language in a similar way, then the psychiatrist insists that the troubled and troubling person is a literal patient who is literally ill, with the literal disease called *schizophrenia.*

Today, the literalization of the metaphor of mental illness—with schizophrenia, ironically, as its paradigm—is so entrenched that, like an accepted religious doctrine, people either do not see the literalized metaphor at all, or if they do see it, they prefer to look the other way. The views of Seymour Kety, quoted earlier in this chapter, are illustrative:

> Diabetes mellitus is analogous to schizophrenia in many ways. Both are symptom clusters or syndromes, one described by somatic and biochemical abnormalities, the other by psychological. Each may have many etiologies and show a range of intensity from severe and debilitating to latent or borderline. There is also evidence that genetic and environmental influences operate in the development of both. The medical model seems to be quite as appropriate for the one as for the other.[36]

Note that Kety first analogizes somatic and psychological *symptom clusters* much as the doctrine of transubstantiation analogizes Jesus' body and the consecrated host, and then proceeds to treat them as if they were the same sorts of things. As a result, he misinterprets what is meant by a metaphor, treating a metaphorical disease as a disease instead of as a metaphor. This is an absurd mistake few of us would make if the word used metaphorically was not as weighty as the word *disease.*

For example, no one thinks that a mixture of orange juice and vodka is a type of tool for tightening and loosening screws. Let me briefly explain. By *screwdriver* we ordinarily mean a tool used by carpenters; we also give this name to a drink made of orange juice and vodka. Clearly, saying that the drink is a *metaphoric screwdriver* is not saying that it is some other kind of screwdriver; it is saying that it is *not a screwdriver at all.* Similarly, if I say that mental illness is a metaphorical illness, I am not saying that it is some other kind of illness; I am saying that it is not an illness at all. I emphasize this in the hope of transcending the usual psychiatric misunderstanding of, and rejoinders to, my assertion that mental illness is a metaphor, often phrased thus: "What difference does it make what you call mental illness (schizophrenia, bipolar illness, etc.)? Regardless of what *you* call it, *we* know it is an illness (just like paresis; soon we shall identify its somatic basis in the brain)." Such a rejoinder misses my point: It is like saying that it does not matter what you call a mixture of orange juice and vodka, because I know that it is an instrument for fastening and loosening screws. (If that is not yet apparent to some skeptics, it soon will be, when the drink called *screwdriver* will be shown to be a real screwdriver.) Placing mental illness as metaphor in the same class as mental illness as abnormal behavior is like placing the screwdriver as drink in the same class as the screwdriver as tool—which would lead us to sell metaphorical screwdrivers in hardware stores, and literal screwdrivers in bars.

Literalized Metaphor as Social Convention

Why do people, even if they recognize the difference between symbol and the object it symbolizes, often treat literalized metaphors as if they were the thing the metaphor names? For example, non-Catholics, and even many Catholics, recognize that bread and wine are not the body and blood of a man long dead who is said to be a deity. In certain situations, however, they all behave, Catholics more often than non-Catholics, as if the symbol were the thing symbolized. Why do people act this way? Catholics do so mainly because this is what establishes their identity as Catholics. Non-Catholics do so mainly because it is— say, in a church—the polite thing to do.

Although psychiatrists insist that mental diseases are real diseases, and although many persons do not believe this, most people much of the time act as if they did. They also recognize that disagreements are personal and social events usually called *conflicts* and are not the symptoms of undemonstrated and undemonstrable pathological processes in synapses in the central nervous system. In certain situations, however, they all behave, psychiatrists more often than nonpsychiatrists, as if the symbol were the thing symbolized—that is, as if schizophrenia were actually like syphilis and depression like diabetes. The question is: Why do people act like this? Psychiatrists do so mainly because this is what establishes their identity as physicians. Nonpsychiatrists do so mainly because, as a rule, it is the polite and proper thing to do in our society lest one risk revealing oneself as stupid or sick.

A Further Lesson from Language

Many people rightly fear being manipulated by the slick and deceptive use of words, especially when it comes to matters they think they understand as well as they want to. Hence the frequently expressed belief: "I don't care what you call it, I know this is X" (where X might stand for a thing or idea). When this sentiment characterizes a person's attitude toward an abstract noun—such as *democracy* or *mental illness*—then we have a problem if we try to change his mind, which, as such a person himself admits, is closed. Assuming that no one who has read this far has a closed mind about diseases of the mind, I want to offer a brief digression into linguistic analysis in order to further enrich our grasp of what it means to view mental illness as a metaphor.

When we say that someone has a closed mind, everyone recognizes that the mind is not, literally, an area or space, that may be closed or open. Accordingly, people do not expect chauffeurs to drive through an open mind. But they do expect psychiatrists to cure a sick mind.

How can a mind be sick? How can a foot be sick, or a tiger be sick, or a tree be sick, or the economy be sick, or a joke be sick? Is there *anything* that cannot be sick? Perhaps we best begin with a brief analysis of the words *sick* and *ill*.

The terms *ill* and *sick* are often used interchangeably. For example, we say, "Jones has pneumonia, he is quite ill." We can just as well say, "Jones has pneumonia, he is quite sick." However, *ill* has a history and a scope that have nothing to do with medicine or disease: it then means, roughly, bad, unfortunate, tragic, or something of that sort. For example, we can speak of ill will or ill fate, but we cannot speak of sick will or sick fate. Moreover, we can speak of ill health but cannot substitute sick as an adjective for health.

On the other hand, *ill* has a more restricted implication than *sick*, so that there are many instances in which we can use the latter term but not the former. For example, we don't say, "The tiger is ill," or "The tree is ill," but we do say, "The tiger is sick," or "The tree is sick." Revealingly, the strict use of *ill* is restricted to persons; not even body parts or organs may be ill, although they may be sick. We don't say, "His hand is ill," or "He has an ill hand," but we say "His hand is sick," or "He has a sick hand." If we want to convey the idea of ill about an animal, a part of the human body, or even an abstract noun, then we use *sick*. Thus, we can say about a person that "His liver is sick," and we can also say that a cat or a car, a television set or a joke, or even a whole society is sick. None of them can be ill, however.

Qualifying *ill* and *sick* with *mentally* introduces new possibilities and limitations into how those terms can be used and what they mean. Interestingly, *mentally ill* and *mentally sick* tend to function linguistically very much as the metaphorically *sick* functions and not at all as does the literally *sick* or *ill*. (By *metaphorically sick*, I mean that the person uses it to express disapproval or dislike of the referent or attributes some sort of malfunctioning or wrongness to it, whereas by *literally sick* or *ill*, I mean that the person uses it to express the specific idea of some sort of bodily disorder or medical disease.)

The literally or medically *sick* occurs in all tenses and moods and with all sorts of time modifiers; the metaphorically or mentally *sick* does not. For example, we can say all of the following: "Jones is sick; he cannot work." "Jones was sick; he could not work." "Jones has been sick; he has not been working." "Jones had been sick; he missed a lot of work." "Jones will be sick; he will not be at work." "Don't get sick, Jones; you don't want to miss work."

When metaphorically *sick* is used explicitly, it has a much more restricted range of tenses. We can say, "The joke is sick," or "The joke was sick." But it would be weird to say, "The joke has been sick," or "The joke will be sick." And it would be absurd to say, "The joke is often sick."

The psychiatrically or mentally *sick*, which I have long contended is covertly metaphorical, has the same restricted range of use as does the overtly metaphorical *sick*. Thus, we can say, "Jones is mentally sick (or ill); he shot the president." But it would be wrong, as well as odd, to say, "When Jones will be mentally sick, he will shoot the president." (If we thought this about Jones, we would say he *is* mentally sick.) It would be odder still to say, "Don't get mentally sick, Jones, you don't want to shoot the president." Humorous as that sounds, the psychiatric and witty dimensions of *mentally sick* would become indistinguishable were we to say, "Jones is mentally sick today; he shoots the president," or "Jones is often mentally sick; he shoots a lot of presidents."

Some of these differences between *sick* and *mentally sick* stem from the fact that we tend to use *sick* to describe conditions and *mentally sick* to describe characteristics, and that we usually attribute more permanence to the latter than to the former. Thus, Jones may have pneumonia and may recover from it. Hence, we say, "Jones is sick," and "Jones was sick." But if Jones is an American, so long as Jones is alive, we cannot in the same way say, "Jones is an American," and "Jones was an American" (for the latter generally means not that he is no longer an American but that he is no longer alive; it may also mean, of course, that Jones has renounced or lost his American citizenship).

CONTENTIONS AND REFUTATIONS

To further sharpen what I mean when I assert that *mental illness is a metaphor*, let us now consider the principal arguments with which psychiatrists and others typically try to refute this contention.

"He Acts Sick, He Looks Sick, He Is Sick"

One such refutation goes something like this: "Here is a man who is hallucinating and has delusions. He has no money, no place to go, his family rejects him. He has been in several mental hospitals and psychiatrists have repeatedly diagnosed him as suffering from schizophrenia. You mean to tell me he is not sick?" Note that to describe a person as having hallucinations and delusions, and as having been diagnosed as schizophrenic is, in effect, the same as saying that he is sick, but without identifying the criteria for illness. So we must ask, by what criterion is this person sick? If literal illness is identifiable bodily disease, then, having hallucinations or delusions and being called schizophrenic are simply irrelevant to ascertaining whether or not a person is sick.

A comparison will make the point clear. Suppose a person were to say: "Look at this cute animal. Doesn't he look just like a baby bear? He is a Teddy-bear. People call him a koala bear. You mean to tell me he is not a bear?" The koala bear is, however, not a bear, but a marsupial. Calling it a bear is a mistake. The same sort of error may be committed by a child who, upon being taken to see a whale, exclaims: "What a huge fish!"

If Not Mentally Sick, then Mentally Healthy

Another closely related rebuttal rests on the way people unwittingly entrap themselves, and try to entrap me, into the consequences of the language of mental illness. Thus, when I assert that a person psychiatrists consider to be mentally ill is not ill, my critics assume that I consider him to be mentally healthy. This rejoinder is hurled against my views in an astonishingly mindless manner, as the following example illustrates: "It is *clinical evidence* (detailed investigative reports, case histories, etc.) showing that a representative sample of such putative neurotics are *completely healthy* that Szasz . . . fails to offer his readers" (emphasis added).[37]

This is sheer nonsense. Again, a historical example will quickly show why. At the height of the Inquisition, a Christian was seen as either a faithful Catholic or a heretic. At that time, when a Christian acted in a religiously deviant fashion, he was called a heretic. We would not now consider such a person a heretic, but neither would we consider him a faithful Catholic. Likewise, it does not follow that by rejecting the concept of mental illness, one commits oneself to the view that those now considered mentally ill are mentally healthy. I reject both concepts and terms as false labels for social conformity and deviance, social competence and incompetence, and other behavioral characteristics.

Treating Metaphoric Illness as Illness

Still another argument, seemingly more sophisticated and scientific, goes like this: "We, psychiatrists, follow the medical approach to mental illness. We believe this is the correct approach. There are others [and here the author or speaker may or may not mention me by name] who prefer the social approach. But they are wrong because . . . ." The advocates of this argument then go on to cite studies about the genetic determinants of schizophrenia and the effectiveness of drugs in controlling this disease.

I am often confronted with this argument, sometimes by reporters or others from the news media, and have concluded that it is founded on so successful a distortion of my position that it is virtually impossible to counter it. For if a well-meaning questioner does not see the point on which this riddle turns, no amount of fresh explanation about the mythology of mental illness is likely to make him see it. Still, I try to answer it, along this line. Let us go back four hundred years. People then believed in witches, and the official explanation of witchcraft was theological. Suppose someone had come along and said: "There are no witches. *Witch* is only a name we now attach to poor and helpless people, usually women." Would it be proper to call this person's views a *social approach* to witches, as opposed to the official theological approach to them? Of course not. How can a person have any kind of an approach to X if he believes that X does not exist? (X may here stand for witches, unicorns, the devil, God, or mental illness.) What the disbeliever in witches offers is not a social approach to witches, but a philosophical analysis and ethical critique of the idea of witch and the practices it generates and justifies. Since everyone now knows that there are no witches, no explanation of their nonexistence is necessary. However, since everyone now knows that there are mental diseases, no explanation of their nonexistence can be convincing. The reason why professionals who speak like this, and lay people who hear them speak, know that I must be wrong lies, in this case, not so much in inattention to what constitutes a disease, as in an unshakable presumption that the term *mental illness* (or *schizophrenia*) is the name of a real disease.

Rejecting Bodily Lesion as a Criterion of Illness

Among my more thoughtful critics must be counted Sir Martin Roth, a professor of psychiatry at the University of Cambridge and a leading contemporary British psychiatrist. Roth's argument flows from his premise that my definition of disease in unacceptable. "Of course," he concedes, "if illness is a matter of lumps, lesions, and germs most schizophrenics are perfectly healthy. But such a definition of disease would be repudiated even by physicians."[38] As I have shown, however, this is not so; pathologists define disease exactly as I do (or rather vice versa); and nonpsychiatric physicians often adhere to the pathologist's criteria, except insofar as mental diseases are concerned.

What, then, is Roth's criterion of literal illness? He does not have one. Instead, he claims all of life for psychiatry with the seemingly humane and disarming assertion that psychiatry ". . . is primarily concerned with mental suffering, its mitigation and prevention irrespective of cause."[39] Roth's strict orthodoxy may account for his being so irritated by my irreverent heterodoxy. "Szasz's meteoric rise, his growing influence and world renown are not, therefore, unexpected," he writes begrudgingly. "The reasons are perhaps to be found in the verdict, 'I think that bad philosophers may have a certain influence, good philosophers never.'"[40] Surely, such a quip falls far short of British standards of intellectual debating. Paradoxically, Roth's most serious criticism comes closest to what I consider to be one of my most important claims:

> The attitude of the law and the legal profession to psychiatry and mental disorder has been transformed by the writings of Thomas Szasz . . . . He is obsessed by the need he feels for psychiatric patients, psychotic or neurotic, to be accepted by all of us as human beings of no less value than ourselves, and therefore not ill.[41]

Roth seems to object to my proposal that we accept persons denominated as mental patients "as human beings of no less value than ourselves." However, instead of telling us why we should not do so, he merely adds ". . . and therefore not ill." I assume Roth does this to make my views seem absurd. But I think his tactic backfires: We accept patients with polio and Parkinsonism as fully human, *albeit ill*; why, then, should we not also accept patients with psychosis as fully human, *albeit ill?* Why should illness negate moral agency? Roth never engages the argument.

Charles Krauthammer, a psychiatrist turned social commentator, rejects bodily lesion as a criterion of illness. First, however, he summarizes the practical consequences of my work:

> As a polemicist, Szasz has no peer. He has succeeded in focusing attention on the loose and easy quality of psychiatric definitions, on the destructive and indelible stigma that often accompanies psychiatric diagnosis, and on the unique and easily corrupted power that psychiatry has been granted. He has spawned an entire movement of anti-psychiatry, complete with schools, sages and schisms. Ripples from his abolitionist crusade against commitment laws are only now being felt. Self-help groups and legal defense funds for mental patients have sprung up throughout the country. . . . Szasz deserves much of the credit.[42]

Nevertheless, Krauthammer considers my argument fundamentally flawed. Few people are aware, he writes, "that the entire argument depends on an unusual definition of illness. The only real illness, Szasz says, is a bodily lesion."[43] As I have shown (Chapter 1), there is nothing unusual about this definition.

Krauthammer notes, and I agree, that "Bodily abnormality simply is not the same as illness." In addition, a judgment—made by individuals (patients), experts (physicians), professional organizations (medical societies), and political entities (governments)—is required to transform a *deviation* (from a biological or other norm) into a *disease.* "Many epileptics," Krauthammer observes, "have no detectable brain lesions or brain wave abnormality. On the other hand, many perfectly normal people, when screened, turn out to have abnormal brain waves. According to Szasz's criterion, the former are well, the latter diseased."[44] That is not correct. These examples do not defeat my argument, as Krauthammer claims. I do not contend that persons exhibiting genuine epileptic seizures or suffering from migraine (another of Krauthammer's examples) are well. I view such persons as having bodily diseases without presently demonstrable pathoanatomical or pathophysiological correlates or lesions: in other words, they suffer from what I call *putative diseases.* Nor do I claim that persons with abnormal brain waves but without any other signs or symptoms of epilepsy are necessarily ill or have a disease; I claim only that such persons exhibit deviations from certain biological norms—in this case the norms defined by electroencephalography. The relationship between proven violations of biological norms (bodily lesions) and diseases is similar to the relationship between proven violations of legal norms (lawbreaking) and crime. Terms such as *illness* (or *disease*) and *crime* imply not only that certain phenomena or events have been observed or exist but also that it is socially legitimate to *classify* them in a particular way, or to give them certain *names*. It is an empirical question whether a deviation identified by means of mechanical, electrical, or chemical tests—for example, by sphygmomanometry (blood pressure measurements) or electroencephalography (measurement of brain waves)—is relevant to human health. If it is relevant—as in the case of blood pressure—then the abnormal measurement itself may reasonably be said to be, or signify the presence of, a disease; if it is not relevant—as in the case of brain waves—then the abnormal measurement is not enough for such a conclusion. Some tests are better than others, just as some people are richer or smarter than others.

The Specter of Conspiracy

A decidedly less thoughtful refutation of my views rests on the mistaken belief that a myth is something invented by one group of persons to confuse or persecute another. As a result I am viewed as a "conspiracy theorist" who blames psychiatrists for inventing insanity. Many critics have adopted this view, including some mental health professionals who, having made mental patient advocacy their career, seem to believe that doing their job properly requires accepting the proposition that mental illness is a bona fide disease. For example, Larry Gostin, the legal director of MIND (a mental patient advocacy group in Britain) writes: ". . . there is a deep intuitive recognition of the existence of insanity . . . . There is a common sense acceptance that madness is not a myth invented by medicine."[45] However, intuitive recognition and commonsense acceptance do not count for much in trying to understand why Negro slaves should be counted as three-fifths rather than five-fifths human, or why certain criminals should be treated as mad rather than as bad.

Getting Personal . . .

Another rather unimaginative counterargument goes like this: "So you think mental illness is not real. Try telling that to a catatonic patient in a mental hospital or to his mother." Since I do not try to tell anything to anyone who does not ask my advice or opinion, and since catatonic patients and their relatives convinced of the reality of mental illness usually do not ask for my opinion, the injunction is moot. If a person thinks that one can lose one's mind just as one can lose one's car keys, why should I try to tell him about the metaphoric uses of the word *lose* and the tragedies it can mask when used as an adjective to qualify a man's mind?

In a more personal vein, some psychiatrists criticize me for being too liberal (libertarian), while others accuse me of being too authoritarian. For example, Donald Klein, a professor of psychiatry at Columbia University, writes:

> Authoritarians, on the other hand, claiming that mental illness is a myth, condemn assaultive paranoids to jail and suicidal depressives to death. I believe that their real covert agenda is the promulgation of a heartless individualism whose target is not the malingerer or the criminal disguised as mentally ill, but the poor, disadvantaged, and socially deprived.[46]

Although Klein never mentions my name and does not list any of my publications in his references, I take this to be his reply to my views. Klein does not bother to explain why individuals who assault others should not be punished, nor why punishing them by means of psychiatric sanctions is necessarily or self-evidently superior, as a social policy, to punishing them by means of criminal sanctions. The proposition that *not coercing* an individual whom psychiatrists call *suicidal* is synonymous with condemning him to death is now so intrinsic a part of the language of psychiatry that psychiatrists do not even notice what they are saying or, if they do notice it, are proud of it. Clearly, when a person embracing psychiatric coercion calls another who eschews such coercion *authoritarian*, then we are in the presence of a profound transvaluation of our values and transformation of our language.

Does Klein offer a defense of psychiatric coercion? Not really, since he views it as self-evidently necessary and useful. "Does anyone believe," he asks, "that if commitment were outlawed the FBI would be better controlled?"[47] It would be uncharitable, and perhaps risky as well, to comment on Klein's choice of words, since another critic states that I overestimate the importance of words:

> Szasz may be revealing the presence and influence of a belief that words can actually create and destroy. [He then cites several of my aphorisms ostensibly supporting this interpretation, and continues] . . . to believe that words can be used to create or destroy is to believe in *word magic:* something which, as psychoanalysts have learned, is typical at the age of two or so, but which becomes increasingly unusual thereafter.[48]

Other critics say more explicitly that my views are the symptoms of mental illness. "Dr. Thomas Szasz," declares a psychiatrist, "is widely recognized in authoritative medical circles for his paranoiac utterances of psychiatry."[49]

Miscellaneous Refutations

Nathaniel Laor, a professor of psychiatry at Yale, is a careful and conscientious commentator on my writings, but he sometimes misconstrues my views and then criticizes the misconstruction. For example, he writes: "Thomas S. Szasz is an uncompromising thinker and a brave psychiatrist . . . . For him, suffering and sorrow cannot serve as signs and symptoms for medical disease entity—only organic markers could serve this function."[50] This is correct and complimentary. But then Laor significantly misstates my views:

> Take away the suffering and no disease entity remains. Thus, says Szasz, mental illness is a mere myth or, at best, a mere metaphor. . . . Hence, it is by claiming the mentally ill to be always autonomous, that is always free of specific (pathological) organic constraints and free to determine their own goals that Szasz excludes the mentally ill from the realm of medicine and renders them always responsible.[51]

But I do not claim that persons denominated as mentally ill are "always free of specific (pathological) organic constraints": I clearly allow for the possibility that, like anyone else, such persons may suffer from undetected diseases. Moreover, it is not because I believe that so-called mentally ill persons are "always autonomous" that I want to treat them as responsible moral agents: I clearly state that since somatic pathology per se is not a sufficient condition for depriving a bodily ill person of moral agency, it should not be a sufficient condition in the case of a mentally ill person either.

Laor's misunderstanding of the concept of autonomy leads him, as it does many people, to being unable to distinguish between caring and coercing. "Out of respect for the individual's alleged autonomy," he writes, "Szasz requires we stand by while people drop dead on the streets."[52] It is not clear why Laor thinks I am opposed to someone *offering* money, food, or lodging to poor people—or anything else the generous donor thinks the recipient needs or wants. Indeed, although I am not enthusiastic about it, I willingly support a social policy whereby an agency of the State would *offer* food, shelter, and other services to people in need, provided that those delivering the services would be effectively prevented from coercing those who receive them.

Credit for the most absurd counterargument goes to Samuel Guze, who, in his zeal, bases his reasoning on his ignorance. The word *disease* he asserts, has no literal meaning or use at all: "Disease is . . . a metaphoric concept. It may be said that there is no such thing as a disease. . . . The concept of disease may be a 'myth.'"[53] Imitation may be the highest form of flattery, but this is going too far. Perhaps because he is a psychiatrist, Guze seems to believe that the word *disease* has only rhetorical uses and can have no descriptive meaning at all.

In contrast to the foregoing refutations, most of which miss their mark by a mile or more, I now want to mention an argument that is cogent, albeit deceptive. No sooner did I suggest, almost 30 years ago, that mental illness is not a real disease, than psychiatrists started to say that I am partially right because (for example) hysteria is, indeed, not a real disease, but schizophrenia, of course, is. Since then, with increasing frequency, psychiatrists have discovered or decided that this or that formerly recognized mental illness—for example, homosexuality—is not a mental illness. (In DSM-III not only has the term *neurosis* been dropped but so also has the term *mental illness;* it was replaced by *mental disorder.*) Such claims attract much media attention and support, I believe because they simultaneously assert and deny the validity of the concept of mental illness: By asserting that X is not a mental illness, the speaker ostensibly informs us about the nature of X, while implying that although X is not a mental disease, Y and Z are. Again, the criterion for what constitutes illness or mental illness remains unexamined and unchallenged.

This argument is tactically sound. By sacrificing some outlying positions, the defenders of a besieged army can retreat to the safety of their fortress: in this way, the defenders of the proposition that mental illness, exemplified by schizophrenia, is a brain disease get away unharmed—without having to prove their case.

Finally, my suggestion that mental illnesses are not bona fide diseases—that they are personal problems in living—was immediately and instinctively viewed, especially by psychiatrists, as an attempt to redistribute the wealth inherent in insanity. This is a false, though not entirely unjustifiable, interpretation. Speaking of so-called mental illnesses as problems in living does not imply that these problems are, ipso facto, the property of psychologists. Indeed, I have made it clear from the beginning of my work that the issue of control or ownership of conduct—healthy or sick, sane or insane—is an integral part of the problem of so-called mental illness; that in order to come to grips with these problems we must decide whether we value freedom more than health or vice versa; and that I, placing freedom above health, advocate returning health and illness, mental health and mental illness, to their rightful owners—the so-called patients and mental patients, the persons who possess (or are said to suffer from) these conditions.

Because the various criticisms I have just reviewed overlap and pivot around two important issues, I now want to rephrase them, and my responses to them.

Some critics say that I am wrong because what we now call mental diseases may yet be shown to be caused, at least in some cases, by subtle pathophysiological processes in the body—in particular, by disorders in the molecular chemistry of the brain—that we do not yet know how to measure or record. Nevertheless, such processes, like those responsible for the psychoses associated with paresis or pellagra, exist, and it is only because of the present state of our knowledge, or rather ignorance, that we cannot properly diagnose them. Actually, such an advance in the science and technology of medical diagnosis would only add to the list of literal diseases and would not in the slightest impair the validity of my argument that when we call certain kinds of disapproved behaviors mental diseases, we are using the word *disease* metaphorically. This objection to my views, which actually represents just another instance of biological reductionism, misses the point I try to make; to uphold it would be like upholding the view that because certain canvases thought to be forged Renoirs prove to be, on closer study, genuine, all forged masterpieces are genuine. If there are real or literal diseases, there must also be others that are fake or metaphorical.

Other critics say that I am wrong, not because I say that mental illnesses are unlike bodily illnesses (an assertion with which they claim to agree), nor because I say that involuntary hospitalization or treatment is no more justified for so-called mental illness than it is for bodily illness (a moral principle with which they also claim to be in sympathy), but because the term *mental illness* often designates a phenomenologically identifiable and hence valid category of conduct. But I do not deny that. I have never maintained that the conduct of a depressed or elated person is the same as that of a person who is contented and even-tempered or that the conduct of a person who claims to be Jesus or Napoleon is the same as that of one who makes no such false claims. I simply prefer not to place deviance in the category of disease.

PSYCHIATRIC INTERVENTION: LITERAL OR METAPHORICAL TREATMENT?

Although common sense—which sometimes affirms timeless truths, and sometimes egregious errors—is not a reliable guide to reality, we must always pay heed to it. As common sense tells us that where there is smoke, there is fire, so it also tells us that where there is treatment—allegedly, or ostensibly, or seemingly effective treatment—there is disease. As I noted earlier, psychiatrists often rest their claim that mental illness is a neurochemical disease on the fact that they treat it as if it were such a disease; and lay people often believe that mental illness is a real disease because *it* is being treated by psychiatrists. Accordingly, I now want to say something about psychiatric treatment, an idea that stands in the same relation to psychiatric illness as a key stands to a lock. As the idea of a lock implies that of a key and vice versa, so the idea of mental illness implies that of mental treatment and vice versa. Hence, if there is no mental illness, there can be no such thing as mental treatment. What, then, is it that psychiatrists do when they dispense what they call *psychiatric treatments* or practice what they call *psychotherapy?* My answer is: They dispense pseudomedical, metaphorical treatments. Let me briefly explain what I mean.

Psychiatric Interventions as Metaphorical Treatments

There are three reasons for holding that psychiatric treatments are metaphorical treatments. First, if the conditions psychiatrists seek to cure are not literal diseases, then the procedures they use to influence them cannot be literal treatments. For sick economies, the cures must be metaphorical, which is not to say that the level of employment is not real or does not affect the economy. Similarly, drugs and dialogues are real and may indeed help people said to be mentally ill: but this proves not that mental diseases are literal maladies, but only that mental treatments can be effective interventions.

Second, we must again face the fact that psychiatric treatments are often imposed on persons against their will. If a surgeon operates on a competent adult without the patient's consent, the intervention, even if curative, constitutes assault and battery. We make this judgment because our conventional concept of treatment condenses two very important ideas: namely, that a medical treatment is an intervention believed to help a condition called a *disease,* and that it is desired and consented to by the person who has the disease. *Logically,* if there is no disease, there can be no treatment: no treatment can *exist. Legally,* if there is no consent (not necessarily the patient's), there can be no treatment: treatment may not be *given.* Moreover, there are many diseases for which there are no treatments. To be sure, there is always something the doctor can do, and something the patient wants done—and that something is conventionally called *treatment.* Similarly, there are many consensual relations between psychiatrists and patients: psychiatrists give and mental patients receive certain things and those interventions are conventionally called *mental* or *psychiatric treatments.* Psychotherapies in general, and psychoanalysis in particular, exemplify this class of interventions. Just what are they? Are they properly called treatments? I believe the answer is no.

Finally, then, we must consider the nature of so-called psychotherapeutic procedures, the paradigmatic interventions psychiatrists provide for voluntary patients. There are many kinds of psychotherapies. I shall use individual psychotherapy as my model. Since this procedure consists basically of a confidential conversation between two people, it can be therapeutic only in a metaphorical sense. In the eighteenth century, when people spoke of the *cure of souls,* everyone knew that the diseases such cures were supposed to heal were spiritual, that the therapists were clerical, and that the cures were metaphorical.[54] Today—with the soul securely displaced by the mind, and the mind securely subsumed as a function of the brain—people speak of the *cure of minds,* and everyone knows that the diseases the psychiatrist treats are similar to ordinary medical diseases, that the therapists who administer such treatments are bona fide physicians, and that the cures are the results of literal treatments. In short, mental illness and mental treatment are symmetrical and indeed symbiotic ideas. The extension of the idea of somatic therapy into psychotherapy and the metaphorization of personal influence as therapy coincide with the extension of pathology into psychopathology and the metaphorization of personal problems as mental diseases.*

In this connection, I want to say something more about the psychiatric treatment now most in fashion—namely the use of so-called neuroleptic, psychotropic, or antipsychotic drugs. Because of the social circumstances in which psychiatrist and mental patient typically encounter each other, it is impossible to know whether most people now receiving so-called psychopharmacological therapy really want to take psychiatric drugs. That psychiatrists want to give patients such drugs is clear. Indeed, the allegedly therapeutic powers of these drugs is now

---

*The result is a comic multiplication of psychotherapies and of psychotherapists making comic claims—all of it being taken seriously. For example, T. Byram Karasu, a professor of psychiatry at Cornell Medical Center in New York, is quoted as stating, at a recent meeting of the Association for the Advancement for Psychotherapy, that there are now "250 to 450 varieties of psychotherapy competing for dwindling health dollars" and that "psychotherapy . . . helped more people with mental illness than coronary bypass helped patients with angina."[55]

used as a fresh justification for psychiatric coercion, as the following statement, excerpted from a legal brief filed by the American College of Neuropsychopharmacology, illustrates:

> The vast majority of patients committed to an institution, especially a state-run facility, need some form of drug therapy. . . . Psychotic disease alters the minds of afflicted patients; antipsychotic medication is mind restorative. . . . It would be a clinical error to deny a schizophrenic patient an antipsychotic drug. . . . antipsychotic drugs are the single best available treatment for schizophrenia. . . . The commitment of a patient to a state psychiatric facility includes an implicit prescription for active treatment rather than mere custodial care. Proper medical treatment of psychotic patients has come to necessarily include the use of antipsychotic drugs. . . . Concerning the medical treatment of rational patients, the philosophy of a person being his own judge as to whether treatment is justified is a laudable goal. . . . For severely ill psychiatric patients, however, this model of the individual rationally balancing the risks and benefits of antipsychotic medication fails.[56]

As my objections to coerced psychiatric treatments are a matter of long record by now, my views on the deplorable practice of forcibly drugging mental patients should be clear without further comment. At the same time, it must be remembered that many people willingly submit to psychiatric treatments of all sorts and eagerly take psychiatric drugs such as Valium, Haldol, or Lithium. A supporter of conventional psychiatric wisdom might therefore ask: "Doesn't that prove that mental patients find relief in these treatments?" And if they do, it may seem like a small step to conclude that people so treated and helped suffer from a genuine illness. But let us see just what inference we should more correctly draw from the fact that many people willingly take psychotropic drugs and are said to be helped by them.

Most people, mental patients included, like to take drugs. If they must seek out and pay for the drug—as people must now seek out and pay for alcohol and cigarettes, marijuana and heroin—then, ipso facto, that proves that they like to take that drug. Whether such drugs can, in a meaningful sense, be said to help those who take them cannot be answered without first answering the question: Help them achieve what goal? Satisfy what craving or need? Of course, we can use the word *help* in effect as a tautology inferring help from the subject's own repeated acts of drug taking. Obviously, that is not a medical or scientific standard for determining therapeutic effectiveness. Furthermore, since there are no objective standards or measures for determining improvement or deterioration in mental disease, as there are, say, in diabetes or hypertension, the assertion that a particular drug helps a patient is nothing but an assertion or claim. There are many possibilities along this line: for example, a person may claim to feel better after taking Haldol or Lithium because, in fact, he feels better; or his wife may say he is better, because she feels better; or his psychiatrist may say he is better, because he feels better. However, none of this proves that the alleged condition for which the patient was getting or taking Haldol, and which is now said to be "improved because of Haldol," is a bona fide (literal) illness. Our criterion for literal, medical illness, as I emphasized at the beginning of this book, is pathoanatomical and pathophysiological. We do not infer the presence of medical illness from the fact that after taking a drug, a person, called a *patient* claims to feel better, or from the fact that someone else claims he acts better. Hence, the alleged effectiveness of psychiatric drugs is no better evidence for the existence or reality of mental-disease-*qua*-brain-disease than was the alleged effectiveness of electroshock or lobotomy (whose inventor received the Nobel Prize).

THE PROBLEM OF DEFINITION RECONSIDERED

Writers on mental illness, law, and psychiatry are wont to engage in endless debates about what constitutes illness or mental illness. These exercises invariably focus on the question of whether we should define these classes broadly or narrowly. This approach is a kind of shadow boxing: it avoids the core issue, namely, the distinction between the literal and metaphorical uses of words. As we saw, definitions of mental illness range from the view that mental illness is proven or putative brain disease, a narrow definition, to the view that it is the human condition itself, a broad definition. To my knowledge, no modern authority addressing this subject has been willing to look at the problem through the resolving lenses of literal/metaphorical meaning. But looking at mental diseases without those lenses is like looking at orthopedic diseases without x-rays: We miss more than we see.

Literalizing the Medical Metaphor

One of my aims in the earlier chapters has been to offer literal definitions of having an *illness* and being a *patient*. If we accept these definitions—even if only for the sake of clarifying our understanding of the scope and function of medicine and psychiatry—then we can conclude that illness and mental illness, patient and mental patient, doctor and psychiatrist, medical hospital and mental hospital stand in the same relation to one another as a literal (biological) father stands to a metaphoric (theological) father or priest. If there is no literal meaning of the word *father*, there can be no metaphorical meaning of it either; people might then be led to believe that further theological research could demonstrate that the fatherhood of priests is just as real as that of genuine (biological) fathers.

Psychiatry rests precisely on such a conflation and confusion of literal and metaphorical meanings—that is, on the metaphoric conversion of problems in living into illnesses and on the literalization of the metaphor of illness. In the Mass and through the priest, bread and wine are miraculously transformed into the body and blood of Jesus. Denying that transformation and insisting that the consecrated bread and wine are nothing but bread and wine used to be regarded as religious heresy. *Mutatis mutandis*, in modern society and through the psychiatrist, human difficulties are scientifically transformed into medical diseases. Sophisticated moderns may doubt the transubstantiation of bread and wine into the body and blood of Christ, but they do not doubt the transubstantiation of deviance into disease. Indeed, denying this miraculous transformation and insisting that psychiatrically diagnosed personal and social problems are nothing but personal and social problems is now regarded as scientific heresy. This is the reason, I believe, why even scholars at ease with the idea of metaphor and aware of the analogical nature of mental illness still give it a medical meaning. For example, Herbert Fingarette states:

> One thing is plain: the notion of mental disease is understood against the background notion of disease in the realm of physical disorders. There are deep analogies at work here; and no doubt other related pairs of terms reflect the same sort of analogy: "sound mind" and "sound body," "physical health" and "mental health," "physical breakdown" and "mental breakdown."[57]

Fingarette goes on to argue that insanity and mental illness are not medical concepts and states: "It is plain that at the heart of the issue of insanity . . . lies the notion of rationality."[58] I cite this example, out of a great many similar statements in the literature, to illustrate that established academics and intellectuals can now be counted on to support and validate the medical myths of the psychiatrist, just as, not so long ago, they could be counted on to support and validate the religious myths of the priest. James Turner's observation concerning the development of religious unbelief is pertinent in this connection. "Unbelief in God," he writes, "thus required so extreme an estrangement from 'obvious reality' as to be, if not strictly impossible, practically so for medieval men and women."[59] The same, I believe, is now true for unbelief in mental illness.*

Let us make no mistake about it: It is one thing to place different bodily diseases—for example, arthritis and glaucoma—in the same class, and quite another to place bodily diseases and mental diseases in the same class. In the former case, we build a category on the basis of a clearly and carefully defined criterion for membership in it, namely, a pathoanatomical or pathophysiological lesion. This is why arthritis and glaucoma are both diseases, although they do *not look alike.* However, if we place bodily diseases and mental diseases in the same class, we build a category without a clear or carefully defined criterion for membership in it, on the basis that its members *look alike.* Diabetes and depression are both diseases because they both cause suffering; eagles and bats are both birds because they both fly. The logical error of making such a *category mistake,* as the British philosopher Gilbert Ryle called it, is clear enough.[61] However, the confusions so caused in the specific instance of *mental illness* are not and are therefore worth briefly restating:

1. *What is it?* What is the event, phenomenon, quality, or thing we are talking about when we call it mental illness? The answer is: *It* might be a brain disease, as in neurosyphilis; or disapproved behavior, as in depression or depravity (crime); or the attribution of irrationality, irresponsibility, and insanity to an adversary, as in calling a public figure *schizophrenic.*

2. *What should we call it?* What name should we attach to the event, phenomenon, quality, or thing we are observing and describing? The answer is: We can call *it* psychopathology, insanity, or mental illness; madness or genius; conflict, deviance, or disagreement; psychiatric scapegoating and victimization; or, simply, human behavior.

3. *How should we treat it?* What personal attitude and social policy should we adopt toward the event, phenomenon, quality, or thing? The answer is: We can treat *it* as an illness, provided the person who has it approves; or as a mental illness, regardless of whether or not the person who has it approves; or as deviance or crime, and punish it; or as admirable behavior or artistic achievement, and reward it; or as

---

*Indeed, not only is unbelief in mental illness now practically impossible for ordinary men and women, but so is unbelief in any abstract noun modified by adjectives such as *mental, psychic,* or *psychiatric.* Thus, in April 1986, an American jury awarded $1 million in compensation to a woman "who claimed that a hospital CAT scan had damaged her psychic powers."[60] Why not? If a person's *mental* health can be damaged, so can his *psychic* powers.

behavior requiring us to adjust our actions to it, as any other behavior does; or as something uninteresting and of no concern to us.

The mythology of mental illness and the rituals of psychiatry now make it virtually impossible for professional and layman alike to distinguish between phenomenon, label, and policy. This explains, for example, the persistent but erroneous belief that if persons now diagnosed as schizophrenic were shown to be suffering from diseases of the brain, that would justify and make possible their involuntary treatment. However, persons suffering from diseases of the central nervous system are not, and legally cannot be, treated against their will. Thus, even if persons diagnosed as schizophrenic were suffering from a demonstrable brain disease, treating them involuntarily would still require that they be declared insane as well. Truly, mental illness is like a genie we have summoned to help us solve our problems: now, *he* is the problem. Much time will pass and much suffering will be inflicted and endured before we shall succeed in getting him back into his bottle.

6

MENTAL ILLNESS AND THE PROBLEM OF IMITATION

*But besides real diseases we are subject to many that are only
imaginary for which physicians have invented imaginary cures:
these have their several names, and so have the drugs that are
proper for them . . . .*

—Jonathan Swift (1726)[1]

One of the most interesting and important characteristics we possess as
human beings is our immense talent for *imitation*. (This talent is, of
course, not limited to human beings). We *learn* our mother tongue, and
much else besides, by such a process.

The ability to imitate is an inherent and inherited part of our basic
behavioral repertoire: as such, it is neither good nor bad. Our vast
vocabulary for describing different kinds of imitations—for example,
aping, duplicating, copying, counterfeiting, faking, feigning, impersonating, malingering, mimicking, pretending, repeating, simulating—is eloquent testimony that, like almost anything we do, imitating
may serve many aims and be deemed either good or bad depending on
the observer's interests and values. Imitating illness may thus be a
problem for one person (the physician), and a *solution* for another (the
would-be patient). We must keep in mind, too, that every item in the

repertoire of the doctor-patient relationship can be imitated. In short, we should be as sensitive to the differences between real doctors and false doctors, or real treatments and false treatments, as we are to the differences between real diseases and factitious diseases, or real patients and malingerers.

To imitate something—a pattern of sounds, called *language;* a masterpiece or text, called a *copy;* a precious gem, called *paste*—we must have an original or a model of it. Obviously, if there is no *original* or *real* X, there can be no *imitation* or *copy* of X. If there is no truth, there can be no lie. This is one of the reasons why I took care to clarify at the outset what we mean by the term *illness* and to offer an original model of it.

Since the idea of illness comprises undesirable anatomical and physiological processes as well as certain characteristic behaviors we exhibit when we are ill, it is possible to imitate both illness and the behavior of ill persons. In fact, nothing is easier. I am not sure what children learn first: to speak or to malinger.* After all, what could be easier than to pretend that we hurt even if we do not?

What should we make of the fact that healthy persons often pretend to be ill? How should we interpret the phenomenon that used to be called *malingering* but which psychiatrists now call *factitious illness?* Before trying to answer these questions, let me diagnose and dispose of a troublesome problem concerning the contemporary medical posture toward malingering.

MALINGERING RECONSIDERED

The idea of malingering or pretending to be ill presupposes an idea of illness. Obviously, a person cannot copy or counterfeit an act or an object without being familiar with it—whether *it* be money, a famous painting, being ill, or curing illness. To put it the simplest possible way: Lying presupposes knowing the truth (or what one thinks is the truth); the person ignorant of the truth uttering a falsehood is said to be erring, not lying.

These are important considerations in relation to the problem of imitating illness or mental illness, because if we do not know what illness is, or do not want to attach a clear meaning to the term, then we shall be unable to distinguish real illness from counterfeit illness. Indeed, this is

---

*I was once told the story of a nine-month-old baby who developed a chronic unexplained cough. She did not speak yet. It was midwinter and both mother and father had for months suffered from an annoying upper respiratory infection which made them cough. After repeated careful examinations of the little girl, the pediatrician concluded that the baby had learned to cough.

why, as I shall show in a moment, physicians were much clearer about malingering at the beginning of modern medicine, when the business of diagnosing and treating disease was a nascent craft, than they are today, when medicine is a triumphant ideology.

In the not so good nor so old days of medicine, doctors could do little to cure disease but were confident that there was a distinction—however difficult it might be to make sometimes—between persons who were truly sick, and those who were not but pretended to be, whom they called *malingerers.* Of course, those days are gone. I look back on them not in nostalgia but in the expectation they can teach us something. What they can teach us is this.

Insofar as we define disease as a condition of the body, and insofar as we infer its existence from the sick person's behavior, it must be possible to *imitate being sick.* Everyone knows that. How, then, can we be sure whether a person who complains of pain speaks the truth? Whether he really experiences pain or only pretends to feel pain? Whether he feels a negligible discomfort and exaggerates it into an unbearable suffering? Worse still, how can we be sure whether such a complaint signifies only an unpleasant personal experience of no particular medical import, or the presence of an underlying disease requiring prompt treatment, such as an acutely inflamed appendix? How can we *ever be sure* whether a complaint is only a complaint or a symptom of an underlying disease? Obviously, there can be *no certainty* in such matters. But that does not mean that imitating illness does not exist, or that it is particularly difficult to distinguish a person who is ill from one who is not.

The imitation of illness, however, poses a serious problem, and not only for physicians but also for parents, teachers, businessmen, judges, all of us. Perhaps the most important problem is that we must take a definite, initial stand on the distinction between real and fake diseases and real and fake patients. Moreover, we have only two options. One option, which is old, is to distinguish between persons who are truly ill and those who are not, between honest patients and dishonest malingerers—and to accept the former but not the latter as persons deserving medical care and the benefits of the sick role. The dangers that lie that way are familiar and I shall not belabor them.

The other option, popular today, is to downplay the distinction between persons with demonstrable bodily diseases and those without them (it is impossible to ignore this distinction completely), to define both types of complainants as ill—and to accept both types of persons as deserving of medical care and the benefits of the sick role. The danger in this case is that we legitimize both of these types of persons as bona fide patients suffering from bona fide diseases—eliminating the distinction between truly ill persons and malingerers, while creating certain novel distinctions, namely, between persons suffering from *bodily* illnesses, *mental* illnesses, and *factitious* illness. The consequences of this choice are, in my opinion, even more disastrous—especially for our political freedoms and public safety—than are the consequences of the first choice. Moreover, this choice entails the embarrassing logical absurdity of defining and treating both real diseases and fake diseases as real diseases.

Is a malingered, faked, imitated, factitious illness a *condition*, an illness or mental illness, we deliberately or otherwise cause ourselves *to have?* Or is it an act of deliberately or otherwise assuming the *role* of patient or mental patient, not because we are ill but because we want to be patients? The relationship between having an illness (diabetes) and faking illness (a nondiabetic person injecting himself with insulin)—or between being a patient brought to the emergency room with a skull fracture, and impersonating the patient role (presenting oneself in the emergency room with complaints of renal colic and offering a specimen of urine with blood in it drawn from our own finger)—is of the same type as the relationship between an *original* and its *imitation* (real money and counterfeit). Asserting that real illness and factitious illness are both *real* illnesses is like saying that a Picasso and its copy are both Picassos. The present medical and psychiatric posture toward the conditions called *factitious illnesses* embodies precisely this absurdity: "Malingering," explains Kurt Eissler, a prominent Viennese-American psychoanalyst and the Director of the ill-famed Freud Archives, "is always the sign of a disease, often more severe than a neurotic disorder. . . . The diagnosis should never be made but by the psychiatrist."[2]

After reviewing the recent psychiatric literature on simulating insanity, George G. Hay, a British psychiatrist, similarly concludes that "Usually the simulation of schizophrenia is simply the prodromal phase of genuine illness . . . . The majority of such patients will be suffering from the early stages of a genuine psychosis and should be managed accordingly."[3] Evidently, Hay sees no self-contradiction in the proposition that the imitation of schizophrenia is itself genuine schizophrenia. This situation illustrates what the epistemologist of psychiatry is up against.

How did we get to this point in the history of psychiatry and in the cultural history of the West, where illness and counterfeit illness are both accepted and viewed as illnesses of the same kind, or as identical? Or where counterfeit illness is viewed as even more serious an illness than the illness it counterfeits? I shall try to show how we got here by scrutinizing both the patient's pretendings of being ill and the doctor's pretendings of curing.

PRETENDING TO BE ILL

For the reasons I have just mentioned, it should not surprise us that at the dawn of modern medicine—when professionals and educated laymen alike began to realize that diseases, such as smallpox or dropsy, are dysfunctions of the body—the distinction between sickness and malingering was much clearer than it is today. The following example illustrates this point. In the sixteenth century, there were frequent episodes of maniacal dancing, typically occurring in public. These frenzies—spreading from group to group and city to city like the plague, and called *dance epidemics* or *St. Vitus' dance*—were thought to be due to a contagion such as caused epidemics of infectious diseases.

Paracelsus (1493–1541), considered to be one of the first modern physicians, disagreed: He attributed St. Vitus' dance to "the irrational power of imagination and belief"—surely, a remarkably perceptive way of describing it—and asserted that it is "nothing but an imaginative sickness arising frequently in women from a voluptuous urge to dance."[4] Today, psychiatrists call such phenomena *mass hysteria*, or the results of *brainwashing*, or, most pretentiously of all, *factitious illness*—and the editors of *The New York Times* and *Science* recognize these pathetic psychiatric imitations of medical diagnoses as the names of bona fide diseases.

Molière on Malingering

The most marvelously lucid and prescient presentation of imitating both illness and curing—the two typically going hand in hand—is, I suspect, Molière's *A Doctor in Spite of Himself.* Written in 1666, this comedy lays bare, in the simplest and most direct way possible, what modern psychiatrists and psychoanalysts pretentiously call the *psychodynamics of conversion hysteria.* Actually, Molière shows us something far more important, namely, that what we now call mental illness is a false problem of our modern scientific age—of an age in which we see complicated *problems* where what stares us in the face are obvious *solutions:* in short, what seems to us a mysterious mental-physical malady, Molière understood as—well, I shall let him speak for himself.

The scenes I want to present begin with Sganarelle, a woodcutter impersonating a physician, being called upon to treat Lucinde, a young girl who has lost her voice. Even before Sganarelle sees his patient, Molière, through the mouth of Jacqueline, a friend of Lucinde's father, Géronte, tells us what Charcot and Freud supposedly discovered more than 200 years later:

Jacqueline: The best doctor you could give your daughter—to my way of thinking—would be a strapping young man for a husband, one as she had a fancy for.[5]

What was an ordinary and obvious fact to Molière and his audience in the seventeenth century, thus became, in the nineteenth century, a mysterious malady, called hysteria, while its solution became, in our own day, a marvelous medical remedy, called *sex therapy*.[6] How right and prophetic Molière was when he remarked that "Once you have the cap and gown [of the doctor], all you need do is open your mouth. Whatever nonsense you talk becomes wisdom and all the rubbish, good sense."[7]

But let us return to Sganarelle. He arrives at Géronte's house and Lucinde is brought in to meet him. He asks her: "What's wrong with you?" She replies by gesturings.

Sganarelle: I don't understand you. What the deuce language is this?

Géronte: That's exactly the trouble, sir. She's lost the power of speech and so far no one has been able to find what the reason is. It has caused her marriage to be postponed.

Sganarelle: But why?

Géronte: The man she is to marry wishes to wait until she's recovered.

Sganarelle: But who is this idiot who doesn't want his wife to be dumb. Would to God mine had the same trouble! I shouldn't be wanting her cured.[8]

In a few lines, the whole meaning of this charade—this mental illness—is laid bare: Lucinde does not want to marry the man her father picked out for her and has succeeded in having the wedding postponed. Sganarelle shows us that a wife's silence may be a curse or a blessing. And through it all, Molière reveals that dumbness such as Lucinde's may be a blemish or blessing—or, in our terms, the symptom of an illness which Géronte may want cured but Lucinde may not. Of course, Molière makes no bones about Lucinde's faking being dumb, just as Sganarelle fakes being a doctor. Léandre, the young man Lucinde wants to marry, sums it up as follows (speaking to Sganarelle):

Léandre: I wanted to tell you that this illness which you are here to cure is all put on. The doctors have done the usual diagnosis and they've not hesitated to say how it arose. According to some, from the brain or the bowels, according to others from the spleen or the liver, but the fact is that the real cause is love. Lucinde only assumed the symptoms in order to avoid being forced into a marriage with a man she detests.[9]

Soon Sganarelle cures Lucinde, who, having regained her voice, expresses herself only too clearly.

Lucinde: [To Géronte] No paternal authority can make me marry against my will.

Géronte: I have—

Lucinde: I'll never submit to such tyranny . . . I'll shut myself up in a convent rather than marry a man I don't love.

Géronte: Oh, what a torrent of words. There's no doing anything with her. (To Sganarelle). I implore you, sir—make her dumb again.

Sganarelle: That's the one thing I can't do. The only thing I can do to help you is make you deaf if you like.[10]

It would be gilding the lily to offer any comment on this exchange. I will say, however, that we have made progress since Molière. Psychiatrists now know how to make a Lucinde dumb again.

Pretending to Be Mentally Ill

Psychiatry has a dual character and a correspondingly dual origin. One part—the older and most important—originates from the seventeenth century, with the incarceration of insane persons in madhouses. The madmen and madwomen so treated—the furiously insane and the homicidal and suicidal maniacs—presented behaviors very different from those of medically sick persons; they acted *crazy*, not *sick*. Hence, these persons were not regarded as malingerers—that is, as healthy persons who pretended to be sick. Thus began asylum care and the insane asylum, which became psychiatry and the institutional psychiatric system as we now know them.

Another part of psychiatry can be traced to a quite different origin, namely, to the separation, in the nineteenth century, of neurological diseases such as general paresis and multiple sclerosis, from mental diseases, such as dementia praecox and hysteria. In contrast to the asylum doctors who cared for incarcerated madmen and madwomen, the neuropsychiatrists—typically professors in medical schools—were part neuropathologists and part clinicians whose task was to distinguish persons with bona fide diseases of the nervous system from persons without such diseases whose symptoms, however, *resembled* those of the former group of patients. For example, a young woman complained of inability to stand and loss of vision: Was she suffering from multiple sclerosis or was she merely pretending to be unable to stand and see? Another had seizures: were they due to epilepsy or not? From this medical-social matrix grew the second, more recent part of psychiatry—the part that comprised hysteria and neurosis, hypnosis and psychotherapy, and whose patients and practitioners were generally located without, rather than within, the mental hospital. (See Table 6.1.)

The most important single figure in the development of this branch of psychiatry was Jean-Martin Charcot (1825–1893), a French neurologist, who was the first to describe and identify several neurological diseases and is also credited with having claimed or discovered hysteria as a bona fide disease, and hypnosis as a bond fide treatment for it. I suggest that we view hysteria as a pretense of being ill, the patient lying by means of bodily gestures rather than with words alone (although words too are typically employed); and that we view hypnosis as the pretense of curing, the physician lying by means of medical gestures (although he, too, uses words as well). It will be worth our while to briefly review the evidence for this interpretation.

Georges Guillain, a student of Charcot's who himself became a famous neurologist, has told us, in no uncertain terms, that the poor women on whom Charcot made his original discoveries of hysteria were coached to malinger—that is, to pretend that they were epileptics:

> In 1899, about six years after Charcot's death, I [writes Guillain] saw as a young intern at the Salpêtrière the old patients of Charcot who were still hospitalized. Many of the women, who were excellent comedians, when they were offered a slight pecuniary remuneration, imitated perfectly the major hysteric crises of former times.[11]

Who was fooling whom? The daisy-chain went like this: Charcot's assistants and the poor patients they trained were fooling Charcot, Charcot was fooling his medical colleagues, and the medical profession was fooling the public. The result was that, in the end, everyone accepted simulated illness as (real) mental illness, and mental illness as (real) bodily illness.[12]

The idea of a real—that is, bodily—disease as a scientific concept is

TABLE 6.1. Psychiatry, Mental Illness, Mental Treatment: A Historical Schema

Social setting and scope of psychiatry	Institutional psychiatry Insane asylum Major mental illnesses (psychoses)	Outpatient psychiatry Physician's office or patient's home Minor mental illnesses (neuroses)
Historical paradigm of problem/illness	Homicidal frenzy or mania; murder, suicide: madness	Fake pains, paralyses, and blindness; counterfeit illness: malingering
Nature of danger or problem	Danger of homicide and suicide: acute threats to family and society	Disability of agent: chronic burden to self and family
Medical-legal conceptualization and response		
Seventeenth century	Birth of institutional psychiatry: insanity; incarceration in insane asylum	Not yet viewed as the business of the mad-doctor (psychiatrist); physician treats malingerer, much as he does other patients
Nineteenth century	Dementia praecox; mental hospitalization; institutional psychiatry becomes the cornerstone of the psychiatric profession	Birth of psychotherapy: fake illness (malingering) becomes hysteria and the paradigm of neurosis; fake treatment (charlatanry) becomes hypnosis and the paradigm of psychotherapy
Today	Paradigm diagnosis: schizophrenia; paradigm treatment: involuntary mental hospitalization and coerced drug treatment	Malingering/hysteria becomes factitious illness (or personality disorder); drug treatment, family therapy, hospitalization, sex therapy, and countless other interventions all legitimized as bona fide medical treatments

the product of the morgue, the autopsy table, and the pathological laboratory: it was by examining dead bodies and their organs, tissues, and cells that physicians discovered various diseases and distinguished one such disease from another. That is not how mental diseases were discovered. The idea of mental illness is, as I have tried to show, the product of the insane asylum as theater.* This model must be taken seriously. Like any theater, the madhouse comprised not only actors and audience but also playwright and stage manager. It was by placing certain persons on the stages of insane asylums and watching their performances that physicians—as well as lay people to a degree unknown in the rest of medicine—discovered various mental diseases and distinguished one such disease from another.

The theatrical atmosphere of the early insane asylum—where, like freaks in a circus, *mad* men and *mad* women were actually exhibited and expected to perform—is familiar to anyone conversant with the history of psychiatry.[14] However, what is much less well known is that the discovery of *mental* illness, *in the modern sense of that term*, also occurred in that setting. I refer to the closing decades of the nineteenth century when, largely as a result of the work of the great French neurologists, diseases of the nervous system were separated from mental diseases, grand mal epilepsy serving as the model of neurological illness, and its imitation, *grande hystérie,* as the model of mental illness. (Hypnosis was then thought to be a means for inducing hysterical seizures as well as for curing them.) This was the scene, as described by the famous physician-author, Axel Munthe:

> I seldom failed to attend Professor Charcot's famous *Leçons du Mardi* in the Salpêtrière, just then chiefly devoted to his *grande hystérie* and to hypnotism. The huge amphitheatre was filled to the last place with a multi-coloured audience drawn from tout Paris, authors, journalists, leading actors and actresses, fashionable demimondaines, all full of morbid curiosity to witness the startling phenomena of hypnotism almost forgotten since the days of Mesmer and Braid.[15]

It seems to me that there is something very wrong with this scene—wrong, that is, if we consider how bodily diseases were discovered and studied. Obviously this is not the sort of setting in which, say, Rudolf Virchow or Paul Ehrlich worked and made their discoveries. Instead—let us make no mistake about it—this is the setting of the faith healer,

---

*The same sort of contextual genesis characterized the appearance and display of diabolical possession. "A conspicuous feature of cases of possession about which details survive," writes Keith Thomas, "is that they frequently originated in a religious environment."[13]

the charlatan, the circus performer, perhaps even of the political demagogue on his way up the political ladder from talking to killing. What is remarkable about all this, moreover, is that the diseases and cures of psychiatry continue to be discovered and presented in this way. Television producers and newscasters continue to regale the public with the astounding performances of mentally ill patients and their miraculous cures. Gripping anecdotes and shocking scenes—of devastating disability and dramatic recovery—fill the screens, the newspapers, magazines, and even psychiatric journals: These are legitimate methods for presenting life as theater, but are totally irrelevant to, and inappropriate for, a scientific effort to understand the human body as a material object.

The upshot was that from about 1900 until the Second World War, physicians, psychiatrists, and lawyers recognized hysteria and malingering as two distinct and separate conditions, the first an illness, the second not. However, since the difference between them was that the former was supposedly due to unconscious and the latter to conscious motives, there was no objective or reliable way of telling them apart. Still, some psychiatric texts continued, despite a fast-growing confusion between malingering and hysteria, to discuss malingering in a surprisingly reasonable, traditional way. For example, in 1969, in the tenth edition of the British text, *Henderson and Gillespie's Textbook of Psychiatry*, malingering is presented under the heading of "Hysteria and Simulation":

> To distinguish sharply between hysteria and simulation is often arbitrary. Simulation is the voluntary production of symptoms by an individual who has full knowledge of their voluntary origin. In hysteria there is typically no such knowledge . . . . Kretschmer rightly pointed out, however, that the criteria "conscious or unconscious?" will not serve to distinguish simulation from hysteria, for not all of the motives of the healthy mind are conscious, and not all hysterical ones are unconscious.[16]

Ernst Kretschmer (1888–1964) was right but did not go far enough: The adjectives *conscious-unconscious (voluntary-involuntary)* are ostensibly explanatory, but are actually strategic (see Chapter 9). Nevertheless, authoritative texts—for example, the *Encyclopedia of Psychology*—continue to define malingering by emphasizing that it is "the *voluntary* production and presentation of false or grossly exaggerated physical or psychological symptoms" (emphasis in the original),[17] as if anyone could distinguish voluntary from involuntary production of symptoms, or as if anyone could *present* a symptom involuntarily. The attempt to distinguish between voluntary versus involuntary, or conscious versus unconscious self-production of symptoms or lesions seems to me a potentially bottomless source of confusion. Surely, most people who smoke or overeat do not intend to make themselves sick with the symptoms and signs of atherosclerosis. Yet, insofar as that disease may, partly or wholly, be due to the consequences of such behaviors, it might be necessary to classify it as a type of malingering, a pretty absurd conclusion. I believe it would make more sense to view, say atherosclerosis, if it is indeed self-induced, as self-induced (or *autogenic;*) and then try to understand how and why people, deliberately or otherwise, give themselves this disease. Since health is not the only value in life, many autogenic diseases may be the results of trade-offs we more or less willingly make—for example, between experiencing the pleasures of eating certain foods or smoking cigarettes and risking the discomfort and disability of certain diseases.

Pretending to Be Insane

It should be noted that most of the literature on malingering concerns persons imitating being *ill*, not being *insane*. Indeed, if insanity does not exist—if, as I contend, mental illness is a metaphorical illness—how can it be imitated? The answer is that what a person imitates is *not insanity* but the *role of the insane person:* since acting crazy cannot be distinguished from being crazy, the person who wants to be taken for a madman has only to act like one. In this connection, the following vignette from Bleuler's original study of schizophrenia is of particular interest. Considering schizophrenia as a bona fide disease—but without biological markers, as we would now say—Bleuler believed that it was possible to simulate schizophrenia, just as it was possible to simulate other diseases. But how did he distinguish between real schizophrenia and its imitation? Here is how:

> A very special sort of unconscious disease simulation was shown by a patient who was accused by her supervisor of being crazy. From that moment on, she behaved as if she were "crazy"; while still living at home, she insisted that the house janitor was an attendant of an insane asylum; refused to take food; etc. After one tube-feeding, there was a sudden cure.[18]

Tube-feeding, especially when unnecessary and unjustified as in the foregoing case, is of course simply a method of torture rationalized as treatment. Bleuler's handling of this patient and his unashamed description of it should serve as a stark reminder that people, especially physicians, have long understood that, as Samuel Taylor Coleridge (1772–1834) put it: "Real pain alone cures us of imaginary ills. We feel a thousand miseries till . . . we feel misery."[19] It is this principle that has inspired the time-honored practice of curing the imaginary torments of the madman with the real tortures of the mad-doctor.

The brief passage previously cited illustrates several other important points. It reveals, for example, that there was no real distinction, in Bleuler's mind, between the ensemble of human behaviors he considered to be schizophrenia and the imitation of that ensemble: for had this woman not recovered from the tube-feeding, but, on the contrary, exhibited even more stubborn negativism, he would no doubt have concluded that she was a typical schizophrenic. However, since she was cured—schizophrenia then being characterized by being incurable—she was a malingerer.

Finally, this vignette illustrates how much more free and justified psychiatrists then felt to punish patients they thought were malingering than they do now, when psychiatric punishments are carefully concealed as treatments. Obviously, since there is no immediate need to tube-feed a person who has just stopped eating, this highly unpleasant procedure was a pretty transparent form of torture—though not too bad a torture by current standards. It is worth adding that despite considering this patient as having been a malingerer, Bleuler speaks of having cured her—surely a deplorable euphemism for what happened. (Although many words in Bleuler's book are placed between quotation marks, the word *cure* in the sentence previously quoted is not one of them.)

While deception pervades all human endeavors, it is expected to pervade some more than others: for example, politics and religion (unless one is devoutly religious) more, and science and medicine less. Because I see the very nature of what we mean by mental illness as inherently deceptive, so long as we do not recognize this, the methods we use in an effort to cope with it are bound to be deceptive also. Thus, a good deal of what passes for research in psychiatry is also fundamentally fraudulent—not infrequently based on admittedly deceptive premises and procedures.

For example, in 1972, David Rosenhan, a professor of psychology at Stanford University, set out to deliberately deceive a number of hospital psychiatrists. Rosenhan and several associates assumed the role of mental patients—they called themselves *pseudopatients*—by pretending to hear voices: they called up mental hospital psychiatrists, complained of this symptom, and gained admission to the hospital. Once inside the insane asylum, regardless of how sane the pseudopatients acted, they continued to be regarded as crazy. "With the exception of myself (I was the first pseudopatient and my presence was known to the hospital administrator and chief psychologist, and, so far as I can tell, to them alone)," writes Rosenhan, "the presence of the pseudopatients and the nature of the research program was not known to the hospital staff."[20] This deception was supposedly necessitated by the problem to be investigated. "However distasteful such concealment is, it was a necessary first step to examining certain questions," explains Rosenhan. The questions he wanted explained were: "If sanity and insanity exist, how shall we know them?" and ". . . whether the sane can be distinguished from the insane (and whether the insane can be distinguished from each other)."[21] The trouble is that this so-called experiment was not premised on concealment—as are double-blind studies—but rather on deception: the researchers impersonated psychotics and deliberately lied to the psychiatrists whose help they ostensibly solicited. Nevertheless, this study was accepted for publication in *Science* and hailed as an important piece of research, supposedly proving the labeling theory of mental illness and the unreliability of the psychiatric-diagnostic process. To me it proves only that it is easy to deceive people, especially when they want to be deceived.

PRETENDING TO BE POSSESSED AND DISPOSSESSED

Today people believe that mental illness exists and is real: hence arises the problem of distinguishing real cases of mental illness from simulated cases of it. It may surprise the contemporary reader that, not so many years ago, when people believed that diabolical possession existed and was real, they faced a similar problem: namely, having to distinguish real cases of possession from simulated cases of it.

How, people may now wonder, could anyone pretend to be possessed or a witch? This question reveals how uneasy and uncertain we are about distinguishing between what the sociologists call the *social construction of reality* and what, let us just say, is a more solid, scientifically constructed reality. Actually, what the former term means is simply something like this: If a person, P, believes in X and thinks he is X, and if virtually everyone in his society also believes in X and legitimizes P as X, then P *is* X. For example, Peter Berger and Thomas Luckmann, in their authoritative exposition of this perspective, write: "Rural Haitians *are* possessed and New York intellectuals *are* neurotic" (emphasis in the original).[22] Well, yes and no, as I try to show throughout this book. Actually, the fact that someone thinks he is possessed, or insane, or a leader with God-given powers, together with the fact that most other members of society agree with him, establishes that person's identity as what he claims it to be only in a very limited, or soft, sense of this word (which Berger and Luckmann recognize). For our present purposes it suffices to note, however, that when belief in demonic possession was as dominant and popular as belief in psychosis is now, the authorities charged with dealing with possessed persons had problems concerning pretended possession very similar to those that authorities now have dealing with pretended insanity.

Sad but true, a person's life can be so drab, his motivation so seemingly perverse, that sometimes he will pretend to be anyone or anything, so long as it promises to dramatize or end his existence. Thus, when people believed in demonic possession and witchcraft, it was not unusual for individuals to pretend that they were possessed or were witches: for example, lonely, old women sometimes did so in order to be put to death, an option that, for obvious reasons, they viewed as morally preferable to committing suicide.*

In his masterful study, *Religion and the Decline of Magic,* Keith Thomas tells of several women in sixteenth-century England who "were punished for fraudulently simulating the symptoms of possession . . . ."[23] He also chronicles the cases of persons faking diabolical possession and of judges, revolted by the severity of the law against witchcraft, exposing them as impostors and acquitting them of the charge of witchcraft. One such judge, Sir John Holt, Lord Chief Justice (1689–1710), Thomas tells us,

> presided over some eleven successive acquittals, and secured the conviction of the impostor for pretending to be afflicted with witchcraft . . . . "By his questions and manner of hemming up the evidence," remarked an observer, "he seemed to me to believe nothing of witchery at all!" His example was followed by his colleagues. Mr. Justice Powell, presiding over the trial of Jane Wenham in 1712, is said . . . to have greeted the more sensational testimony with the cheerful remark that there was no law against flying; he took prompt steps to arrange for her reprieve.[24]

It seems that we shall have to wait until the next, or even some later, century before a judge dismisses a petition for commitment by cheerfully declaring that there is no law against having delusions or hallucinations,

---

*It is worth noting in this connection that except for the Bible, the most important medieval book was titled *Imitatio Christi,* or *The Imitation of Christ.* Written some time between 1390 and 1440 and attributed to Thomas à Kempis, the book enjoins people to emulate Christ's life as the true purpose of human life. No doubt, it is easier simply to declare that one is the Savior than to conduct oneself as He lived. But surely He would be surprised to learn that doing so is an illness called *schizophrenia.*

or against believing that one is Jesus, or against claiming that one can communicate with the FBI through the fillings in one's teeth.

Still, as Thomas emphasizes, statutes against witchcraft "made it difficult for judges to be liberal. As Lord Chief Justice North complained to the Secretary of State in 1682, 'we cannot reprieve them without appearing to deny the very being of witches, which . . . is contrary to law.'"[25] This complaint is a good example of the fact that legal fictions control those who judge no less than those who are judged—which, perhaps, is one of the reasons why such fictions endure so long, despite disbelief in them from above, and displeasure over them from below.

Moreover, since possession could, in both principle and practice, be cured by dispossession, some exorcists, not surprisingly, coached persons to simulate being possessed so as to then be able to dispossess them—a scenario later faithfully reenacted in the relationship between hysteric and hypnotist. Thomas records the story of such an exorcist who coached women to simulate being possessed, and who was subsequently "convicted by the High Commission as an impostor who had trained his patients to simulate the now conventional symptoms of the disorder in order to demonstrate his curative skills. Some of the most notable clergy of the day had been assistants at his dispossessions . . . ."[26] This was so embarrassing that the subsequent controversy raised questions about the "possibility of diabolical possession and the status of the cure by prayer and fasting."[27]

However, since most people wanted to believe in miracles, whether they tranquilized or horrified, they continued to believe in them. There were exceptions, of course, such as Thomas Hobbes (1588–1679), who denounced the "pretences of exorcism and conjuration of phantasms."[28] Though a devout Christian—or, as he insisted, because of it—he denounced the Roman Catholic Mass as also a pretense: "But when, by such words [the priest's consecration] the nature of or quality of the thing itself, is pretended to be changed it is not consecration, but either an extraordinary work of God, or a vain and impious conjuration." Such conjuration, he hastened to add, is "contrary to the testimony of man's sight, and of all the rest of his senses."[29] I similarly insist that the claim that the phenomena we now call mental illnesses are illnesses like cancer and heart disease is contrary to the testimony of man's sight, and of all the rest of his senses.

To summarize: When, as in the Middle Ages, virtually everyone believed in possession, there arose the following phenomena and problems: Some people pretended to be possessed; some pretended to cure possession; hence, it was necessary to distinguish real cases and cures of possession from pretended cases and cures of it; and, finally, some persons denied the officially acclaimed doctrine of the miraculous transformation of bread and wine into the body and blood of the Savior.

Similarly, when, as now, virtually everyone believes in mental illness, there arise the following phenomena and problems: Some people pretend to be insane; some pretend to cure insanity; hence, it is necessary to distinguish real cases and cures of insanity from pretended cases and cures of it; and, finally, some persons deny the officially acclaimed doctrine of the miraculous transformation of personal problems into psychiatric diseases.

PRETENDING TO CURE

Malingering is feigning illness: it is what the healthy person does when he pretends to be ill. What is the corresponding pretending on the part of the healer or physician? How do we view the nonphysician pretending to be a physician? Or the physician who, without the faintest idea of what ails the patient or how to help him, pretends to diagnose and cure him?

The nonphysician who pretends to be a doctor is, of course, called a *quack*. However, the physician who pretends to diagnose without really knowing what ails the patient, and to cure him without really knowing how, is not necessarily categorized negatively: to be sure, he may be discredited as a charlatan; but, more often than not, he is accredited, merely because he is a bona fide physician, as a bona fide healer.

Indeed, perhaps nothing illustrates more dramatically the profound bias built into our language than the definitions of, and the meaning we ordinarily attach to, the terms *malingering* and *placebo*. Actually, malingering is a something—a false complaint of illness—that a patient gives to a physician; whereas a placebo is also a something—a false promise of treatment—that a physician *gives* to a patient. Where is the bias? It is in the way we use these terms.

Descriptively, *malingering* and *placebo* both refer to an *act of imitation* and a *counterfeited object*—pretending to be ill and a simulated illness in one case, pretending to be prescribing a treatment and a simulated treatment in the other. To state it more fully: The malingerer is a person who plays the role of sick patient, who pretends to be ill, and who presents doctors with faked symptoms and signs of illness; whereas the prescriber of a placebo is a person who plays the role of physician-healer, pretends to be trying to help a genuinely ill patient, and provides the patient with the faked accoutrements of a supposedly needed pharmacologically active therapeutic agent. Of course, this is not at all the way these symmetrical acts of imitation are defined or understood in ordinary discourse.

Webster's defines *malingering* as "feigning illness," which implies not only that there is an identifiable and meaningful difference between real illness and fake illness, but also that the imitator is up to some mischief. By contrast, *placebo* is defined as "a medicine given merely to satisfy a patient," which implies not only that it is a bona fide medicine (therapy), but also that the physician prescribing it is engaged in a praiseworthy enterprise.

The vast political imbalance between the roles of patient and doctor—symbolized by *malingering* doing the work of a bad word, and *placebo* that of a good one—point to a delicate issue: namely, that throughout the entire history of medicine—from Hippocrates to our day—the physician's proper role has been seen as resembling that of the politician rather than that of the scientist. By this I mean simply that, as Plato had advocated, since both the politician and the physician labor in a good cause, they should be permitted to lie. The ethic of truth-telling characterizing science has thus been alien, if indeed not inimical, to the ethics of medicine. I touch here on a large subject whose importance for the entire practice of medicine—in all of its reaches and ramifications—cannot be overemphasized. However, it is a subject I cannot pursue further here. Suffice it for us to note that in her book on *Lying*, philosopher Sissela Bok devotes an entire chapter to the way doctors deceive patients and comments cogently on "deception as therapy." She emphasizes that principles and oaths of medical ethics have never placed any value on the doctor's veracity toward the patient. "The Hippocratic Oath," she observes, "makes no mention of truthfulness to patients about their condition, prognosis, or treatment. Other early codes and prayers are equally silent on the subject."[30] The Nuremberg Code and the Principles of Medical Ethics of the American Medical Association also make no reference to truthfulness.

It makes no sense, however, to gnash our teeth over this, assuming we despise medical despotism concealed as therapeutic paternalism. The only thing that makes sense is to bring this matter to the attention of the public. It is all too clear that unless a particular patient has reason to believe that his physician is, and will be, truthful with him, he has no reason or duty to be truthful with the physician; sadly, it will probably be in the patient's best interest not to be so. The litigious posture patients have come to assume toward physicians may in no small part be due to this unjustifiable imbalance—concerning the expectation to tell the truth—between doctor and patient. If a physician wants to help his patient—especially in our day of undreamt-of possibilities for doing so—he has no need to resort to fraud or force vis-à-vis the patient. His knowledge and skills are enough. More than ever before, the physician could now let himself be guided by the principle that "a word to the wise is sufficient." If the patient does not want to take the physician's word, why should that matter to the physician? Or vice versa? Neither doctor nor patient ought to use, or tolerate the use of, fraud or force in their relationship to each other. On the other hand, if the patient lies to the doctor, and vice versa, if both parties accept the lies as truths, and if both then manipulate each other with escalating strategies of deception and counterdeception, then the result will be that the medical situation will continue on its precipitously downhill course, each party trying to con, rather than to cooperate with, the other. The fact that today psychiatrists, physicians, and even the general public accept both real and faked illnesses as bona fide diseases, and both real and faked treatments as bona fide treatments, is a symptom of the malignant power—ideologically even more than politically—that the medical profession now wields over the mind of modern man. This power is also largely responsible for the profound conceptual confusion that pervades our health care system and the economic and legal chaos toward which, as a practical enterprise, it seems to be heading. To see how we got where we are now, it might help to briefly review the history of the physician's—or rather, for the sake of economy, the psychiatrist's—pretending to cure.

Psychiatry: Pretending to Cure

Study of the writings of the pioneer psychiatrists clearly shows that they viewed insane patients as deceivers, and themselves as counterdeceivers. Indeed, they saw the essence of the patient's illness in his succeeding to deceive himself and in his trying to deceive the doctor as well; similarly, they saw the essence of the doctor's cure in his succeeding to undeceive the patient, which fully justified the use of appropriate methods of counterdeception. Thus were insane and untruthful patients to be restored to sanity and truthfulness.

It would be no exaggeration to say that, at the beginning of the nineteenth century, the asylum doctor regarded the madman as insane because he lied, and that he believed the madman lied because he was insane; similarly, the asylum doctor regarded himself as sane because, as a man of reason and a scientist, he told the truth even when he lied, because he lied not to lie but only to bring the patient to the truth. "Lying," asserted Benjamin Rush (1745–1813), the father of American psychiatry, "is a corporeal disease. . . . Persons thus diseased cannot speak the truth upon any subject."[31] Shamelessly, Rush articulated the modern psychiatrist's credo—that the madman is irrational because he disagrees with the psychiatrist:

> There was a time when these things [criticism of his opinions and actions] irritated and distressed me, but now I hear and see them with the same indifference and pity that I hear the ravings and witness the antic gestures of my deranged patients in our Hospital. We often hear of "prisoners at large." The majority of mankind are madmen at large.[32]

Convinced that his patients were self-deceived and deceiving, he enthusiastically advocated deceiving them in order to cure them:

> If our patient imagines he has a living animal in his body, and he cannot be reasoned out of a belief of it, medicines must be given to destroy it; and if an animal, such as he supposes to be in his body, should be secretly conveyed into his close stool, the deception would be a justifiable one, if it served to cure him of his disease.[33]

In addition to the coercion implicit in incarcerating his patients, deception formed the very foundations of Rush's efforts to treat them. Here is another example of one of his cures:

> Cures of patients, who suppose themselves to be glass, may be easily performed by pulling a chair, upon which they are about to sit, from under them, and afterward showing them a large collection of pieces of glass as the fragments of their bodies.[34]

It's a pathetic scene. Rush's patients are convinced that they have living animals in their bodies (they might have had intestinal parasites) or that they are made of glass (surely a fine poetic way of saying one is weak and vulnerable)—and for that Rush diagnoses them as insane. At the same time, Rush convinces himself that insanity is a disease of the brain (not of the mind), and yet believes that he can cure it by means of such childish stratagems.

The psychiatric scene has not changed very much since those days. The patients still often propound lies—claims and metaphors; and the psychiatrists still often propound counterlies—diagnoses and treatments. Much of modern psychiatry consists of a compounding of these prevarications—the lies steadily concealed by a ceaseless relabeling of the patient's deceptions as new diseases, and the psychiatrist's as new treatments. Nor, as I now want to quickly show, are psychiatric research and teaching free of the pervasive dishonesty that, as I see it, is an inevitable consequence, and must become an integral part, of any enterprise based on nothing but deception and coercion.

Pretending to Do Research and Teach

The following example illustrates not only the pervasiveness of deception in psychiatry, but also its acceptance by psychiatrists as legitimate and indeed scientific, provided the pretender is a psychiatrist.

Attending the annual meeting of the American Psychiatric Association in Atlanta, in May 1978, Natalie Shainess, a well-known psychoanalyst in New York City, arrived late in the evening at the Omni Hotel. "I was unpacking," she writes, "when my phone rang about 11:30 P.M. Wondering who might be calling at that hour, I picked up the phone receiver to hear a man's voice say, 'Would you like us to send up a gentleman to pleasure you?'" Offended by the offer, Shainess interrogated the hotel manager about the incident, only to learn that *"a member of the American Psychiatric Association* was conducting a piece of sex *research* and had arranged for 25 women arriving alone to receive this call" (emphasis added).[35] By representing himself as a scientific investigator, the unidentified psychiatrist deceived not only his victims, but also the hotel manager. The American Psychiatric Association never exposed the identity of this impostor.

Perhaps the ultimate in psychiatric pretendings is the pretense, perpetrated by certain psychiatric educators, of presenting pseudo-instruction about mental illness. In 1972, independently of David Rosenhan's scheme to deceive psychiatrists by means of pseudopatients, Donald Naftulin, a University of Southern California psychiatrist, devised a scheme to deceive mental health educators by means of a pseudopsychiatrist. The result was predictable: just as psychiatrists were unable to distinguish pseudopatients from real patients, so mental health educators were unable to distinguish pseudopsychiatrist from real psychiatrist. In fact, the pseudopsychiatrist was rated an outstanding psychiatrist. The purpose of this experiment, according to the investigators,

> was to determine if there was a correlation between a student's satisfaction with a lecturer and the degree of cognitive knowledge required . . . . We hypothesized that given a sufficiently impressive lecture paradigm, even experienced educators participating in a new learning experience can be seduced into feeling satisfied that they have learned, despite irrelevant, conflicting, and meaningless content by the lecturer.[36]

To this end, the team hired a professional actor "who looked distinguished and sounded authoritative," named him Dr. Myron L. Fox, bestowed upon him the persona of "an authority on the application of mathematics to human behaviour," created a bogus curriculum vitae, and coached him in a speech entitled "Mathematical Game Theory as Applied to Physician Education." The experimenters coached "Dr. Fox" to teach "charismatically and non-substantively on a topic about which he knew nothing," instructing him to use double-talk and other trickery in the question-and-answer period and to intersperse the nonsense "with parenthetical humour and meaningless references to unrelated topics." The lecture was first presented to a group of 11 psychiatrists, psychologists, and social work educators and was videotaped. The tape was then shown to a group of 11 psychiatrists, psychologists, and psychiatric social workers, and finally to a group of 33 educators and administrators taking a graduate course in educational philosophy. All 55 subjects were asked to answer a questionnaire evaluating their response to the lecture. The audience loved "Dr. Fox." All respondents had significantly more favorable than unfavorable responses. One even believed he had read Dr. Fox's publications. Among the subjective responses quoted by the investigators were the following: "Excellent presentation, enjoyed listening . . . Good analysis of the subject . . . Knowledgeable."[37]

What does this experiment about the "pseudopsychiatrist as educator" prove? To Naftulin and his colleagues,[38] it proves that "if a lecturer talks at a group, with no participation permitted to the group [a question-and-answer period was, however, permitted] then a mellifluous, trained actor might do just as well, possibly better than, an uncharismatic physician."* That is not what it proves to me. Like the Rosenhan pseudopatient study, the Naftulin pseudopsychiatrist study proves only that when it comes to the institutionalized deception of psychiatry, observers trained in mental health are unable to distinguish fake fakes from real fakes— not exactly a surprising conclusion. As if to support this contention, Naftulin and his coworkers offer this conclusion, couched in the appropriate gobbledygook: "[The] study supports the possibility of training actors to give legitimate lectures as an innovative educational approach toward student-perceived satisfaction with the learning process."[39] The authors do not explain why medical students or their parents would want to pay

---

*This observation, by a group of respected academics, is similar to Hitler's famous remark that, in politics, a big lie works better than a small one. Hitler did not mention truth at all; he knew it was useless for capturing crowds and was therefore not interested in it. In the main, psychiatrists and psychiatric patients exhibit the same thirst for big mental health lies as do crowds of disaffected people thirsting for the redemptive messages of messiahs, whether religious or political.

the huge tuition fees charged by medical schools to listen to actors talk about nonexistent subjects. No doubt they envision a system of psychiatric education patterned in the tradition of psychiatric diagnosis and treatment—true facts being mendaciously misdescribed every step of the way.

PATIENT AND DOCTOR AS LIARS: RECAPITULATION AND REVIEW

As I have tried to show, impersonating the patient role, feigning illness, and malingering all refer to a type of verbal (or nonverbal) behavior we ordinarily call *lying.* Curiously, it is now taboo to use the word *lying* in connection with both mental patients and psychiatrists. We act as if we believed that psychiatrists are too honest ever to lie, and that mental patients are somehow too sick to lie and hence can do so only *unconsciously.* The fact that even as intrepid a thinker as Barrows Dunham repeats this empty slogan, like some sacred incantation, suggests how heretical it now is to say that mental patients lie. "Lunatics," he writes, "deceive themselves, but they do not do it consciously, and so do not lie."[40] Elsewhere, Dunham reveals that he sees lying, by mental patients and others, rather more clearly:

> Organizations [he writes] thus feel the same need to distort reality which lunatics privately feel; they feel it, indeed, rather more strongly than lunatics. . . . For, in organizational lying, the moral deterrent has been removed: the liar effects his lie (so it seems), not from self-interest but from loyalty to the group. There is even a kind of self-sacrifice about it: the organizational liar surrenders his integrity to the common good.[41]

The behavior of the loyal psychiatrist, especially in connection with the definition of mental illness (see Chapter 3), exemplifies what Barrows calls *organizational lying.* Of course, it is obvious that all human beings lie some of the time—and that some lie more often than others, and some more dramatically or bizarrely than others. Not so long ago, intelligent people generally believed that physicians and lunatics lied more often and more brazenly than others; now they believe—and are expected to believe—that these two groups of persons never lie.

Contemporary opinion regarding lying by mental patients and psychiatrists thus represents a complete reversal of the opinion that prevailed less than 200 years ago. As we saw, it was then widely held that while all human beings lied, madmen and physicians were cheats on an especially grand scale. Today, the mental patient is treated as if he had completely *lost his ability to lie;* while the psychiatrist is treated as if *he could not lie,* because his lies, being therapeutically motivated, are not really lies at all.

From Malingering to Hysteria, from Quackery to Psychotherapy

Assuming that persons lie and that mental patients and psychiatrists are persons, we should expect them to lie also. Indeed they do. When Mesmerism—and its inventor, Franz Anton Mesmer (1734–1815)—flourished, critical observers had no trouble regarding the sufferers as malingerers and the healers as mountebanks. "There are," observed Benjamin Franklin, "no greater liars than quacks—except for their patients."[42] Franklin knew this to be the case partly because he was levelheaded and partly because he had been a member of the French Royal Commission, appointed by Louis XVI in 1784, charged with investigating Mesmer's cures by means of "animal magnetism." The Commission concluded, in aphoristically terse French: *"L'imagination fait tout; le magnetism nul"* ("Imagination is everything; magnetism nothing").[43] Franklin was not fooled: "As to animal magnetism so much talked of," he wrote, "I must doubt its existence . . . . I cannot but fear that the expectation of great advantage from this method of treating disease will prove a delusion."[44] Actually, it was precisely because the performances of both malingerers and magnetizers smelled so badly of deception that they were renamed and reconceptualized: what began as cheating and lying ended up as bona fide diseases and treatments.

Although physicians probably lie more often than patients, their lies have traditionally been excused, and even extolled, on the ground that they serve the patient's interest rather than the doctor's. This, of course, is paternalism at its most invincible: The liar not only lies but, because his aims are noble, demands a license for his mendacity. The pillars of society thus not only grant the doctor the right to lie but authenticate his lies as truths. This is why the patient's lies about being sick were first seen as malingering, then as hysteria, and now as various types of mental diseases—all blemishes, if not on the patient's character then on his mental health (appropriately enough, this has turned out to be a distinction without much of a difference); and why the physician's lies about being able to cure, condemned and ridiculed as quackery in the eighteenth century, soon became respected as hypnosis, and are now glorified as the scientific treatment of mental illness. Since the story of the evolution of pretended illnesses is more familiar than that of pretended treatments,

I herewith offer a brief list of the latter. In Molière's day, the doctor who conned his malingering patients—or his genuinely sick patients, for that matter—was viewed as a crook and a quack; by the end of the eighteenth century, thanks to Mesmer, he was, at least for a time, seen as a miracle-worker, curing by means of *animal magnetism,* later called *Mesmerism;* by the middle of the nineteenth century, he was more successfully mystified and glorified as a *hypnotist;* today, he is regarded as practicing scientific *psychotherapy.* *

Why do I call hypnosis a lie? Isn't it a real and effective treatment? It is ironic that physicians claimed, and people came to believe, that hypnosis was a *real,* legitimate treatment—because it *worked.* To do what? To dispel the patient's pains. But didn't the patient's lie—his hysterical complaint that he feels pain—also *work?* Didn't it convince relatives, employers, and doctors that the patient was *truly* disabled and diseased? After all, what is the classic paradigm of malingering? The patient plaintively asserting that he feels pain, is paralyzed, or is blind. And what is the corresponding paradigm of mental healing? The doctor authoritatively commanding: "Your pain is gone, you can walk, you can see." At the height of their popularity around the turn of the last century, these twin lies were named, respectively, *hysteria* and *hypnosis.* They are real in the same sense in which possession and exorcism were real—that is, as social constructs.

This might be the proper place for me to add a further remark on the problem of whether a malingerer's imitation of illness is conscious or unconscious. One of the most effective psychiatric selling points behind the idea of hysteria as something other—and more real—than feigning illness was the claim that the patient was not conscious of what he was doing. I submit that this is just another way of saying that liars are generally more convincing if they believe their own lies than if they do not: clearly liars who do not believe their own lies have to be *good actors,* whereas those who do believe their own lies need only to be *good cowards.* The same considerations apply, of course, to the physician's lies about curing. Mesmer believed in animal magnetism, the nineteenth-century French hypnotists believed in hypnotism, Breuer believed in catharsis, and Freud believed in psychoanalysis: this is why they were so effective

---

*The term *psychotherapy* is barely 100 years old.[45] Moreover, Daniel Hack Tuke (1827–1895), the English psychiatrist who introduced it in 1872, intended it to mean something quite different from what we now mean by it. Tuke defined *psychotherapeutics* (which was the original form of the word) as the "treatment of disease by the influence of the mind on the body." In other words, Tuke used the term to identify what he considered to be a particular method for treating *bodily illness;* whereas we now use it principally to identify a particular method for treating *mental illness.*

in persuading others that these purely interpersonal relations were, in fact, bona fide treatments that effectively cured bona fide diseases.

Much of this may seem obvious. It is, indeed, obvious to me. It has long been obvious to playwrights and novelists. And it may be obvious to the reader—especially after he has read this far. Actually the suspicion that mental illness is a form of malingering, a pretense of being ill, has plagued psychiatrists for a long time and only recently have they convinced themselves that their patients are truly ill. However, they have never convinced the man of letters. "Neurosis," observed Marcel Proust, "has an absolute genius for malingering. There is no illness which it cannot counterfeit perfectly . . . . If it is capable of deceiving the doctor, how should it fail to deceive the patient?"[46] Replacing the illness with the treatment, Sartre remarked that "psychoanalysis substitutes for the notion of bad faith, the idea of a lie without a liar."[47] These aphoristic observations are, of course, couched in figurative language: Proust and Sartre knew perfectly well that neither neurosis nor psychoanalysis can counterfeit or lie; only a person can do that.

Let us see now why physicians regard persons who lie about being ill as bona fide patients suffering from bona fide illnesses. Understanding their reasoning and justifications will perhaps explain why physicians, especially psychiatrists, who lie about diseases and treatments regard themselves as bona fide researchers, discoverers, diagnosticians, and therapists.

ILLNESS: CONFUSING PHENOMENON, CAUSE, AND CONSEQUENCE

Since the imitation of illness depends on an understanding of, and agreement on, what the thing is that is being imitated, we must periodically come back to square one, namely, to our definition of the core concept of illness. The canons of science, not to mention common sense, require that, regardless of how we choose to identify illness, our criteria be phenomenological. In other words, we must define illness in terms of what we can see, hear, or measure, that is, in terms of something material and observable. As I showed earlier, confusing and equating illness as a *phenomenon* with its actual or alleged *cause* (etiology), or its actual or possible or probable *consequence* (disability, death) is a typical tactic of psychiatric propaganda as well as a fertile source of misunderstanding about what is a *real illness* as against a *false illness* (or a *mental illness*).

A confused commingling of phenomenon, cause, and consequence characterizes much of the writings of psychiatrists purporting to prove that mental illnesses are diseases. For example schizophrenia is said to be a disease because it is *caused* by a genetic-metabolic defect, a schizophrenogenic mother, or a sick society. Almost any cause will do. Psychiatrists who write this way mislead the reader into tacitly accepting that schizophrenia—whatever it is—is a disease and that our only problem is how to cure or prevent it. Similarly, alcoholism is said to be a disease because it *results* in cirrhosis of the liver and death; anorexia nervosa is a disease because it *results* in cachexia and death; and so forth. Again, instead of establishing, by phenomenological criteria, that drinking or self-starvation are diseases, persons who write this way mislead people into tacitly accepting that they are, and that our only problem is how to cure or prevent them. The following paragraph is illustrative:

> The attitude of people who deny the very existence of mental disease [writes Guze] include a number of different strands . . . . First, we have the contention that disease does not exist in the absence of some *anatomic or physiologic abnormality*—which, of course, cannot be demonstrated in most kinds of mental illness. The answer, known to most physicians, is that the *cause* of not a few general medical disorders, hypertension being a good example, also has eluded us (emphasis added).[48]

Note the author's casual switch from disease as phenomenon, identified by anatomical and physiological criteria (absent in mental illness), to disease as effect, identified by etiological criteria (present in mental illness). Like all loyal psychiatrists, Guze refuses to be bound by an objectively identifiable criterion of illness. Instead, he simply declares that certain behaviors constitute illnesses and then speculates about their causes and dramatizes their consequences. "Acute depression [and] acute anxiety," for example, are illnesses, writes Guze. How does he know this? By "know[ing] that these 'deviations' can incapacitate or even (as with the suicidal depressive) destroy the sufferer."[49] So, of course, can famine and war.

Fictitious and Factitious Illness: Pretending to Be Ill and Producing Illness

The confusion of bodily illness with the patient role is now equally pervasive in medicine and psychiatry. For example, in 1984 the prestigious British medical journal *The Lancet* published an article by Roy Meadow, a pediatrician, titled "Fictitious epilepsy." Meadow describes 36 cases of faked seizures, never questioning that persons who claim to have nonexistent seizures or induce seizures in others or themselves are ill and in need of medical attention:

Fictitious epilepsy is not rare . . . . It is not surprising that false epilepsy is common, for it is easy to fabricate. . . . One bonus that came the way of many of these families was considerable support from social services by way of attendance allowances, nursery places, privileged car parking, free school meals, and disability allowances. At least one family has ended up with more than £100 per week in allowances as a result of false illness.[50]

The language Meadow uses to describe his observations cripples his thinking and predetermines his conclusion. He refers to "extensive investigation and treatment for epilepsy because of false *seizures* invented or induced by a relative," and asserts that "for 18 children recurrent seizures were the only *false illness*" (emphasis added).[51] Actually, in most of the cases reported, relatives made *false claims* about their children having had seizures; properly speaking, these reporters were *lying* and the children had *no disease* at all. The claim that one's child has seizures when he does not is no different, logically and grammatically, than the claim that one's basement is full of gold or water when it is not.

In a few of the cases reported, relatives induced seizures in children by partially suffocating them with a hand, pillow, or plastic bag; properly speaking, these malefactors were assaulting their victims, causing them to have *real seizures*. Nevertheless, the author consistently refers to these phenomena also as *false seizures;* not once does Meadow speak of *assault, injury,* or the *deliberate causation of real illness.*

Obviously, human behavior is one of the most important causes or sources of illness. People injure others and make them ill in countless ways, for example, by boxing, reckless driving, exposure to toxic environments, war. Similarly, people injure themselves and make themselves ill in countless ways, for example, by eating too much or too little, ingesting toxic chemicals, exposing themselves to grave risks, cutting, and shooting themselves. In other words, some diseases—for example, hemophilia or systemic lupus erythematosus—happen to people without their participation or volition. Others—for example, the cachexia of anorexia nervosa or the self-mutilation of a psychotic—are the results of certain habits or are purposefully self-induced. In addition, certain persons who are not ill want to be treated as if they were, and therefore imitate being ill and try to assume the role of patient. In the vast literature on malingering, these two quite different phenomena—that is, *pretending to be sick* by faking the appearance of illness and *making oneself sick* by causing real illness—are hopelessly combined and confused, as the following example illustrates.

A recent article titled "Factitious illness: An exploration in ethics," published in *Perspectives in Biology and Medicine,* begins with the vignettes of three patients exhibiting what the authors call *factitious illnesses:* a woman hospitalized for fever due to systematic self-injections of her own saliva; a nondiabetic woman with hypoglycemia due to repeated self-injections of insulin; and a woman who sought medical care for stones in her urine that proved to be her mother's gallstones.[52] In my opinion, the behavior of all three of these persons constitutes malingering; however, the condition of the first two women, who have produced real, identifiable lesions in themselves, differs radically from that of the third woman, who has merely impersonated or played the patient role.

Perhaps all this is obvious. However, it is not the way authors interpret their own observations. Although they say that they recognize the phenomenon of malingering, they insist that none of their patients is a malingerer. This makes sense only if we assume that they are more interested in legitimizing these claimants as patients, their problems as diseases, and themselves as diagnosticians than they are in understanding the phenomena they address. According to the authors, the difference between malingering and factitious illness is

> that, while factitious illness is often chronic, malingering is usually situation specific. Furthermore, although malingering is motivated by manifest secondary gains, in factitious illness there are no apparent goals other than the bizarre psychological significance of being a patient.[53]

This is what happens when physicians fail to distinguish between illness as a demonstrable bodily abnormality and the sick role as a social construct and status. But this confusion cannot be due to stupidity. More likely it is due to the simple fact, so memorably satirized by Molière, that doctors need patients. Real patients—that is, persons with demonstrable bodily diseases seeking medical help—are of course the best. But if they are in short supply, any other kind will do. Thus, fake patients, healthy persons who pretend to be ill, can and must—because they are mentally ill—be treated as (mental) patients; while persons who literally make themselves ill but do not want to be patients can and must—because they are dangerously ill—be treated as (involuntary) patients.

PRETENDING TO BE ILL AND MAKING ONESELF ILL

In modern, Western societies, people often claim to be ill when they are not: that is, they pretend to be ill or offer illness as an excuse or white lie. For example, people plead a minor illness, in person or more often over the telephone, to avoid an unpleasant social obligation or to stay away from work. Witnessing such behavior, children learn from an early age that they, too, may be able to avoid going to school or other unpleasant duties by complaining of an upset stomach or headache. As they get older, they learn more sophisticated methods of malingering, such as producing a fever by placing the thermometer near a light bulb.

We must be clear about what this sort of malingering is and is not: It is the assertion of false or fraudulent complaints about the body—that is, *misinformation;* it is not the production of a bodily lesion—that is, *illness.* In other words, such persons define themselves as ill and assume, usually for a brief period, the sick role. They play being ill the same way children play being doctor or fireman or actors play Hamlet.

A completely different situation, also called malingering, is involved in the case of a person who assumes the sick role not by making false or fraudulent complaints about his body, but by actually making himself ill. In the first case, a healthy person complains about feeling and being ill—for example, by *faking the pain of renal colic.* In the second case, a healthy person makes himself ill and then presents evidence of actual illness—for example, *an amputated penis.* Clearly, the diseases we inflict on ourselves are just as real as the diseases others inflict on us or that afflict us without the deliberate intervention of human agents. Whether or not a person has a disease does *not depend*—and *should not be made to depend*—on what causes it, although understanding its causation is very important and inevitably influences our attitude toward it.

Autogenic, or Self-Induced, Illnesses

Although malingering has traditionally been viewed as a psychiatric problem, physicians and even medical philosophers now generally accept the proposition that pretending to be ill and producing illness by injuring oneself—*both now called factitious illnesses*—are all bona fide diseases. Since this view rests on, and embodies, a commingling of the concepts of bodily lesion and the role of patient—ideas I am anxious to distinguish from one another—I should, at this point, like to propose a terminological and conceptual clarification.

To begin with, what characterizes so-called factitious illnesses is that they are self-induced; accordingly, I shall call them *autogenic* diseases. Secondly, the term *factitious illness* is unsatisfactory for another, even more important, reason—namely, because, strictly speaking, some factitious illnesses are *not illnesses* at all, but merely impersonations of the patient role; whereas certain others are *not factitious* because the patients exhibit lesions every bit as real as those exhibited by patients with

TABLE 6.2. Types of Autogenic Illness (Factitious Illness, Malingering)

Complaint	Lesion	Phenomenon and Its Interpretation
+	+	Production of self-injury with complaint: for example, self-inflicted gunshot wound in soldier who wants to avoid hazardous duty; factitious illness with lesion and desire to be a patient.
+	−	Faking being ill without self-injury: for example, false complaint of stomachache by child wishing to avoid going to school; factitious illness with desire to be a patient but without lesion.
−	+	Production of self-injury (directly or indirectly) without complaint: for example, a young man who amputates his penis (schizophrenia), or a young woman who starves herself (anorexia nervosa); factitious illness with lesion but without desire to be a patient.
−	−	No faking of being ill, no production of self-injury, no factitious illness, no patient.

nonfactitious illnesses. Finally, because autogenic diseases are produced by, and are diagnosed on the basis of, two independently variable factors—namely, false complaints of being ill and the self-induction (directly or indirectly) of actual lesions of bodily illness—we can readily distinguish three quite different kinds of problems now lumped together as factitious illnesses. (See Table 6.2.)

Perhaps the best way to illustrate what I have just described abstractly is by considering the simplest cause of illness and death in a human being (or any living thing): namely, depriving the organism or person of food. Clearly, a person may suffer the ill effects of starvation, such as malnutrition and death, for several quite different reasons: he may be a prisoner of war deprived of food; he may be a civilian prisoner on a hunger strike as a form of political protest; or he may starve himself for certain personal reasons. In each of these cases, the result of prolonged starvation is the same: disease and death. In the first case, the disease is considered to be inflicted on the subject by his captors. In the second case, although the starvation might be regarded as self-inflicted, it is not likely to be viewed as a form of malingering and its consequences are accepted as real diseases. Sometimes authorities accept such behavior as a legitimate political act and the prisoner is allowed, in effect, to kill himself; at other times, the authorities refuse to accept such behavior and forcibly feed (treat) the prisoner. In the third case, medical and psychiatric authorities refuse to regard the starvation as deliberately self-induced; instead, they define the subject as a patient suffering from a disease called *anorexia nervosa* which, they claim, causes the food-avoidance.

These examples illustrate how our perception of a phenomenon may be colored and confused by the way medical or political authorities treat them and the names they give them. When an Irish Republican Army prisoner in a British jail starves himself, no one claims that he suffers from *anorexia politica* and that his self-starvation is anything other than a personal choice; however, when a young woman in America starves herself, psychiatrists claim—and everyone concurs—that she suffers from *anorexia nervosa* and that her self-starvation is not a personal choice but the result of a serious mental illness.

One more example—illustrating the intimate connections between faking disease, self-induced disease, and mental disease—should suffice. In wartime it is not unusual for a soldier to suffer a bullet wound. If the wound is inflicted by the enemy, the soldier is considered to be a hero and is decorated. If, on the other hand, the wound is self-inflicted, then the soldier is considered to be a malingerer and may be imprisoned or even executed. *Surgically, a bullet wound* is a bullet wound, regardless of how it is acquired; whereas *legally, a person with a bullet wound* may be an assailant, the victim of an assailant, his own victim, or an innocent bystander.

In sum, illness, defined as a lesion, is a phenomenon that may be caused by many agencies, among them pathogenic microorganisms, poisons, accidents, other people, or the subject/patient himself. I suggest that we designate self-induced diseases (lesions) as *autogenic*. Such phenomena must be distinguished from the impersonations of the patient role by persons who are neither suffering from an illness nor making themselves ill.

The concept of autogenesis offers a precise criterion for identifying self-induced bodily conditions that physicians regard as diseases and thus allow us to see the similarities as well as the differences between various diseases, some now classified as factitious and others not. For example, in Charcot's day the paradigmatic autogenic disease was grand hysteria, while today it is anorexia nervosa. I classify both as autogenic because both are entirely self-induced or self-willed by the patient: that is how they resemble each other. Yet each differs from the other in that the person who pretends to have seizures imitates being ill, whereas the person who starves herself makes herself ill: the former runs the risk of perishing existentially through chronic hospital dependency, while the latter runs the risk of perishing biologically through malnutrition and inanition. In short, like the whale and the cow that resemble each other in the way they bear and feed their young, and differ in that one lives in the oceans and the other does not—so Charcot's hysteria and the DSM-III's anorectic resemble each other in the way they make themselves the objects of medical attention, but differ in that one wants to be the object of such attention and the other does not.

Malingering: Lesion and Role

As this analysis demonstrates, there are two entirely different kinds of behaviors that physicians regard as malingering, each resulting in a different kind of situation. One type of behavior consists of pretending to be ill by faking symptoms or signs of illness and seeking the care of physicians and hospitals; the other consists of producing self-injury or making oneself ill by an acute act or a chronic habit but not seeking, or even actively avoiding, the services of physicians and hospitals. Not surprisingly, both types of behaviors, as well as the persons who engage in them, make doctors angry, but for very different reasons: the first type of person because he is (as the physician sees it) healthy but *wants to be a patient*; the second type, because he is (as the physician sees it) sick, but *does not want to be a patient*. Feeling deceived in the first case, and frustrated in the second, the physician feels justified in retaliating. How he punishes the patient changes with medical fashions.

For example, as recently as 1957, a feature article in the *Journal of the American Medical Association* described persons who impersonate sick patients as an "economic threat" to hospitals and an "extreme nuisance" to doctors, and proposed that they be punished by "permanent custodial care . . . in a mental hospital."[54] The logic was sound: Fake illness requires fake treatment. It has since become both more expensive and more difficult to incarcerate persons indefinitely in mental hospitals, which is perhaps one of the reasons why malingerers of this type are now punished merely with stigmatizing psychiatric diagnoses and psychiatric drugs.

The second type of behavior—exemplified by the person who eats too much or too little—makes doctors feel frustrated by the fact that an individual whom physicians regard as a sick patient refuses to be a patient. Like the Russian intellectual who rejects and resists the Soviet ideology and is therefore called a (political) *refusenik*, the medically sick nonpatient rejects and resists the medical ideology and might therefore also be called a (medical) *refusenik*. And once again, the doctor's punishment fits the nonpatient's crime: the nonpatient is forced to become a patient. Indeed the deceptive-coercive treatment of autogenic diseases—such as

drug abuse, chemical dependency, alcoholism, smoking, anorexia nervosa, obesity—is now one of the fastest growing segments of the medical
industry.

Why do I emphasize these seemingly obvious distinctions? Because
psychiatry stands or falls on its ability and power to confuse and obliterate them. As we have seen, psychiatrists begin by confusing the differences between bodily illnesses and mental illnesses: they insist that
mental illnesses *are* bodily illnesses, that they are *like* bodily illnesses,
and that they are also *different from* bodily illnesses. Next, psychiatrists
confuse the differences between a bodily lesion and the patient role:
they insist that assuming the patient role in the absence of illness *is*
itself an illness. According to the APA, the "diagnosis of a Factitious
Disorder always implies psychopathology, most often a severe personality disorder."[55] But if it is psychiatrically correct to conclude that a
person who says he is ill is ill only because he claims he is, then it is also
correct to conclude that a person who says he is the Emperor of China is
the Emperor of China because he claims he is. Of course, psychiatrists
stop short before reaching that conclusion, and for an obvious reason:
they have a vested interest in illnesses, real or false, but have no vested
interest in personal identities. Thus, when a person assumes a false
identity—for example, by claiming that he is Jesus—the psychiatrists
do not say that he is Jesus; they say he is having a delusion and is sick.
The point of the game, after all, is not to agree with the patient, but to
authenticate an illness.

I might add that when it comes to faking illnesses, psychiatrists
indulge their patients and themselves equally. Thus when the professional manufacturers of madness fabricate mental illnesses—as they
have done in the past with masturbatory insanity and homosexuality
and more recently with pathological gambling and paraphilic rapism—
their colleagues eagerly authenticate these fabrications as real diseases.
There is an important exception to this rule, however: it applies only to
psychiatrists who serve the same ideological and political master. This
is why American and Russian psychiatrists often differ in psychiatric
diagnoses in general and on the psychopathology of specific patients in
particular. Moreover, as if they hadn't created enough confusion already by claiming that healthy persons who assume the sick role are ill
and by treating nonlesions as if they were lesions, psychiatrists now
also claim that real lesions are not real lesions if they are self-inflicted.
Under the caption of "Factitious Disorders with Physical Symptoms,"
DSM-III offers this astonishing denial of the reality of real lesions: "The
essential feature is the presentation of *physical symptoms that are not
real.* The presentation may be . . . self-inflicted, as in the production

of abscesses by injection of saliva into the skin."[56] If such abscesses are not real abscesses, then persons who kill themselves are not really dead, a conclusion characteristic of current psychiatric logic.*

SIMULATING AND DISSIMULATING INSANITY

We are ready now to consider psychiatry's classic twin riddles, namely, the problems of sane persons pretending to be insane and vice versa. The former is usually called *feigning insanity,* the latter, *dissimulating insanity.* Both terms imply that just as a rich person can pretend to be a poor person and vice versa, so a sane person can pretend to be an insane person and vice versa. The trouble, once again, is that since there are no objective tests for ascertaining whether a person is mentally healthy or mentally sick, there can be no way of determining or knowing whether he is *really insane* or only *feigning insanity* and whether he is *really sane* or merely *dissimulating insanity.* This is one of the reasons why psychiatrists love the idea of simulating-dissimulating insanity so much: regardless of what their examinations reveal or what they say, they cannot be proven wrong.

In order to solve these riddles, it is necessary to situate them in the social contexts in which they typically arise. The riddle of whether *insanity is real or simulated* arises typically when, for example, a person in the military service feigns, or is suspected of feigning, insanity (in order to be separated from the service): the serviceman claims, by word or deed, that he is crazy, while the authorities who have power over him claim he is not. The opposite riddle, namely whether *sanity is real or the product of successful dissimulation of insanity,* arises typically when, for example, a previously normal and perhaps even greatly admired person commits a shocking crime: those in authority over him may now claim that his embarrassing behavior proves not only his present insanity but also that he had been insane in the past and that his seemingly sane

---

*Scrutinizing the way psychiatrists conceptualize faking illness reveals, perhaps more clearly than anything else, the fakeries of psychiatry. Consider in this connection a Congressional committee's estimate that one of 50 practicing physicians in the United States today is an impostor.[57] Surely this suggests that physicians are not particularly adept at distinguishing real doctors from fake ones—a fact that does not inspire confidence in their ability to distinguish real patients from fake ones. Moreover, even if physicians identify a person as faking illness, psychiatrists, as we saw, immediately diagnose him as suffering from a factitious illness. But if the person who pretends to be ill is considered to be a bona fide patient having a *factitious illness,* why is the person who pretends to be a doctor not considered to be a bona fide physician offering *factitious therapy?*

behavior was merely the result of his successful dissimulation of insanity. The subject, if still alive, is likely to insist that he is sane and has always been perfectly sane.

How are these conflicting claims resolved? The way all such conflicting claims in psychiatry (and, of course, not in psychiatry alone) are resolved—by the stronger party imposing his will on the weaker one. The result, in the first instance, is that the subject's claim to insanity is disconfirmed and he is officially declared to be sane; while in the second instance, the subject's claim to sanity is disconfirmed and he is officially declared to be insane. I shall illustrate both of these scenarios.

Simulating Insanity

In the aftermath of the war in Vietnam many ex-servicemen reported difficulties in personal adjustment which they attributed to the stress of military action endured in that unpopular war. Psychiatrists recognize this as a type of mental illness and call it "Posttraumatic Stress Disorder" (abbreviated as PTSD). If this condition is defined as being due to the stress of military service, it would seem that if a person who had never been in Vietnam claimed to be suffering from PTSD due to service in Vietnam, his claim would not constitute an illness. But it does. Psychiatrists regard "Factitious PTSD" also as an illness that "can and must be diagnosed, has an etiology, and requires appropriate treatment."[58]

Edward Lynn and Mark Belza, two psychiatrists at the VA Medical Center in Reno, Nevada, have published a report on "seven cases of factitious PTSD . . . found among veterans who were never in combat, and, in some cases, were never in Vietnam."[59] In the authors' experience, this is not a rare ailment: During a five-month period, in a 20-bed psychiatric unit with an average daily census of only 14, the authors observed seven such cases. After discussing "the etiologies of the disorder and the underlying psychopathology and . . . recommendations for diagnosis and treatment," the authors conclude: "Clearly, then, our first responsibility is to develop an awareness of factitious PTSD . . . for until we do, patients with such disorders will not receive appropriate care."[60] To conclude that persons who lie about having been made mentally ill in Vietnam are liars is, evidently, not among the responsibilities of contemporary American psychiatrists.

The eagerness with which psychiatrists—and even district attorneys and judges—accept fabricated stories of stress in Vietnam as genuine mental diseases is illustrated by the case of a man named Samuel Lockett. Accused of several robberies in Brooklyn in 1983, he pleaded not guilty by reason of insanity, claiming "that he was suffering from Vietnam Stress Syndrome." His claim was accepted not only by numerous psychiatrists but also by Brooklyn District Attorney Elizabeth Holtzman and New York State Supreme Court Justice Michael Juvilier. It was later discovered that Lockett was never in Vietnam.[61]

Dissimulating Insanity

Dissimulating insanity, also known as simulating sanity, is the mirror image of the situation we have just considered: the subject wants to appear sane but others discredit him as insane. The stories of some sensational crimes in recent American history give us a ringside seat from which to watch this spectacle. The first such story I shall present is that of one of the most celebrated crazy murderers of recent years— namely, the story of David Berkowitz, also known as the Son of Sam. I offer this case because although Berkowitz seemed patently, totally insane *after* he was apprehended, his supposedly severe mental illness completely escaped detection *during* the many years preceding his capture.

The Son of Sam, as may be recalled, was a young man named David Berkowitz who terrorized New York City in 1976 and 1977 by killing six people and wounding seven others. At the time of his trial, Berkowitz justified the killings by claiming that he was carrying out the orders of demons and a dog. Barely 18 months later, Berkowitz insisted that his crazy behavior had been a sham. "Quite frankly," he told an Associated Press reporter who visited him in the Attica (New York) prison, "this is fictitious, it is invented, it is a lie. There were no real demons, no talking dogs, no Satanic henchmen. I made it all up."[62]

Confronted with Berkowitz's claim that he had faked insanity, Daniel Schwartz, who headed the team of psychiatrists who had examined Berkowitz and testified that he was psychotic, said: "[If] it [the story of demonic possession] was an act, it was an all-time winner." Schwartz explained that he believed Berkowitz's story because it was "so convincing and had so much peripheral validation."[63] That, of, course, is nonsense. He accepted Berkowitz's wild story because by authenticating Berkowitz as a crazy psychotic, Schwartz in effect legitimized himself as a caring psychiatrist.

In August, 1980, in an interview with the *Buffalo Evening News*, Berkowitz reiterated his claim that,

he is not now and never was mentally ill. . . . noticeably thinner than in 1977, he insists he was not mentally ill when he was in the Army, not when he was firing a gun at nameless faces in New York's dark lovers' lanes, not when he was being examined by psychiatrists, and not when he was screaming out in the courtroom.[64]

Some of the things Berkowitz told the *Buffalo Evening News* reporter are worth repeating here. "The tapes," Berkowitz explained, "are authentic in that I said those things [demons impelling him to kill, etc.] but they are not authentic because I was feigning and malingering."[65] Berkowitz maintained that he was faking insanity to allay his guilt for the killings. Perhaps. And perhaps he was doing it also for the dramatic attention his claims attracted. In any case, Berkowitz has petitioned the courts for a hearing to declare him competent to manage his affairs. (He had been declared incompetent and assigned a conservator.) Indeed, the *Evening News* reporter who spoke at length with Berkowitz found him to be quite sane:

> If clear, articulate responses and conversation coupled with normal amounts of smiling and laughter and the appreciation of nuances of good and evil concepts are signs of competency, then David Berkowitz is all there.[66]

Frances Mills—chief of psychiatric services at the Attica correctional facility, who sees Berkowitz almost daily—agrees: "I have never found him psychotic."[67] Another Attica official described Berkowitz as "crazy as a fox."[68]

None of this matters. After concluding that "Berkowitz acted like a sane man and talked like a sane man," the *Evening News* reporter ends with the characteristic caveat of our psychiatric age: "Yet what is one to think of someone who for no visible reason shot at 15 people he didn't know, killing six of them, injuring seven and missing two?"[69] One thinks, of course, that such a person was insane, is presently insane, and will always be insane.

My second example—the story of the Reverend Jim Jones, the minister who presided over the once-famed people's paradise in Guyana and then went on to murder every member of the group he could lay his hands on—is more complicated. Although this story offers the same cautionary tale concerning the question, "Who is really insane?" as does Berkowitz's, the Jones story is more complex, and perhaps also more instructive because, despite his remarkable utterances and behavior, Jones was never diagnosed as mentally ill while he was alive; the diagnosis that he was psychotic was made only posthumously. Of course, it was not based, as one might expect in the case of a brain disease, on what pathologists discovered in his brain; instead, it was based entirely on what his followers, friends, and political supporters discovered to be in their own best interest.

The story, briefly, is this. Jim Jones, the founder of Jonestown, had been a duly consecrated priest of a respected Christian denomination and the object of praise and admiration by the high and mighty in American politics and public life. He was also the cold-blooded murderer of 900 men, women, and children.

James Warren Jones was born on May 13, 1931, in a small town in Indiana. As a child he liked to play minister, his first flock being animals. According to Kenneth Wooden's story of Jonestown, as a boy, Jones "frequently took in animals, cared for them, won their trust, then killed them and gave them elaborate funerals, with candles and all the accoutrements."[70]

In 1964, Jones was ordained a minister in the Protestant denomination called "Disciples of Christ." The following year, he and his followers moved to California. In San Francisco, Jones advertised himself with fliers that read, in part, as follows:

PASTOR JIM JONES/PROPHET—saves lives of total strangers with his predictions. Scores will be present to give medical documentation of the amazing healing . . . Healer of cancerous diseases doctors called "incurable" . . .

SPECIAL NOTICE: This message of God proclaims Apostolic Social Justice of Equality and PROVES his message by divine SIGNS and wonders.[71]

With the proven formula of claiming to help the helpless—especially blacks, children, the aged, and the poor—Jones quickly amassed a fortune by funneling their Social Security benefits to himself. At the same time, with the aid of the media, he succeeded in creating an image of himself as a humanitarian, a healer, and a defender of civil rights. Consider just a few of the accolades heaped upon him.

In April 1975, Religion in American Life, a national interfaith organization, named him one of the 100 most outstanding clergymen in the nation.[72] In the same year, the San Francisco newspaper, *Sun Reporter*— owned by Carlton Goodlett, a black physician who became Jones's personal doctor—presented him with a citizen's Merit Award for his dedication to social justice. A year later, the *Los Angeles Herald* bestowed upon him its "Humanitarian of the Year" award. In September, 1976, Jones supported Jimmy Carter's candidacy for president and dined in private with Mrs. Rosalynn Carter in San Francisco. Subsequently, Mrs. Carter heaped praise on Jones. Among those who endorsed Jones during his early years in California were Hubert Humphrey, Jane Fonda, Walter Mondale, and many others.[73]

Was this the same man who, on November 18, 1978, murdered 900 men, women, and children? Of course not. It couldn't have been. So the story had to be quickly rewritten.

As soon as the news of the massacre hit the wires, it was taken for granted—by psychiatrists, politicians, the press, the public—that Jones was, and had for some time been, crazy, insane, psychotic. Political columnist Patrick J. Buchanan's rhetorical query was typical: "Why wasn't the Secret Service alerted to keep Mrs. Carter miles away from a certifiable madman like the Rev. Jim Jones?"[74] (Mrs. Carter had met Jones two years earlier.)

Distinguished American psychiatrists quickly volunteered to suggest that the murdered as well as the murderer were really *good people to whom something terrible had happened*. Opined Thomas Ungerleider, a professor of psychiatry at the University of California at Los Angeles: "I believe it was the jungle. The members got no feedback from the outside world. They did not read *Time* magazine or watch the news at night."[75] Alvin Poussaint, a professor of psychiatry at Harvard and one of the leading black psychiatrists in America, offered this interpretation: "We cannot in good conscience fault the mission of the rank-and-file because of the *acute psychosis* of their leader. . . . The humanitarian experiment itself was not a failure, the Reverend Jones was" (emphasis added).[76] Leading commentators in the press agreed, but framed their diagnoses in simpler terms. The Reverend Jones, concluded James Reston of *The New York Times*, was "an obviously demented man."[77]

But it was not so obvious when Jones was alive. One of Jones's lawyers, Mark Lane—an attorney of considerable notoriety and an expert on conspiracies and madness in high places—served as Jones's trusted counselor right up to the very moment of the mass murder. Lane must thus have considered his client to be sane, at least sane enough to be his client. However, as soon as Lane got away from Guyana he described Jones as a "paranoid murderer."[78]

Charles Garry, Jones's other legal advisor, also liked the insanity theory. Before the massacre, he heaped praise on Jones and his commune. The camp, he asserted, was "a beautiful jewel. There is no racism, no sexism, no ageism, no elitism, no hunger." After the massacre, he was equally well informed. "I am convinced," he declared, that "this guy was stark, raving mad."[79] I shall try to show that the description of Jones's concentration camp as a beautiful jewel and of Jones as a madman are equally untrue.

Moreover, even after the massacre, Carlton Goodlett, the influential black physician-newspaper owner, insisted that "Jones was involved in a brilliant experiment in Guyana . . . ," and added: "The deserters from the church had come to me, but they were just a neurotic fringe." After the story in *New West* magazine appeared in 1977—this was the exposé that led to Jones's flight from San Francisco to Guyana, and ultimately to the end of his experiment—Goodlett complained that the reporters got their information from "malcontents, psychoneurotics, and, in some instances, provocateurs—probably Establishment agents."[80]

Clearly, Jones was someone to reckon with. Kenneth Wooden documents the veritable torrent of complaints lodged against Jones, especially during the last three years of his reign, all of which, because of Jones's political connections, were either ignored or killed. He writes:

> Many of the survivors of the People's Temple were bitter toward the President and Mrs. Carter as well. After Jim Jones' highly publicized meeting with Mrs. Carter and his public endorsement of her husband, a number of ex-members wrote the First Lady. Mickey Touchette [a survivor] remembered: "We told her what he was doing and what was involved and what kind of a man he was, and she turned a deaf ear to us."[81]

Mrs. Carter, it should be recalled, was Honorary Chairperson of the President's Commission on Mental Health and ranked mental health as her foremost concern. She embraced Jim Jones as a fellow soldier in the war on mental illness and helped to consolidate Jones's image as a great healer, successful in "rehabilitating drug abusers."

The facts are embarrassing, indeed. Numerous authorities colluded with Jones in his criminal activities and stand convicted by the evidence, such as the large quantity of arms and ammunition that had been sent to Guyana from the United States—all illegally.

Finally, perhaps the supreme irony of this story lies in a pair of contradictions I have not yet even mentioned. Jones, the man who goes down in history as one of the greatest mass *poisoners* the world has ever seen, was hailed, while alive, as a heroic fighter in the struggle against what we mendaciously call *drug abuse*—that is, the self-administration of drugs, especially illegal drugs. In addition, Jones, the man who practiced mass *homicide*, preached and protested against *suicide*—that is, self-determined death. On Memorial Day in 1977— only 18 months before he murdered his followers—Jones led a delegation of People's Temple members on a march onto the Golden Gate Bridge in San Francisco, demanding that the city build a suicide barrier there.[82]

Was Jones the supremely sane humanitarian, seeking to lift up the oppressed—as everyone who mattered saw him before the Jonestown massacre? Or was he an insane tyrant, seeking to imprison and murder his victims—which is how everyone who matters has seen him ever since? I think both questions are foolish. Consider only a few of the reports about Jones's behavior during the period when he was generally regarded not merely as normal, but as morally superior: Jones insisted that he, and he alone, be addressed as Father; he was married, kept several mistresses, and "had sex" with numerous women and men in the commune. Everyone in the commune had to "confess publicly" that he or she was a homosexual. Several times before the final butchery, he conducted rehearsals of the communal carnage. He claimed that he was Jesus, could cure cancer, and ordered pages torn from Bibles to be used as toilet paper.

I conclude that Jones wanted to appear as if he were a savior like Jesus, that his followers wanted him to appear in that light, and that that was the foundation on which Jonestown was built.

Why was Jones never diagnosed as mentally ill, insane, or psychotic during his lifetime? If Jones was psychotic when he ordered Congressman Leo Ryan's murder and the mass murder-suicide of his followers, why didn't anyone in the Ryan party or any of the visiting journalists observe any sign of mental illness in Jones? The answer, I submit, is briefly this. Jones never presented himself as crazy or in need of psychiatric help and neither did anyone else ever present him in that way. On the contrary, he defined himself as a devout religious leader, a compassionate Christian whose only goal in life was to help the poor, the sick, and the downtrodden. He also claimed to be a devoted family man and numerous courts authenticated him as a father not only to his own children but to many orphans as well. In short, Jones had never cast himself in the role of a person with mental problems; no one had ever impugned his sanity; and most importantly, his own physician, lawyers, fellow churchmen, prominent politicians, and the press all legitimized him as a completely normal, mentally healthy person: this, I believe, is why he always appeared sane to everyone who met him. Because of its sheer simplicity, this answer may strike most people as unsatisfactory or wrong; but the evidence strongly supports it.

INSANITY: APPEARANCE OR REALITY?

Berkowitz's serial claims—first of insanity, then of sanity—raise the question always asked in such cases, namely: Was he pretending to be insane, or was he really insane? The form of this question implies that *feigning insanity* and *being insane* are two distinct and separate conditions. I believe that is not so. It only seems so because we give a literal interpretation to the metaphoric illness we call insanity.

Imitating Real Illness and Imitating Fake Illness

Feigning bleeding from a peptic ulcer and bleeding from a peptic ulcer are two different conditions: the former consists of an act—namely, the impersonation of a person who bleeds from a peptic ulcer; whereas the latter consists of a display of an objectively verifiable bodily condition—namely, bleeding from an ulceration of the stomach or duodenum. By contrast, feigning insanity and being insane are not two different conditions, but are one and the same thing: both consist of the insane acts of a person or moral agent.

As I have tried to show in earlier chapters, mental illness is an *action*, not a *lesion*. As Shakespeare showed—and I agree with him—it is also an *act*, in the sense of a theatrical impersonation. But if being psychotic is like playing Hamlet, then feigning being psychotic is like feigning playing Hamlet, which would be the same as playing Hamlet. The point is that Hamlet is nothing but a role. No one *is*, or can *be*, Hamlet. An actor who plays Hamlet and an actor who impersonates an actor who plays Hamlet (there is a potentially infinite regress here) are both playing Hamlet. Similarly, a person who *is psychotic* and another who *merely pretends to be psychotic* are both *acting* crazy, both will *appear* to be crazy, and both will be *diagnosed* by psychiatrists as crazy.

Of course, there are many different reasons why people act crazy, just as there are many different reasons why actors are actors; but these reasons or motives do not affect the *phenomenon* we see and observe—which is an *act* that we call *insanity* or *psychosis*.

In short, the question whether Berkowitz was psychotic or was only pretending to be psychotic poses a pseudoproblem: the fact is that Berkowitz was deceitful and dishonest. This was clear in the theatrical dramatization of his madness—specifically, in his claim that he was not *David Berkowitz* but the *Son of Sam*. He might as well have listed himself on the playbill as *Jack the Ripper*. It was perfectly obvious who he *really was*. Whether Berkowitz was trying to deceive us, himself, or both, we cannot readily determine and may even be unknowable. In any case, it has no bearing on the view I am proposing. Nor has the *intentionality* or *conscious awareness* with which Berkowitz was pretending have any bearing on it (see Chapter 7). I allude here to some of my critics' attempts to rebut my argument by asserting that persons who commit such crimes are not *fully conscious* of their actions; in short, that such imitations are *unconscious*. But that, too, is beside the point. Imitation is imitation, regardless of the actor's awareness of his behavior, his reasons for it, or his intention for performing it.

It is worth noting here, at least in passing, that the imitation of mental states is of interest not only to psychiatrists and other interpreters of our (secular) criminal and mental health laws, but also to theologians and other interpreters of the (Roman Catholic) Canon Law. For example, Canon 1101, titled "Simulation of Matrimonial Consent," is devoted entirely to an analysis of the problem of simulation as it relates to the "internal consent of the mind" of the party contracting to marry.[83] Unlike psychiatrists, priests interpret the simulation of consent not as a manifestation of "factitious consent" but as a manifestation of the simulator's true intent to withhold consent. In addition, the priests also emphasize that simulation is not the sort of thing one can observe: "Since simulation involves an internal act, its external proof is difficult. Basically, simulation involves a person's taking a definite stand contrary to the Church's view of marriage."[84]

Mental Illness as Deception and Counterdeception

Suppose we grant, for the sake of advancing the argument, that behavior such as Berkowitz displayed by pretending to be the Son of Sam is a type of deception. What have we proved? Obviously, deception is not the same as what we call a psychosis. Actors, politicians, people in all walks of life also engage in deceptions. So deception is not enough for generating a diagnosis of psychosis. In addition, a certain kind of response from psychiatrists, lawyers, and judges is also required: Specifically, what is required is a counterdeception, couched in the language of psychiatry, that fits, like a-hand-in-a-glove, the subject's deception. The subject— viewed as a *patient*—asserts that he is not bad, because his act was *compelled*—by God or demons. The psychiatrist—viewed as a *medical scientist*—asserts that the patient is, indeed, not bad, because his act was *caused* by his psychosis. The crux of such a diagnosis thus lies in the smoothly meshing combination of a reciprocal deception and counterdeception and its official—medical, legal, and social—acceptance and accreditation as *disease* and *diagnosis.* *

The case of the Son of Sam illustrates beautifully this meshing pattern

---

*It is this last-mentioned element that has led some observers to speak of a *labeling theory* of mental illness.[85] Since everything in science, and indeed in everyday life, is labeled one way or another, the phrase *labeling theory* seems to me a trite term for a trivial idea.

of *deception* and *counterdeception* and its legitimation as *psychosis* and *psychiatric diagnosis*. Berkowitz's *behavior*—consisting of an obviously staged caricature of the behavior of a crazed maniac—was officially accepted as a *psychosis;* and the psychiatrist's *behavior*—consisting of a similarly staged caricature of a doctor examining a patient—was officially accepted as a *diagnostic determination*. What is invariably overlooked in situations of this sort is that every person observing or participating, whether as actor or audience, in a situation of this sort has a choice: he is free to accept the stereotyped psychiatric story now conventionally regarded as the correct explanation, or to reject it and formulate his own explanation. The following interpretation seems to me particularly plausible.

When adults view a child playing fireman, they interpret his behavior as playing fireman. Similarly, an observer of the Berkowitz trial—especially a newspaper reporter—could, in principle, have interpreted Berkowitz's behavior as that of a person impersonating (playing the role of) a madman claiming to be controlled by demons; and he could have interpreted the forensic psychiatrist's behavior as that of a person impersonating (playing the role of) a doctor diagnosing a dangerous and mysterious disease. The point is that virtually no one today chooses such an interpretation: not the defendant, not the defense attorney, not the psychiatrist testifying for the defense, not the prosecuting attorney, not the psychiatrist testifying for the prosecution, not the judge, not the reporters—not anyone! Obviously, I am suggesting just such an interpretation: namely, that Berkowitz *chose to kill* and *chose to act crazy*, and that the authorities *chose to define him as psychotic*. Now Berkowitz says he is no longer interested in killing people, and some of the psychiatrists say they are no longer interested in defining him as psychotic. But if Berkowitz was so sick, how did he get cured? I raise this question here only to show how the mendacity that psychosis is a disease is matched by the mendacity that it can be cured. Like anyone else, a psychotic person, can, of course, change his behavior. But abandoning a career of killing people is not a cure, just as embracing such a career is not a disease.

What can we learn from a story such as that of David Berkowitz? We can learn that although it is impossible *to fake having a mental illness*, it is possible, indeed it is quite easy, *to assume the role of mental patient by acting crazy*. Since a person who acts crazy is usually regarded as crazy or having a mental illness, it is, ipso facto, impossible to distinguish a person who *is crazy* from one who *only pretends to be crazy*.

To repeat, Hamlet is the name of a fictitious person and of a role. When the play *Hamlet* is performed, an actor plays Hamlet. An actor imitating an actor playing Hamlet would still be playing Hamlet. Thus, it is sensible to say that a person *plays the role* of Hamlet—or *the role* of a mental patient—well or poorly, convincingly or unconvincingly, but it is stupid, indeed nonsensical, to say that a person *imitates* the role of Hamlet or the role of a mental patient. I have called attention earlier to the corresponding phenomenon in relation to bodily illness, namely, that just as *a lesion is always real*, regardless of whether it is inflicted on the patient's body by another person, the patient himself, or some other impersonal agency—so a *role is always real*, regardless of whether others approve or disapprove of the actor's motives for assuming it. In short, a person can perform a role well or poorly, successfully or unsuccessfully, with or without the approval of certain authorities; in any case, *the role he plays is his role.* C. S. Lewis anticipated what I am trying to say here when he warned that "All mortals turn into the things they are pretending to be."[86]

7

MENTAL ILLNESS AND THE PROBLEM OF INTENTIONALITY

I cannot help myself at all, for he [the demon] uses my limbs and organs, my neck, my tongue, and my lungs . . . .
                                                    —*The Malleus Maleficarum*[1]

Although we regard some human actions as obviously intentional and some bodily movements as clearly unintentional, the meaning of the terms *intentional* and *unintentional* is often vague and uncertain, open to different interpretations. This terminological opacity is characteristic of our entire vocabulary for describing and explaining human behavior: It applies also to words such as *deliberate, voluntary,* and *conscious,* and their antonyms; and it reflects our pervasive ambivalence about human existence. Is life an opportunity or a burden—a sunlit arena where we exercise choice and shape outcome or a dark dungeon where we must plod as the slaves of superior forces?

INTENTIONALITY: A CLASSIC PSYCHIATRIC CONUNDRUM

The psychiatric enterprise has long been bedeviled by trying to answer the seemingly reasonable question: Did Jones *intend* to do what he did?

This problem was further complicated when the psychoanalysts arrived on the scene and demanded to know: Did Jones *consciously intend* to do what he did?

In this chapter I shall try to show that—except when bodily movements are demonstrably the results of neuromuscular discharges—we use the terms *intentional* and *unintentional* to praise or blame an actor rather than to simply describe or explain his behavior.* Before undertaking a systematic inquiry into the relations between the ideas of insanity and intentionality, I shall sketch four brief vignettes to better illustrate the problem.

Some Typical Cases of Intending and Nonintending

1. Smith is developing a slowly growing malignant tumor in his left motor cortex. After complaining of headaches and visual problems for several weeks, he suffers a grand mal seizure while having dinner with his wife in a restaurant. Subsequent diagnostic studies and a neurosurgical operation confirm the diagnosis. Knowing this, it would be absurd to say that "Smith *decided* to throw a fit." This is an obvious (and uninteresting) sense in which we can say that Smith's seizure was unintended or involuntary.

2. Smith is invited to join an office party celebrating the birthday of a fellow worker. The person in charge of the dinner arrangement at the restaurant asks him whether he wants steak or chicken, but Smith, explaining that he is a strict vegetarian, requests a special meal of plain spaghetti and a salad. Knowing this, it would be absurd to say that "Smith *did not really want* to order a meat-free dinner. This is an obvious (and uninteresting) sense in which we could say that Smith's choice was intentional.

Actions or happenings that fall between these two poles are open to interpretation concerning whether or not the actor acted intentionally. Here are two typical examples.

3. Harry is in love with Harriet and marries her. The union proves to be disastrously unhappy for him. He consults a psychoanalyst hoping to understand how or why this happened to him. After many weeks (or months or years or decades) of therapy, the analyst writes a scientific paper in which he explains that "When Harry married Harriet, he *unconsciously chose* a woman who reminded him of his mother (who had dominated him and made him unhappy)." The gist of the analyst's

---

*The analyses of intentionality in this chapter, and of responsibility in the next one, overlap; they are intended to be complementary, each being incomplete without the other.

interpretation is that Harry *did not really intend* to marry a woman who was like his mother but that his *unconscious repetition compulsion* made him do so. This is an essentially theoretical example of choice categorized as unintended happening.

4. Betty feels powerfully attracted to Bill, a handsome athlete much admired by her female friends. She marries Bill, only to discover that he is a bully who enjoys humiliating and beating her. After enduring the role of a battered wife for several years, Betty waits till Bill is soundly asleep one night, pours gasoline on the bed and sets it on fire. Betty comes to trial, pleads *not guilty by reason of insanity,* and is promptly acquitted. This is a supremely practical example of choice categorized as unintended happening.

Caprice and Confusion Concerning Intentionality

The ways in which people, especially members of the legal and psychiatric professions, actually use the yoked-together ideas of intentional/ mentally healthy, nonintentional/mentally ill illustrate their conceptual character and practical importance. For example, the trade in illegal drugs, like any trade, involves two parties, buyer and seller. Psychiatrists insist, and lawyers and legislators agree, that one of these parties—the buyer—is sick, because his behavior is not intentional, the result of an illness called *substance abuse disorder;* and that the other party—the seller—is not sick, because his behavior, called *pushing drugs,* is a deliberate, voluntary act. While this distinction makes sense as social strategy (see Chapter 9), it is patently absurd as an ostensibly phenomenological-scientific discrimination between what is and is not intentional behavior. After all, many persons who sell illegal drugs also use them. Do they have two personalities—one, habitually selling drugs, being bad, the other, habitually using drugs, being ill?

Actually, the distinction the law and psychiatry now make between the practice of selling and using illegal drugs is reminiscent of the distinction the law made not so long ago about bootlegging (liquor) and prostitution. The man who sold whiskey and the woman who sold her sexual services were considered to be criminals. The people who bought these goods and services were not.

Although the ideas of sanity and intentionality, insanity and unintentionality are often coupled, this seemingly necessary correlation need not always apply. Actually, several mental illnesses are described by the psychiatric nosologists themselves as consummately intentional behaviors. For example, in DSM-III *elective mutism* is described as the "continuous refusal to speak in almost all social situations. . . . The refusal to speak is not, however, due to a language insufficiency or another mental disorder";[2] another disease, called *oppositional disorder*, is described as "a pattern of disobedient, negativistic, and provocative opposition to authority figures . . . . The disorder generally causes more distress to those around him or her than to the person himself or herself."[3] In short, although these acts are viewed as intentional, they are nevertheless categorized as mental diseases.

A similar relationship exists between intentionality and insanity in connection with certain dramatically violent acts, which typically prompt the response: "Only an insane person would do such a thing." Examples abound in the daily press. In August 1985, person or persons unknown set fire to a New York subway car used by derelicts as a home. Luckily, no one was killed but 117 persons were injured and traffic was disrupted for a day. Mayor Edward Koch promptly declared that "Anyone who would start this intentionally is a deranged person."[4] Mr. Koch thus offered the conventional definition of an arsonist (a person who deliberately sets a fire) as if it were the definition of a pyromaniac (a person who, strictly speaking, does not set a fire, but where, according to the DSM-III, "fire-setting *results* from a failure to resist an impulse" [emphasis added]).[5] But if a person who sets a fire unintentionally is deranged], as psychiatric textbooks tell us, and if a person who sets a fire intentionally is also deranged, as Mr. Koch tells us, then we would have to believe that all fires are set by deranged persons—a conclusion characteristic of the reasoning of our psychiatrically enlightened intellectual elite.

Is there a way out of this psychiatric-semantic morass? Or must we throw up our hands and conclude that the ideas of intentionality and nonintentionality are invoked to serve precisely the purpose Mr. Koch's psuedoexplanation served—namely, to satisfy the hunger for an explanation of disturbing behavior? When a dramatic incident threatens people's sense of security, any explanation—no matter how nonsensical—is felt to be better than none. Scapegoats fulfill this function. In the past, a Jew or a Communist *did it*. Now, a mentally ill person—or even mental illness—*does it*. Although I believe that this scapegoat model often adequately accounts for the meaning-and-function of mental illness explanations, there is a subtlety and strength to the idea of intentional/unintentional and its relation to the idea of sanity/insanity that is worth exploring further. I shall do so by examining the psychiatric perspective on art, the human activity now paradigmatic of our notion of intentionality.

ART AND INSANITY

Because art is much older than psychiatry, artists have had a big jump on insanity. Indeed, artists, especially poets and writers, have always shown a good deal of interest in madness. As soon as psychiatry appeared on the scene, psychiatrists returned the compliment by showing a keen interest in art. Before long, it became a truism that there is a close—albeit mysterious—connection between madness and art.[6]

The *mad artist*, like the *mad genius*, may be a creation of the human imagination; nevertheless, the figure of the insane artist, like the idea of insanity itself, now seems very real to most people. Although no one can define madness, most people believe that they can tell a madman, especially a mad artist, when they see one. And while people usually disagree vehemently about who is a mad artist—one person's madness is another person's sanity, and vice versa—virtually everyone believes that some artists are mad and some madmen are artists. One person will thus nominate Vaslav Nijinski as an example, another Vincent Van Gogh, and still another Ezra Pound, while each is likely to proclaim the sanity of the other nominees. Although I do not think this is a very satisfactory state of affairs, most people view the examples I have cited (and others like them) as irrefutable evidence of the reality and validity of the construct called the *mad artist*.

If we peer behind the mystifying and mysterious facade of the mad artist, we quickly discover an interesting connection between art and insanity. This connection pivots around the fundamental idea of intentionality—art being viewed as quintessentially intentional, and insanity as quintessentially nonintentional.

How did this peculiarly polarized view develop? Why is it nonsensical to say that an artist *is not responsible* for the music he composed or performed, or the painter for the portrait he painted, or that the madman *is responsible* for his delusions or compulsions, or for killing himself or his wife? The answers to these questions reveal an essential aspect of what we now—in the twentieth century—mean by the concept of mental illness.

Art and *Divine Madness*

As anyone familiar with the history of ideas knows, ancient thinkers entertained quite a different view of the relationship between art and insanity. This is largely because the philosophers of antiquity—for example, Plato and Aristotle—use the word *madness* to mean not an illness but an *illumination:* Madness enhances rather than diminishes a person's dignity and stature as a human being. This is why Plato and Aristotle assert (perhaps take for granted would be more accurate) that poets are mad—that they *must* be mad in order to write good poetry. In *Phaedrus*, Plato writes:

There is a third form of possession or madness, of which the Muses are the source. This seizes a tender, virgin soul and stimulates it to rapt passionate expression, especially in lyric poetry . . . . But if any man comes to the gates of poetry without the madness of the Muses, persuaded that skill alone will make him a good poet, then shall he and his works of sanity with him be brought to nought by the poetry of madness and, behold, their place is nowhere to be found.[7]

Clearly, Plato would have recoiled at the idea that the poet is ill (in our contemporary sense of the word) and therefore not responsible for the work he creates. Instead, what he meant was similar to what we now mean when we say that an artist must possess genius in order to be creative. This interpretation is supported by Plato's assertion in the *Laws:*

'Tis an old story . . . which we poets are always telling with the universal approval of the rest of the world, that when a poet takes his seat on the Muse's tripod, his judgment takes leave of him.[8]

Aristotle's views were similar. According to Abraham Heschel's interesting study of Old Testament prophets, Aristotle takes for granted that the poet "is afflicted with madness," that he is a *manikos*.[9] "The Greek word for prophecy *(mantike),*" Heschel adds, "and the word for madness *(manike)* were really the same, and the letter *t* is only a[n] . . . insertion."[10]

The same sort of idea was expressed by Roman philosophers: "There is no great genius without a touch of madness," asserts Seneca.[11] "No man can be a great poet who is not on fire with passion, and inspired by something like frenzy," declares Cicero.[12] Thus, in Greek and Roman times, the artist, epitomized by the poet, was someone inspired by mysterious powers, a process attributed to and called *frenzy, mania,* or *madness.* None of this, to repeat, meant that the artist was not responsible for his behavior. It meant only that the philosophers of antiquity were acutely aware of what is obvious to anyone familiar with creativity—namely, that there is a sense in which the creative person feels or is *passive* vis-à-vis his urge to create. This sense of passivity—variously characterized as helplessness, inspiration, an irresistible vision or urge—is characteristic of the mental state not only of the inspired artist but also of the person heeding (what he considers) a divine calling or the man and woman in love.

Modern artists, too, have emphasized their passivity vis-à-vis what seem like alien powers, their having to "give in" to inspiration, much as ancient seers had to give in to prophetic visions. "I have written this little work," remarks Goethe about *The Sorrows of Werther,* "almost unconsciously, like a sleep-walker." He then adds this remarkable comment:

No productiveness of the highest kind, no remarkable discovery, no great thought which bears fruit and has results is in the power of anyone . . . . Man must consider them as unexpected gifts from above, as pure children of God . . . . The process savours of the daemonic element which irresistibly does with a man what it pleases and to which he surrenders himself unconsciously while believing that he is acting on his own impulses.[13]

Goethe's imagery and idiom bridge the gap between the old idea of *divine madness* and the new ideas of *artistic inspiration* and *unconscious motivation.*

I must add a note of caution here about the ease with which the element of passivity in artistic creativity may be exaggerated. Although the experience of artistic inspiration may be passive and involuntary, translating it into a work of art—into a social product, so to speak— requires action and will. For example, Beethoven or Mozart might have heard beautiful music in their own heads, but they had to play it before others could hear it, and they had to write it down before others could play it. Again, there are important similarities here between artistic inspiration and mental symptom: each is a private (inner) experience over which the subject does not exercise direct, voluntary control.* But action based on or driven by such an experience requires coordinated control of the musculature as well as choice of audience, placing the action squarely within the sphere of voluntary behavior.

ACTION AND INTENTION

As philosophers have always emphasized, what distinguishes us as human beings from other living things is that we *act.* The idea of the person as moral agent thus presupposes and includes the idea of intentionality. But what, exactly, does it mean to assert that we act? It means realizing that our life is inherently, inexorably, social: We act in the double sense that we behave and perform. "To be isolated," Hannah Arendt emphasizes, "is to be deprived of the capacity to act."[14] Arendt, however, overstates the case. The socially isolated individual—for

---

*Even here, a caveat is necessary. We become, in part, what we do. Accordingly, although a person may have no direct control over certain experiences, he may have indirect control over them. It is unlikely that Mozart would have heard the divine music that made him famous had he never been exposed as a child to music and to playing a musical instrument, and had he not practiced the craft. People who take up smoking cigarettes train themselves, in a manner of speaking, to crave smoking. *Mutatis mutandis,* I believe that people also train themselves (and/or are trained by others) to have experiences we call *mental symptoms* and *mental illness.*

example, the shipwrecked person or the social outcast—is deprived of his ability to act only in the sense that he has no opportunity to perform before an audience; he is not deprived of his ability to act in the sense that he retains his capacity to engage in coordinated, goal-directed behavior.

The point is that, in an important sense, everything we do is an act, a performance before others as well as ourselves. To be fully human, a person must thus possess both the *capacity to act* and the *opportunity to perform* before an audience that legitimizes him as capable of acting and worthy of attention. Accordingly, a person can lose or be deprived of his humanity in two basically different, but complementary, ways: by lacking or losing the capacity to act in the sense of ability, which is why children, the very old, and the very sick are often not considered to be (fully) human; or by lacking or being deprived of the opportunity to act in the sense of performing on the stage of life, which is why the mentally ill are often not considered to be (fully) human. Moreover, this is why the powerless— children, unemployed youth, mental patients—are forced either to abandon their performing selves or to resort to dramatic antisocial acts, usually classified as crime or mental illness, to assert them.

Art, Intentionality, and Psychiatry

Viewed as performances by moral agents, both art and madness come down to the words and deeds of persons designated as artists or madmen. How else would we know that a person is an artist, if not for his artistic acts? Or that a person is mad, if not for his mad acts? Clearly, there can be no artist without artistic acts, no madman without mad acts.

From this admittedly circular definition, we can quickly move to examining the words and deeds called *art* and *madness*. Following Susanne Langer, I propose to view art as a nondiscursive or presentational form of self-expression or communication. The term *presentational* is intended to convey the idea that—in contrast to, say, mathematical symbols that represent their referents—presentational forms, such as a photograph or painting, literally present their meaning. As Langer puts it: ". . . *visual forms are not discursive.* They do not present their constituents successively, but simultaneously, so the relations determining a visual structure are grasped in one act of vision."[15] This is why artistic symbols or works of art—such as music, painting, or sculpture—cannot be translated into language. Their sense or meaning is bound to the forms in which they are expressed. In short, art is not, and cannot be, true or false; instead, it is expressive or inexpressive, and it succeeds or fails in proportion as it is or is not expressive.

Furthermore, by definition, art is the result of *deliberate effort* on the part of an artist. *Webster's* defines art as "the power of performing certain actions, esp. as acquired by experience, study, or observation"; and it offers "skill" and "dexterity" as synonyms. In short, art is something a person *does:* it is engaging in an activity that yields a product, called *a work of art.* Hence, calling a work of art *intentional art* would be a tautology, whereas the phrase *unintentional art* would be an oxymoron. Michelangelo chipping away at a block of marble, trying to make it look like his vision of the prophet Moses, is the quintessence of a man *intending* to do something. That the result is also very beautiful must not distract us from an important point, namely, that there may be beauty with or without intention, that there may be art with or without beauty, but that there can be no art without intention. We recognize that beauty is only a part, perhaps a relatively small part, of what we judge to be art when we contemplate the countless natural phenomena we consider to be beautiful but would not regard as works of art: for example, a dramatic sunset or an intricately shaped piece of driftwood. Why is such an object not art? Because it lacks the essential element of art, namely, human intentionality.

These considerations bring us back to madness. By definition, insanity (psychosis) is an illness, or the result of an illness, annulling the so-called patient's capacity to exercise intent. Hence, calling an insane act an *unintentional insane act* would be a tautology, and the phrase *intentional insane act* would be an oxymoron. As against a Michelangelo sculpting a block of marble, a John Hinckley, Jr. shooting President Reagan is (officially, that is) the quintessence of a man *displaying the unintended symptoms of a disease called schizophrenia.* That we judge such an act to be legally nonpunishable is an integral part of this image.

The Social Impact of Art and Insanity

Let us now distinguish between a work of art as an object, say a piece of music or a painting, and its effect on the audience, that is, whether it pleases or displeases. Then let us do the same with madness, distinguishing between insanity as a performance on the stage of life, and its effect on others, that is, whether it pleases or displeases the patient's family, psychiatrists, society. What do we find? We find that the artist does not claim that his work is beautiful or insist that it should move us in some definite way. For example, Michelangelo did not claim that Moses looked like his statue. I emphasize the artist's fundamental noncoerciveness, his offering us a vision instead of attempting to impose one, because I believe it is an essential element of art—and in our unhesitating acceptance of it as the product of the artist's will.

The madman presents us with the opposite reality. The so-called psychotic person is considered to be crazy not only because of what he does, as a physical event, but also because of his own interpretation of why he does it. For example, the typical madman—who is now a stock figure on the evening TV news and on the front pages of the newspapers—is a person who dramatically kills someone and offers an unacceptable explanation for his deed. Hinckley not only shot President Reagan but also explained that he did it to impress Jody Foster. Note that such an ostensibly mad actor treats himself as a moral agent, responsible for his actions: he frames his explanations in terms of motives. However, we so abhor his goal and consider his motive so absurd that we refuse to grant them the logical status of a goal or a motive: thus, we invalidate the actor as a nonagent, the mere object upon which certain causal forces have impinged.

What, exactly, do we find so abhorrent? Clearly, not the deed itself: We understand murder in the family, if the motive is money; we accept the murder of a prominent person, if the motive is political. What we do not accept is the insane criminal's double offense—his adding the insult of his conceited explanation to the injury of his coercive act. This combination of shocking crime and bizarre explanation makes us feel profoundly violated. Our impulse, therefore, is to get rid not only of the actor but also of his act. Killing the criminal accomplishes only the first goal; his deed remains and its meaning may even be intensified by his martyrdom. This is why modern society has developed a more effective method of protecting itself from such injury, namely, declaring the actor insane and locking him up in a madhouse. Herein, then, lies the value of invalidating the other as insane: We protect ourselves not only from being injured physically (by restraining him), but also from being injured spiritually (by labeling his intentions as nonintentional mental symptoms).

Art is of special interest in the spectrum of human activities because we experience it not only as perfectly intentional but also as ideally engaging: Art neither imposes itself upon us, as religion often does, nor does it leave us completely on our own, as pure science typically does. Art affects us, but only with our cooperation and consent. To be sure, since art is persuasive, it may be employed in ways of which we disapprove. But we must not confuse persuasion with coercion. The similarity between art and addictive drugs clarifies this point: each can tempt or seduce us, but each is powerless to affect us unless we actively seek and engage it. Madness, on the other hand, is often (or typically) coercive. Indeed, the principal power and threat of madness lies in its coerciveness, hence the countercoercions of psychiatry.

In short, art and insanity are like the positive and negative images of a photograph: what appears dark/intentional in one, appears light/nonintentional in the other. Our image of the artist, *qua* artist, is that of a person brimming over with intentionality: his artistic product is the embodiment of self-disciplined, self-intended self-expression. Hence, we readily equate the artist with his work. For example, we can look at a canvas by Renoir and say, "This is a Renoir," as if the picture were a veritable clone of its master. In contrast, our image of the madman *qua* madman is that of a person crippled by impaired or absent intentionality: his insane act is the very embodiment of undisciplined, unintended non-self-expression. Hence, we insist on severing the connection between the mentally deranged doer and his deed. For example, we speak of a misbehaving mentally ill person as *not himself,* as if his insane self were completely different from, and unrelated to, his real or normal self.

Actually, these contrasting Jekyll and Hyde images of artist and madman have little to do with facts. Instead, they have to do with our desire and need to describe the most important feature of being human—the fact that we *act*—according to degrees of intentionality. However, the person who truly cannot act, because he lacks or has lost intentionality, is not the madman but the man who is unconscious or paralyzed. In other words, our customary distinction between artist and madman does not identify two *different kinds of human beings,* one of whom acts and the other does not; instead it identifies two *different kinds of ascriptions* to actors and their acts—ascriptions disguised as explanations of behavior and justifications for social policy.

FREUD'S INTERPRETATION OF ART

To put this subject in wider perspective, let us now briefly review Freud's views on this topic. For better or worse, his ideas have shaped not only much of twentieth-century psychiatry but also much of modern art criticism.

Freud was interested in famous artists because they were famous, not because they were artists. That the artist, like everyone else, was "neurotic" was something Freud took for granted, although he pretended that he had discovered this from the artist's motivation for creating works of art.[16] His condescending attitude and outright hostility toward great artists is evident in all his writings touching on art but is perhaps nowhere more obvious than in his following remarks about Leonardo da Vinci:

. . . the great Leonardo remained like a child for the whole of his life in more than one way; the slowness which had all along been conspicuous in Leonardo's work is seen to be a symptom of this inhibition . . . . It was this too which determined the fate of the Last Supper—a fate that was not undeserved.[17]

Actually, Freud acknowledged that he was not interested in art for art's sake, that he was interested in art only as a sign or symptom pointing to something that he considered to be more interesting and important than art itself, that is, the *hidden secret* of the *artistic product* (as Freud always called art). And this, of course, could only be discovered by means of the psychoanalytic method. Furthermore, Freud justifies his analysis of art by postulating a problem, where, in fact, there is none. For example, in the paper cited above he asserts that while different lovers of art say different things about why they admire the Moses of Michelangelo, "none of them says anything that *solves the problem* for the unpretending admirer" (emphasis added).[18] What problem? Note how Freud first plants a secret on the corpse and then, after an elaborately staged psychoanalytic dissection, triumphantly finds it:

In my opinion, what grips us so powerfully can only be the artist's *intention* . . . . But why should the *artist's intention not be capable of being communicated and comprehended in words, like any other fact of mental life?* Perhaps where great works of art are concerned this would never be possible *without the application of psychoanalysis.* The product itself after all must admit of such an analysis . . . . To discover [the artist's] intention, ... I must first find out the meaning and content of what is represented in his work; I must, in other words, be able to interpret it (emphasis added).[19]

What Freud here calls analyzing art and interpreting it is, in fact, deforming art into nonart and hence destroying it. I say this because by asserting that the artist's real intention is not embodied in his product but must be revealed by translating its content into the jargon of psychoanalysis, Freud in effect annihilates the legitimacy of presentational forms. Indeed, there is a close similarity between the psychoanalytic invalidation of art *qua* presentational form, and the psychoanalytic invalidation of abnormal behavior *qua* intentional action. As abnormal behavior is *not really* behavior but an incomplete, symptomatic expression of experience, so art is *not really* art but an incomplete nonverbal expression of experience: each needs to be completed by psychoanalysis, a method that forces them to give up their secrets.

Freud goes further still: he not only robs art precisely of that quality that makes it art (namely, its specially executed presentational form of self-expression and communication), but also actively demeans it by treating art as if it were like madness. "Let us consider," Freud writes, "Shakespeare's masterpiece, *Hamlet*, . . . it was not until the material of the tragedy had been traced back by psychoanalysis to the Oedipus theme that the mystery of its effect was at last explained."[20] This, it seems to me, says more about Freud than about *Hamlet*.

I must add here that Freud never tired of emphasizing that the analyst-analysand relationship is that of superior authority vis-à-vis inferior subject, a view consistent with the verbal imagery embodied in psychoanalytic terminology: the analyst "interprets," while the patient (who disagrees) "resists." Compare and contrast this with the relationship between artist and lover of art. A lover of art is free to dislike Dali or Pound or Bartok without being branded resistant to the artistic pleasure these masters offer. Considerations such as these point to an exquisite connection between the esthetic form of a work of art and its inherently politically noninvasive, noncoercive frame, from which it cannot be severed. Music is music only if you want to listen to it. If you do not, it is noise, even if it is Beethoven's *Fifth* or Mozart's *Jupiter*. Everyone would agree. But that is not the way we view therapy for mental illness: we consider "it" to be therapy, regardless of whether or not the patient consents to, or participates in, the enterprise.

INTENTIONALITY, CRIME, AND JURISPRUDENCE

The psychoanalytic perspective on human behavior has exerted a profound influence not only on artists and art critics but also, indeed especially, on lawyers and jurists. The result has been a veritable tragicomedy, requiring the talents of a Voltaire to do it satirical justice. The story of Judge David Bazelon's absurd experiments with psychiatry in the courtrooms of the District of Columbia has been told by others[21] and I will pass by it in almost complete silence.* Instead I shall briefly cite and comment on the views of James Marshall, another prominent legal scholar: they exemplify what happens when a gullible lawyer drinks too deeply from the poisoned psychoanalytic chalice.

---

*In his Louis D. Brandeis Memorial Lecture for 1960, Bazelon declared: "Would it really be the end of the world if all gaols were turned into hospitals or 'Rehabilitation Centers'"? It would, indeed. Sadly, that end had already arrived in Bazelon's own mind, as he was no longer able or willing to distinguish the offender's intention from the intention of his gaoler: "The offender's purposes [sic] in such a Rehabilitation Center would be to change his personality . . . ."[22]

Psychoanalysis and the Modern Jurist

Marshall devotes an entire book, significantly titled *Intention in Law and Society*, to argue that, in view of the evidence brought to bear on the subject of crime by psychoanalysis, criminals rarely if ever commit crimes intentionally. The book, warmly endorsed by the late Supreme Court Justice William O. Douglas, delivers a remarkable message, as the following quotations illustrate.

"How valid are our legal assumptions about intention and motivation concerning what we know of the unconscious?" asks Marshall.[23] His question is rhetorical. As he sees it, our assumptions are entirely invalid. Not surprisingly, he finds the criminal not responsible for his criminality, and finds society responsible for making the criminal a criminal. Perhaps more than most writers on this subject, Marshall actually seems to believe the nonsense he spouts, especially the view that our "unconscious" is like a gun in our own back: "What a man purposes when in the clutches of his unconscious gives him no more freedom of choice of action than if he were disarmed before another man with a loaded gun."[24]

Unfortunately for this argument, the unconscious is only an abstraction or metaphor, which Marshall here equates, quite literally, with the power that a holdup man with a gun wields over his victim, in order to invoke the classic legal excuse of duress. Although such coercion properly exempts the coerced person from legal responsibility for his criminal acts carried out at the behest of his coercer, it is worth noting that, existentially, even in this situation the actor has free will and choice: he can choose to submit to the man with a gun and carry out his orders, or defy him and risk being killed. The famous postwar Nazi excuse that "I was only following orders," odious though it may be, must be recognized as belonging to the same genus of excuses.

Marshall acknowledges none of this. "Freedom of choice," he asserts without qualification, "is not present when action is dictated principally by unconscious drives."[25] How one knows whether an action is or is not so dictated, he does not tell us. He is satisfied with the conclusion that habitual or repetitive acts are a sure sign that the actor is acting unintentionally. Evidently Marshall has never heard of habits. But he has certainly heard of illness, individual and collective: ". . . the influence of a sick culture can have the psychological effect of depriving the people of choice . . . ."[26]

I have cited Marshall's views on intentionality because they are typical of those of contemporary intellectuals regarded as having a progressive and psychiatrically enlightened attitude toward crime. One of the results of this attitude is that those who subscribe to it tend to hold the criminal increasingly less responsible for his criminality, and the victims increasingly more responsible for (somehow) coercing the victimizer to become a victim of his own criminal career. Writ large, James Burnham rightly saw in this posture "the suicide of the West."[27] Perhaps that fate indeed awaits us. The suicide of the criminal law seems to be upon us already, as the following development suggests.

Negating Intentionality: The Suicide of the Criminal Law

The idea that insanity negates intentionality is now being carried to its absurd, but logical, conclusion by American psychiatrists and lawyers: namely, that we may define any act, even the seemingly most deliberate, as involuntary, simply by defining the actor as insane.

People have always known that a human being, in the process of growing up in a family and society, acquires a conscience—that is, "a sense of consciousness of the moral goodness or blameworthiness of his own conduct, intentions, or character—together with a feeling of obligation to do right or be good" (*Webster's*). Because of the presence of this internal voice in all of us, people have been familiar with the fact, and have never found it very surprising, that the individual who commits a serious crime often feels a compulsion or need to confess it. Some of the greatest works of Western literature deal with this theme.

The entrance of the psychiatric ideologue on the scene of modern history has changed this: he has managed to transform the compulsion to confess into a symptom of mental illness negating intentionality. As a result, should defense counsel claim that the accused was mentally ill when he confessed, the confession may be deemed inadmissible as evidence. I have not made this up: precisely such a scenario was reported recently in *The New York Times:*

> The [U.S. Supreme] Court agreed to hear a prosecutor's appeal . . . suppressing the confession of a murder defendant as *involuntary because he was mentally ill* . . . . The man had approached a police officer on the street in Denver and said he wanted to confess a homicide. The policeman told him of his rights to remain silent and to have a lawyer present. The man said he understood, and proceeded to confess the killing of a 14-year-old girl and to lead police to the scene and to other evidence (emphasis added).[28]

It would be difficult to imagine what other evidence one would need to conclude that this man knew what he was doing: after all, it is not as if he had confessed to a murder and was unable to provide evidence of his guilt except his confession. How, then, did someone get the idea that this man was mad rather than a murderer? Obviously, the killer did not want to talk to a psychiatrist: had he wanted to, he could have sought one out, just as he had sought out a policeman. No doubt, as it is now customary in murder cases in the United States, the authorities arranged for him to "be seen" by a psychiatrist. Sure enough, the killer told the psychiatrists exactly what they expected to hear in such a case: "God's voice had told him to confess." How psychiatrists, lawyers, and judges know that the defendant used the phrase *God's voice* literally, rather than as a metaphor for his conscience, the report in the *Times* does not say.* So much for Raskolnikov. While it may be sad that Dostoevski has been rendered irrelevant by the march of psychiatric science, it is reassuring to realize that Raskolnikov was innocent after all.

THE REDISCOVERY OF INTENTIONALITY

Actually, in this century, two different armies have tried, in the name of science, to destroy the same enemy—namely, the supposedly superstitious belief in free will. One, associated mainly with Sigmund Freud's name, is psychiatry and psychoanalysis. The other, associated mainly with B.F. Skinner's name, is behavioral psychology. Both of these deterministic systems have come under attack by certain psychologists and psychiatrists who, for the lack of a better term, may be grouped together under the name of *will psychologists*. Who are they? The best-known ones are Carl Jung, Ludwig Binswanger, (the later) Otto Rank, Erich Fromm, Abraham Maslow, Rollo May, and Ronald Laing. Marching under banners variously called *Humanistic Psychology, Third Force,* or *Existential Psychiatry/Psychology,* these reactionaries against behavioral scientism agree on one thing only: namely, that intentionality is an essential feature of the human condition, even of the condition of individuals said to be insane.†

---

*Ironically, the same edition of *The New York Times* featured a lengthy report on animal behavior, in which the reader is informed that scientists now recognize "a wide spectrum of devious behaviors in animals. . . . [Certain birds] for example, are using the same signal in two different ways, one honest, one not."[29] Deviousness implies, of course, intention, a term the *Times* finds no difficulty in attaching to the behavior of monkeys: "In nature, the strongest evidence of *intentional,* self-aware deception comes from chimpanzees . . ." (emphasis added).[30] In short, we are asked to believe that chimpanzees possess intentionality, but that adult men and women who mention God's voice do not.

†This generalization must be qualified, however. To my knowledge, not a single will psychologist or existential psychiatrist has criticized the cognitive-ethical absurdities of

Free Will and the New Psychology

Obviously, one need not be a researcher or scientist to discover that people have free will. However, once the proposition that there is no free will becomes officially accepted as the correct, scientific view, legitimized by the research of accredited experts, the counteropinion of lay people ceases to carry much weight; henceforth the opinion-makers of society pay attention only to other, equally reputable scientists, who, preferably on the basis of their own so-called research, come to conflicting conclusions. Hence the ever-changing fashions in psychiatric theories and therapies, somberly supported by self-seeking charlatans contradicting and superseding one another. Otto Rank's career exemplifies this process: for most of his life, Rank was a devout Freudian preaching the gospel of psychic determinism; then he discovered free will and, for the last decade or so of his life, became the high priest of intentionality.[31] In *New Pathways in Psychology,* Colin Wilson popularizes this fallacy, citing contemporary psychiatrists, psychologists, and other experts to support the revolutionary discovery that human beings can exercise choice.[32]

The triviality of the will psychologists' doctrine is perhaps best illustrated by the following dichotomy: The determinists, as we have seen, yoke together the absence of intentionality with the idea of insanity and build their systems on that fiction; whereas the will psychologists— embracing common sense, it must be said in their favor—yoke together the self-evident presence of intentionality in the behavior of a moral agent with the idea of sanity and build their system on that fatuity. While the determinists thus emphasize the powerlessness of will and dwell on the importance of mental illness, exemplified by stereotypy—the will psychologists emphasize the power of will and dwell on the importance of mental health, exemplified by creativity. What the representatives of neither group can or are willing to do is let go of the ideas of mental illness and mental health and the jungle-growth of slogans they have generated. "All the existential psychologists," writes Wilson, "have one thing in common: an attempt to approach the problem of mental illness in a practical rather than a theoretical way . . . ."[33] Exactly! Wilson completely misses the point that what these psychologists have in common with those with whom they ostensibly disagree is that they all believe in mental illness: All of them talk about mental illness, mental health, schizophrenia, and treatment; and all of them accept the legitimacy of

---

the insanity defense or has urged its abolition, raising doubts about the sincerity or seriousness of their belief that persons conventionally regarded as insane possess free will and are therefore responsible for their behavior.

the two paradigmatic psychiatric interventions—involuntary mental hospitalization and the insanity defense. The results are pathetic.

For example, Wilson approvingly cites Maslow's having "been struck by the thought that modern psychology is based on the study of sick people. But since there are more healthy people around than sick people, how can this psychology give a fair idea of the workings of the human mind?"[34] Nonsense. In the first place, according to the faithful Freudians—and Maslow always counted himself as one—virtually everyone is mentally ill; if so, the assertion that there are more mentally healthy than mentally sick people is false. Secondly, if the ideas and interventions of the psychopathologists are questionable or wrong, why accept—as the will psychologists do—the psychopathologists' criteria of mental health and mental illness? The answer is: Because the deterministic and antideterministic psychologists are like two ladies of the night working different sides of the same street. Indeed, several well-known psychotherapists have themselves worked both sides of it. Otto Rank, as I mentioned already, went from devout Freudian disciple to determined anti-Freudian psychologist; Wilhelm Reich, from inspired individual psychotherapist to mindless pseudobiological charlatan; Ronald Laing from antipsychiatrist to anti-antipsychiatrist. In the 1960s Laing celebrated the superior intentionality of the schizophrenic; now he celebrates "my methods of treating schizophrenics . . . ." For good measure, he adds: "To say that a locked ward functions as a prison for noncriminal transgressors is not to say it should not be so . . . . This is not the fault of the psychiatrists, nor necessarily the fault of anyone."[35] Laing's opportunistic self-reversal has become so blatant that even sympathetic reviewers have begun to notice it: "Laing became an anti-Laingian . . . nervously separating from leftwing politics, drugs, mysticism, attacks on the family, even anti-psychiatry."[36] As I have tried to show, Laing is merely the most recent of a long series of psychiatrists advancing diametrically contradictory claims consistently sensationalized as new discoveries.

Finally, although Wilson makes passing references to intentionality and choice, he casts his own views in the traditional vocabulary of psychiatry. "Schizophrenia," he writes, "is a disorder in which the robot takes over from the 'I' . . . ."[37] So much for a critique of mental illness. "The healthy mind," Wilson then explains, "needs 'newness,' 'otherness'. . . ."[38] Note that Wilson places *newness* and *otherness*, not *healthy* or *mind* between quotation marks. So much for distinguishing between literal and metaphorical diseases.

Revealingly, Wilson—like many of the experts he admires—speaks approvingly of psychiatric coercions and closed institutions: he refers to "the remarkable Synanon experiment . . .";[39] says that "The Synanon visit led Maslow to express again his feeling that modern society is sick";[40] and explains that "The reason that insulin or electric shock treatment often works . . . is that it forces the 'I' to make a painful effort and starts the flow of vital energy."[41] Wilson concludes with what he calls a sketch "of my own general phenomenology of mental health."[42] Clearly, there are no significant differences between the positions of the psychiatric-psychological theorists who support the reality of free will and intentionality and of those who oppose it.

Intentionality and Theology

Educated people today are convinced that the dichotomous view of intentionality I have just reviewed, and which forms so important a part of our contemporary notions of sanity and insanity, rests on, and reflects, the recent discoveries of researchers into the mysteries of human behavior. Of course, psychiatrists and lawyers encourage this delusion. But it happens that, once again, we do not have far to look for the prescientific origin of this belief. Before the Enlightenment, when people were comfortable with the idea of an essentially personal deity, they thought of Him as their Maker who exercised perfect control over all His creations. Not a sparrow could fall from a rooftop without God having intended it, was a favorite maxim of the theologians. These experts, who devoted their lives to the study of God, developed the same dichotomous images of intentionality that we now attribute to artist and madman respectively: In the religious version of this theory, those who understood and obeyed God's will the most perfectly—the saints—were viewed as possessing virtually perfect intentionality, acting completely on their own free will; whereas those who succumbed to the devil and fell under his power—persons possessed by demons—were viewed as completely lacking in intentionality, behaving like automatons without any will of their own. This explains why people went to such desperate measures in an effort to exorcise the victims of that terrible affliction. *Plus ça change . . .*

INTENTIONALITY AND THE IDEA OF BEING HUMAN

I have tried to demonstrate the similarities between our modern ideas concerning art and insanity by showing that they represent the two poles or boundaries of our concept of what it means to be human. We view the artist as so rich in intentionality as to be superhuman, and the madman as so poor in intentionality as to be subhuman.* Our crediting the artist with an overabundance of intentionality, and hence humanity, needs no further comment or illustration here; nor does our crediting the madman with an absence of intentionality, and our consequent discrediting of him as a human being.

There is, of course, nothing new about denying the humanity of the other; much of history is but a footnote to it.† Nor is there anything new about affirming and reaffirming the essential humanity of the other, even when doing so requires our painfully empathetic identification with him. Terence (ca. 195–159 B.C.) is credited with having articulated one of the earliest and most succinct formulations of this view: *"Homo sum; humani nil a me alienum puto"* ("I am a man and reckon nothing human alien to me"). This declaration became the credo of the European Enlightenment.

The credo of modern psychiatry is thus an inversion of Terence's: "Nothing human is alien to me" became "Nothing alien is human to me." The alienated person was thus both seen and defined as a person lacking in intentionality, an image that, in turn, gave rise to the birth of the alienist or mad-doctor (later called psychiatrist), who was both seen and defined as an expert on alienation and the keeper of alienated persons. The earliest British cases involving the defense of insanity center on this very issue. For example, in 1812, in the trial of John Bellingham for the murder of Spencer Perceval, first Lord of the Treasury and Chancellor of the Exchequer, James Mansfield, Lord Chief Justice of the Commons Pleas, instructed the jury as follows:

> In another part of the Prisoner's defence . . . it was attempted to be proved that, at the time of the commission of the crime, he was insane. With respect to this the law was extremely clear. If a man were deprived of all power of reasoning, so as not to be able to distinguish whether it was right or wrong to commit the most wicked transaction, he could certainly not do an act against the law. Such a man, so destitute of all power of judgment, *could have no intention at all* (emphasis added).[44]

Clearly, this cannot be so. A person capable of committing a crime must be able to have *some* intention—for example, to load his weapon,

---

*Insofar as the issue of intentionality is concerned, this is, of course, quite absurd. The fact is that, *qua* moral agent, the artist is like anyone else: He is perfectly able to resist anything, except temptation—a quip first made by Oscar Wilde.

†Like the clergymen they displaced, people in the guru business—where psychiatrists now compete with other cult leaders—are fond of finding their foes subhuman. After being expelled from the United States for violating immigration laws, Bhagwan Shree Rajneesh told a news conference in New Delhi: "I don't consider them [Americans] human, they are subhuman."[43]

aim it, wait to fire it until the moment he thinks is right, and so forth. My point can be made more simply, though less elegantly. Among our most basic intentional acts are urinating and defecating. A person who does not wet and soil himself—that is, who demonstrates sufficient control to urinate and defecate in appropriate places—demonstrates, by so acting, that he can and does have intention (at least for delaying or initiating these bodily evacuations). Obviously a person *totally* lacking the capacity to form intention could not do these things. Clearly, however, a *physically* disabled person lacking the capacity to control certain bodily functions by no means necessarily lacks the intention to control them. Considerations such as these suggest, of course, that the lack of intentionality of the insane, like insanity itself, is a legal fiction (see Chapter 11).

In any case, the fiction—or fact, depending on the observer's opinion—of a person incapable of intending is a threat to society, much as a grain of sand is to an oyster: to protect itself, the oyster surrounds the sand with a substance we call a *pearl;* similarly, to protect itself, society surrounds the idea of lack of intentionality with the idea we call *insanity.* As a pearl is not sand, so an insane person is not a person. Johann Christian Heinroth (1773–1843), one of the founders of modern psychiatry, put it this way: "Individuals in this condition [mentally diseased] exist no longer in the human domain, which is the domain of freedom. . . . Rather than resembling animals, which are led by a wholesome instinct, they resemble machines . . . ."[45]

But if some persons are viewed as subhuman, others, perforce, will be seen as superhuman: they are the artists who are so rich in intentionality that their mental makeup, according to Freud, defies psychiatric analysis. Finally, still others will be viewed as possessing a combination of these conflicting characteristics: they are the *mad artists,* whose *pathological genius* forms a subject especially dear to the hearts of psychiatrists.

While this perspective has helped the psychiatrist to stand with one foot planted in medicine and another in the humanities, it has, in my opinion, harmed both medicine and the humanities. Oil and water do not mix; they are better used separately than combined in an unstable homogenized mixture. Claiming to decipher and dignify insanity, psychiatrists have instead deformed it. If they have failed to deform art as well it has not been for lack of trying, but rather because they have been unable to gain the same kind of legal and rhetorical control over art as they long ago gained, and still exercise, over insanity.

8

MENTAL ILLNESS AND THE PROBLEM OF RESPONSIBILITY

Insanity is certainly on the increase in the world, and crime is dying out. . . . Formerly, if you killed a man, it was possible that you were insane —but now, if you . . . kill a man, it is evidence that you are a lunatic.

—*Mark Twain*[1]

So far I have emphasized two crucial distinctions between illness and mental illness, between being a patient and being a mental patient— namely, that bodily diseases are identifiable in terms of pathoanatomical and pathophysiological lesions, whereas mental diseases are not; and that typically a person assumes the role of medical patient voluntarily, whereas the role of mental patient is ascribed to him involuntarily. There is yet another, equally important, difference between these two classes of diseases and roles to which we must now attend, namely, that mental illness, especially if it is deemed to be severe, renders the person suffering from it not (fully) responsible for his actions. This claim is virtually never advanced for bodily illness. To understand mental illness, it is thus necessary to keep in mind its dual reference— to disease, as a condition of the patient as an organic being, and to

237

nonresponsibility, as a moral attribute or legal status of the patient as a person. My criticism of psychiatric ideas and interventions is similarly two-pronged: I object both to categorizing certain behaviors as literal diseases and certain persons as not moral agents.

When we say that an individual acts responsibly we usually mean that he acts with care. Thus a person is considered to be responsible if he takes good care of himself and of those who depend on him. If he endangers himself or others—for example, by drinking too much alcohol or spending too much money—he may be called an *irresponsible father,* a phrase which does not, however, exonerate him from being a bad parent. In such a case, we usually follow the principle that a person is responsible for his being irresponsible. That may sound like a contradiction, but it isn't: the term *irresponsible* functions here merely as a way of expressing our disapproval of a particular behavior.

We also use the term *not responsible* to conceal our strategy toward the person so designated, exemplified in the courtroom scenario where a defendant is acquitted as *not responsible/not guilty* because of insanity. Here the term *not responsible* functions as a vehicle for our judgment that the defendant should be handled differently from persons deemed to be responsible.

THE WAR ON RESPONSIBILITY

Although the idea that insanity may be an excuse for crime is ancient, the insanity defense, as we now know it, is relatively modern: it developed during the nineteenth century, mainly in England and the United States.[2] While the original impetus behind this practice was the desire to soften the harsh impact of capital punishments inflicted mainly on the poorest and most unfortunate members of society, the psychiatric disposition of persons charged with or convicted of crimes quickly became an important mechanism of social control in its own right. The justification for this mechanism lay in the convenient assumption that the criminally insane were irrational and nonresponsible. For example, commenting on the mental state of "lunatic criminals," the great Philippe Pinel declared: "Finally the nervous affection gains over the brain, and then the lunatic is dominated by an irresistible desire for violence . . . ."[3] In the same vein, a psychiatrist testifying at a mid-nineteenth-century English murder trial asserted that the defendant suffered from a "lesion of the will."[4] The judge not only failed to question the metaphoric nature of that claim, but went on to instruct the jury that "If some controlling disease was, in truth, the acting power within him which he could not resist, then he will not be responsible . . . . The question is, whether the prisoner was labouring under that species of insanity . . . ."[5]

In the twentieth century, psychiatrists added a new wrinkle to the nineteenth-century dogma of the nonresponsibility of the insane; namely, the idea of *diminished capacity* to form intent and hence commit certain crimes.[6] As the idea of total insanity annulling criminal responsibility was tailor-made for exculpating those guilty of capital offenses, thus sparing their lives, so the idea of partial insanity diminishing criminal responsibility was tailor-made for mitigating the punishment of those guilty of certain felonies, typically by reducing the offense from first-degree murder to manslaughter.

Today, psychiatrists are constantly called on to determine whether a person is responsible for his illegal actions. Indeed, the phenomenon of psychiatrists *examining* persons to determine whether or not they are responsible is as common a feature of our social landscape as is the phenomenon of physicians examining persons to determine whether or not they are ill. How and why the idea that mental patients are not responsible for some or all of their behavior arose and developed is a long and complicated story. Here it must suffice for us to look back briefly on the two most important sources of this idea—namely, psychiatry and psychoanalysis.

Psychiatry against Responsibility

There have always been individuals who have injured or otherwise disturbed members of their families or other persons. Many such actions or conditions—for example, talking too much or too little, unemployment, vagrancy, self-neglect—were not against the law or, if they were, their control by means of criminal sanctions was impractical or impossible. It has always been necessary, nevertheless, to control persons displaying such disturbing behaviors. Thus, from the seventeenth century onward, confinement in the madhouse became the method modern societies throughout the Western world chose for the purpose of controlling and containing certain troublesome and troubled persons. Of course, the asylum movement, as it became known, had to be rationalized and justified. This was accomplished by the idea of insanity. It was an idea whose time had come: it offered a view of the behavior of certain men and women that was ostensibly both humane and scientific. The crux of the idea can be stated briefly: As diseases of the heart impair its ability to pump blood, so diseases of the mind impair its ability to reason rationally, as a result of which the person—suffering from the disease called *insanity* or *mental illness*—loses his ability to act responsibly. "The insane action or idea," declared the editor of the *British Medical*

Journal in 1875, "as surely springs from a morbid derangement in brain structure, as a bilious attack springs from a morbid condition of the liver. There is no mystery about it; it is a mental manifestation arising from a physical cause . . . ."[7] How did the medical profession reach this remarkable conclusion? Mainly through the work of Henry Maudsley (1835–1918), one of the most celebrated psychiatrists of all times and the acknowledged father of modern British psychiatry.

What made Maudsley such an influential physician and famous psychiatrist? He discovered no new diseases, no new methods for identifying obscure conditions suspected to be diseases, no new treatments for diseases. He did something more important: he legitimized the alienist as a bona fide physician. One of Maudsley's most influential books is revealingly titled *Responsibility in Mental Disease*. In this work, Maudsley argues, in effect, that the insane are not responsible and that only psychiatrists can diagnose insanity. The view that psychiatrists are indispensable for the proper functionings of modern society follows inexorably from these premises. I shall cite some of Maudsley's views to illustrate how the new science of psychiatry went about destroying the old principle of moral agency and personal responsibility.

> It will be a hard matter for those who have not lived among the insane and so become familiar with their ways and feelings to be persuaded, if, without such experience, they ever can, that a man may be mad and yet be free from delusion and exhibit no marked derangement of intelligence. Nevertheless it is a fact that in a certain mental disease a morbid impulse may take such despotic possession of the patient as to drive him, in spite of reason and against his will, to a desperate act of suicide or homicide; like the demoniac of old into whom the unclean spirit entered, he is possessed by a power which forces him to a deed of which he has the utmost dread and horror; and his appeal sometimes to the physician whom he consults with his sore agony, when overwhelmed with a despair of continuing to wrestle successfully with his horrible temptation, is beyond measure sad and pathetic.[8]

This passage presents us with nearly all the moral, medical, linguistic, and legal mystifications that have marked the origin of psychiatry as a modern discipline. Note that Maudsley's example of an insane person is a seemingly perfectly healthy individual who is *tempted* to commit suicide or homicide. Maudsley himself uses the word *temptation* in the last sentence of this passage. In other words, Maudsley is describing a moral conflict: a person is torn between committing suicide or homicide and not committing these acts. He simply identifies the option he approves as sane and the other as insane, and then introduces the idea of *irresistible impulse*, which he claims represents the scientifically correct understanding of the old theological concept of diabolical possession.

That the *evil temptation* and *diabolical possession* of the theologians has simply been renamed the *morbid impulse* of the psychiatrist finds support in the fact that each of these terms is applied only to morally disapproved options or acts. Priests never talked about temptation to do good: sinners were tempted to be sinful, but saints were not tempted to be saintly. Similarly, Maudsley and other psychiatrists never talk about irresistible impulses to do good: the insane are driven by irresistible impulses to commit mayhem and murder, but the sane are not driven by such impulses to love and honor their fellowman.

Moreover, there is an important practical difference between an evil temptation and an irresistible impulse which we must not overlook. Anyone—theologian or layman—could tell whether or not a temptation was evil and was resisted. However, although anyone can tell whether or not an impulse is resisted, if it is not resisted only a psychiatrist can ascertain whether this is because it is irresistible or because the subject chooses not to resist it. Of course, Maudsley had no criteria for distinguishing between irresistible and nonresisted impulses. But the absence of criteria for irresistible impulses impaired his credibility no more than the absence of criteria for mental illness impairs the credibility of the contemporary psychiatrist. Instead of standards and procedures, the psychiatrist can always fall back on dramatic cases exemplifying that which he cannot define: "When a woman after her confinement kills her child, whom she loves tenderly, because she cannot help it, there is no serious disinclination on the part of those who take the legal stand-point to admit that it is not a voluntary act for which she is responsible."[9] By claiming that such a person does not *intend* to do what she in fact does, Maudsley here tries to unseat the time-honored adage that actions speak louder than words. But why not assume that a woman who kills her newborn infant practices the ancient art of infanticide, a practice with which Maudsley must have been thoroughly familiar?

We should note, also, that when Maudsley says that only those "familiar with the ways" of the insane can appreciate the validity of his, Maudsley's explanation, he is telling us that only those who have actively participated in certain grievous moral offenses against innocent persons can arrive at the conclusion he considers a truism. I say this because the persons he calls "familiar with the insane" are the persons responsible for imprisoning them in insane asylums. Among those who alone can understand the true facts of insanity are thus the relatives of the madman who petition and profit from his psychiatric incarceration, the legislators and judges who socially legitimize psychiatric incarceration as a form of protection and treatment, and the psychiatrists who serve as the patient's wardens. In short, Maudsley's reference to familiarity with the insane amounts to his telling us that only those guilty of coercively controlling the mental patient—and who therefore have an intense need to exonerate themselves—will be able to see the innocent victim as the deranged madman he really is; all others, not so implicated, might see the patient as another human being or perhaps even a victim. The phrase *irresistible impulse* thus emerges as a purely strategic, semantic instrument for the use of the institutional psychiatrist and those who want use of the services.

Revealingly, Maudsley argues not only that *irresistible impulses* exist and are real but also that believing in them is compassionate and morally uplifting:

> To hold an insane person responsible for not controlling an insane impulse of the nature of which he is conscious is in some cases just as false in doctrine and as cruel in practice as it would be to hold a man who is convulsed by strychnia responsible for not stopping the convulsions, because he is all the while quite conscious of them.[10]

We have heard all this before: Maudsley compares conscious conduct with chemically induced convulsion and then insists that the metaphor *is* the literal thing. It is important to remember in this connection that the medical claim that personal conduct is *not volitional* was first staked out in relation to acts that were socially disturbing and could conventionally be called *crazy*. Only after that beachhead was secured by psychiatrists in the nineteenth century was the claim extended, by psychoanalysts in the twentieth century, to encompass all behavior. The result is that, today, psychiatrists, psychoanalysts, and lawyers stand together, shoulder to shoulder, in their struggle against personal responsibility. The situation of those who now protest against the corruption of the principle of personal responsibility by Science thus resembles the situation of those who, at the time of the Reformation, protested against its corruption by Religion (see Chapter 10). Then, thoughtful persons began to realize that instead of teaching truth and practicing tolerance, the leaders of the Church taught falsehood and practiced intolerance. Now thoughtful persons are beginning to realize that instead of informing us about illness and protecting our health, leaders of the medical and legal professions are lying to us and are destroying the social and political conditions that are the very prerequisites for our health. The following incident exemplifies this pathogenic therapeutism.

In 1984, Michael Charney, a medical psychoanalyst in Boston, together with a law professor, founded the Tobacco Products Liability

Project "to actively promote product liability lawsuits against tobacco companies." In an interview, Charney explained that he hoped lawsuits "will place the responsibility for smoking-related illnesses squarely on the tobacco industry."[11] In the past, when patients talked like this, they were diagnosed as engaging in *projection*: that is, blaming others for the consequences of their own behavior. Today, when psychiatrists and psychoanalysts talk like this, they are praised for being public-spirited; while they themselves proudly promote the brazen displacement of blame as a method for protecting the public health. I submit that activism such as Charney's—aided and abetted by the APA's legitimizing, with the diagnosis of Tobacco Dependence, the proposition that smoking is an illness—incriminates the American psychiatric profession as guilty, beyond a reasonable doubt, of complicity in the war on responsibility.

Psychoanalysis against Responsibility

As we saw, the idea that an insane person is not responsible for his behavior was firmly established long before Sigmund Freud came on the scene. However, psychiatrists limited their interest to the insane and were willing to concede free will and responsibility to the sane. Freud went further: Intoxicated with the idea of a science of mental life, he insisted that everyone is mentally ill, that every human action is "fully determined," and that no one has free will. He maintained this view with all the ferocity of a religious fanatic, as the following passages illustrate. In *The Psychopathology of Everyday Life* (1901), he writes:

> Many people, as is well known, contest the assumption of complete psychical determinism by appealing to a special feeling of conviction that there is free will. This feeling of conviction exists; and it does not give way before a belief of determinism. Like every normal feeling it must have something to warrant it. But so far as I can observe, it does not manifest itself in the great and important decisions of the will: on these occasions the feeling that we have is rather one of psychical compulsion, and we are glad to invoke it on our behalf. ('Here I stand: I can do no other.') . . . According to our analyses, it is not necessary to dispute the right to the feeling of conviction of having a free will. If the distinction between a conscious and unconscious motivation is taken into account, our feeling of conviction informs us that conscious motivation does not extend to all our motor decisions. . . . what is thus left free by one side receives its motivation from the other side, from the unconscious; and in this way determination in the psychical sphere is still carried out without any gap.[12]

By introducing the idea of *unconscious* psychic determinism—the Rosetta stone of psychoanalytic psychobabble—Freud lays the ground here for viewing mental health on the model of mental illness. Freud's interpretation of Luther's famous exclamation is, of course, both malicious and stupid; his purpose is clear, however—namely, to empty it of all moral content and significance. Instead of making a difficult but terribly important choice, Luther, Freud tells us, is helpless in the face of a *psychical compulsion.*

So fond was Freud of the idea of psychic determinism, and so convinced was he of its importance that, in 1907, he added a new footnote to the foregoing passage, asserting: "These conceptions of the strict determination of apparently arbitrary psychical acts have already borne rich fruit in psychology, and perhaps also in the juridical field."[13] But what is a *psychical act?* A metaphor? Psychobabble? Blurring the distinction between thought and action may be useful for religious or political demagoguery, but is hardly an asset for a psychological theory. Freud returns to the theme of psychic determinism with undiminished enthusiasm in his *Introductory Lectures on Psychoanalysis* (1916–1917). Addressing an unseen audience, he writes:

> If anyone makes a breach of this kind in the determinism of natural events at a single point, it means that he has thrown overboard the whole Weltanschauung of science. Even the Weltanschauung of religion, we may remind him, behaves much more consistently, since it gives an explicit assurance that no sparrow falls from the roof without God's special will . . . . You nourish the illusion of there being such a thing as psychical freedom, and you will not give it up. I am sorry to say I disagree with you categorically over this. . . . Once before I ventured to tell you that you nourish a deeply rooted faith in undetermined psychical events and in free will, but that this is quite unscientific and must yield to the demand of a determinism whose rule extends over mental life. . . . But I am not opposing one faith with another.[14]

Freud's reference to divine determinism is at once incorrect and ironic. In the first place, God's will was not generally used by Christians as a ground for denying personal choice and hence individual responsibility; secondly, Freud seems unaware that his idea of complete psychic determinism—presumably mediated by material processes in the brain—is, itself, simply a scientistic recasting of his caricature of divine determinism. His remark that "I am not opposing one faith with another" is naively self-serving and wholly false, as has been shown often enough. David E. Trueblood, a philosopher, articulates this error as follows:

Science was his [Freud's] religion, and determinism was a cardinal tenet in the creed . . . . What seems so strange to us now is the fact that Freud did not see clearly the logical consequence of his basic assumption. It is easy for us to see now that, whether psychological determinism is true or false, *if* it is true, the entire basis of human responsibility is undermined . . . the doctrine, if taken seriously and in full consistency, undercuts itself. Planning is indeed possible, if the planner is free, while the subjects of the planning are necessitated, but there is no reason whatever to make this exception. *What the planner undertakes has itself been necessitated.* Therefore, on the basis of determinism, genuine planning is impossible. Each does what he must and that is the end of the matter. . . . What is highly important to say is that, insofar as the popular reaction has been one of irresponsibility, it is the result of a sound logical deduction, and in no sense a perversion (emphasis in the original).[15]

Although an entire volume of the *Standard Edition* of Freud's collected works is devoted to an index, there is no entry for *responsibility* in it. True to the faith of the master, his acolytes must have felt that responsibility was so unscientific a concept that it was not worth indexing.*

Although differing in certain ways, old-fashioned asylum psychiatry, psychoanalysis, and modern biological psychiatry thus all agree on the all-important point, that the behavior of the mentally ill person is strictly *determined*: such a person has no free will and is therefore not responsible for his actions. That this psychiatric-psychoanalytic view on responsibility encourages lay people to be irresponsible and physicians to be paternalistic is obvious and requires no further comment. Perhaps because it is less obvious, people often do not realize that relieving a person of his responsibility is tantamount to relieving him, partly or entirely, of his humanity as well. The person who claims that he, not his brother, is responsible for his brother's welfare and happiness, stabs at the very heart of his brother as a person. The philosopher W.G. Maclagan puts it this way:

Any regard that we may show for the happiness of others must also be governed by the recognition that as persons they, like ourselves, have not only a natural interest in their own happiness but a moral interest in values, and thus in the dignity of life: and further, that this latter interest, precisely because values are values and it *is* a moral interest, must by them as by us be accorded a general priority. How, after all, could we more grossly insult our

---

*Actually, like many another ideology or religious system, psychoanalysis preaches a self-contradictory sermon on responsibility. According to the Freudian doctrine, a person is not responsible for his ordinary, everyday actions because they are determined by unconscious forces, but is responsible for accidents and mental symptoms. I have discussed this basic inconsistency in psychoanalytic theory elsewhere.[16]

fellows than by implying, in our treatment of them, that while *we* indeed have such an interest *they do not?*[17]

In short, the psychiatric and psychoanalytic perspectives on human behavior encourage the tactic of treating persons—especially if their behavior is disturbing—as if they were not moral agents. Moreover, this policy is promoted as if it were beneficial both for the persons so treated and the society of which they are a part, and as if it did not, and could not possibly, have any deleterious consequences. In fact, nothing could be further from the truth. The combined psychiatric-psychoanalytic war on responsibility has cost us heavily indeed. Exemplified by the current national crisis in liability insurance—with payments to plaintiffs often premised on psychiatrically supported claims of emotional injury and mental suffering—the disastrous consequences of this war stare us in the face; but we steadfastly refuse to recognize their cause. As an old rabbinic saying has it, no one is so blind as the man who does not want to see.

This is why we never ask: What existential cost do we inflict on the person whose moral agency we withdraw? What existential price do we, as a society, pay for empowering a group of professionals to deprive persons of their status as moral agents and for treating certain psychiatrically identified persons as if they were not moral agents? These questions—and with them the very possibility of debating the potential conflicts between moral agency, medical care, the safety of society, and other values—are now deeply buried under the rhetoric of mental illness and psychiatric paternalism.

NONRESPONSIBILITY AND THE CRIMINAL LAW

Since responsibility and nonresponsibility are ideas whose consequences are primarily moral and legal, it would be foolish to regard them as belonging to another domain or discourse, such as medicine or science. "What," asks Michael S. Moore, a professor of law at the University of Southern California and a frequent commentator on forensic psychiatry, "have people meant by mental illness such that, both on and off juries, they have for centuries excused the otherwise wrongful acts of mentally ill persons?" This is a good question to ask. Moore, who strongly supports the medical pretensions and political powers of psychiatry, answers it as follows: "To be mentally ill is to be seriously irrational . . . why does severely diminished rationality preclude responsibility? . . . [Because] one is a moral agent only if one is a rational agent."[18]

Unfortunately, this is not reasoning but merely substituting one phrase for another. The assertions "Jones is irrational" and "Jones is mentally ill" may seem like two different statements, but are not: actually, they are the same statement couched in two different forms. Since this is often not recognized, a speaker or writer connecting insanity, irrationality, and irresponsibility can easily appear to be introducing an empirical standard into the determination of mental illness, when, in fact, he is doing nothing of the sort.

> If the issue of the definition of mental illness is a moral one [writes Moore] . . . then the legal definition of the phrase should embody those principles that underlie the intuitive judgment that mentally ill human beings are not responsible. . . . It is easy to understand the long-standing historical tendency of the criminal law to analogize the mentally ill to infants and animals. . . . Only when an infant develops sufficiently that his actions are regularly explicable by rationalizing practical syllogism do we begin to see him as a moral agent who can justly be held responsible. The same is true of the mentally ill. . . . [juries] have perceived that madness itself precludes responsibility.[19]

Moore's foregoing argument founders on a combination of circularity and parochialism. Since people "intuitively" infer insanity from irresponsibility and vice versa, reiterating the connection between these two items—indeed, their virtual equivalence in practice—does not help us to go beyond our conventional understanding of these terms. Nor is it helpful or reassuring, in trying to clarify so important a question as who is and who is not a moral agent, to be referred back to "intuitive understanding." Do we need reminding that not long ago the intuitive understanding of vast numbers of people was that women were childlike creatures who could not shoulder the responsibility of the franchise? Or that blacks were childlike people who, for their own good, had to be treated as slaves? Moore's entire reasoning rests on paternalism (although he avoids the term)—that is, on the superior power of the observing and judging person over the person being observed and judged. In politics might makes right, but in moral philosophy, surely, more than might should be required to make rationality. The history of religious warfare should make us realize that the adage "one man's meat is another man's poison" applies to the idea of rationality no less than it does to the idea of the one and only true faith.

Actually, in contemporary psychiatry, especially in its legal applications, the notions insanity, irrationality, incompetence, and irresponsibility are often used interchangeably, as if one were caused by, or could be equated with, another.* Let us therefore now examine the connections between mental illness and nonresponsibility via the concept of mental incompetence.

NONRESPONSIBILITY AS MENTAL INCOMPETENCE

In common usage, *competence* means the ability to perform a particular task well or to act ably in a certain situation. We speak of a person playing tennis or the piano competently, or of being a competent teacher or doctor.

When psychiatrists use the term *competence,* or say that a person is *mentally incompetent,* they imply that only mentally healthy persons are competent. Psychiatric use of the term *competence* thus implies a connection between mental illness and incompetence, the former presumably causing the latter. This is illustrated by the standard forensic-psychiatric practice of psychiatrists testifying in court that a person is mentally ill and is, *therefore,* incompetent. The assertion about incompetence may be articulated separately, as I have just stated it, or may be left as an unarticulated inference anyone familiar with the concept of mental competence would draw from the assertion of mental illness. In short, to say that a person is mentally ill and hence incompetent is a tautology masquerading as a logical inference drawn from a medical determination.

In addition, there is an obvious but seldom noticed difficulty with the idea of nonresponsibility due to psychiatric unfitness—namely, that the class of persons so categorized actually comprises two completely different kinds of human beings. One group is composed of inadequate, unskilled, lazy, or stupid persons—in short, of individuals de facto incompetent and unfit, however relative the meaning might be. The other group is composed of protesters, revolutionaries, persons on strike against their relatives, society, or their own lives—in short, of individuals, often with superior capabilities, unwilling rather than unable to perform competently in life. Because psychiatrists—and people generally—do not differentiate between these two groups, they often attribute unfitness to unwillingness, and unwillingness to unfitness. But how can we tell one from the other? As a practical matter, not very easily. But we can tell when

---

*It must be remembered, moreover, that in tort litigation, where intention is not a necessary ingredient for ascribing responsibility, persons considered to be mentally ill are usually treated the same way as those considered to be mentally healthy.[20] Mental illness is a legal fiction that plays totally different roles in criminal and in civil law (see Chapter 11).

nature or evil men perform their own experiments, creating dire circumstances, like catastrophic conflagrations or concentration camps: then the unfit perish, while most of those who are unwilling rise to the occasion and demonstrate unexpected competence in their struggle for survival. Because the circumstances I allude to involve extreme hardship for people, no civilized society can allow them to be deliberately created for the alleged benefit of certain persons. (In this connection see Chapter 6 for a discussion of malingering.)

Like many key psychiatric words, the terms *competent* and *incompetent* conceal a dispositional strategy behind a descriptive label. Descriptively, the term *incompetent* refers to the designated person's inability to perform certain acts (or all acts) properly or responsibly, and covers much the same idea as do the terms *not responsible* or *irrational.* On the other hand, dispositively, the term *incompetent* refers to social strategies we employ vis-à-vis such persons in order to prevent them from performing certain acts, such as (1) standing trial; (2) committing a crime; (3) managing one's funds; (4) executing a valid will; and (5) being a parent. As a rule, the prohibited acts are narrowly delimited, the incompetent individual being considered competent in other areas: for example, a person declared incompetent to be a parent loses legal custody of his child but continues to be regarded as psychiatrically competent to manage his funds, stand trial, vote, and so forth.

Incompetence as Justification

Why is the idea of mental incompetence now so popular and so readily accepted as a justification for certain social policies? The answer is: Because it is useful for justifying certain social policies. Indeed much of what I have written in this volume about mental illness as a strategic and justificatory concept applies to incompetence as well (see Chapters 8 and 9).

Whenever a person claims *his own incompetence* (for a past action), and when his claim is accepted as valid by the authorities, we are confronted with a clear case of collusion, exemplified by the Canon Law's recognition of "psychic consensual incapacity" as a justification for dissolving the hasty and unhappy union of a young couple.[21] As *Catholic* consensual incapacity annuls *holy* matrimony, so *scientific* psychiatric incapacity annuls *criminal* responsibility.

On the other hand, whenever one person, A, claims that another person, B, is incompetent, we are confronted with a situation from which we can draw two quite different inferences, one more probable than the other. The less probable inference is that A's assertion is true:

in other words, that B is indeed incompetent. The more probable inference is that A's assertion is untrue: in other words, that A wants to paternistically control or coerce B.

Paternalism is, of course, a fundamental feature of many human situations. The presently fashionable practice of depriving people of their right to decide whether or not they should be tried for a crime or treated for a mental illness—because they are mentally incompetent—is but the contemporary version of a practice that can be applied, and has been applied, to many other activities. In the past, it was universally applied to religion. In a theological society, who is considered to be mentally competent to choose his own religion (and repudiate the religion of his ancestors) or no religion at all? "A stock argument for the state teaching of religion," Herbert Spencer cogently noted, "has been that the masses cannot distinguish false religion from true. . . . This alleged *incompetency* on the part of the people has been the reason assigned for all state-interferences whatever" (emphasis added).[22] It is not a coincidence that state interference with religion in the United States today—slight as it is—is based almost entirely on psychiatric arguments. Directed against the new, unconventional religions, pejoratively called *cults,* interference is regularly justified by the contention that so-called cult members are mentally incompetent to decide what the religion of their choice ought to be. Why are they incompetent in this way and how do we know that they are? Because only a mentally ill person joins a cult and because, once a person has joined, he is quickly brainwashed, further impairing his mental capacities.

Of course, in a modern democracy, arguments and policies based on paternalism suffer from a fatal inconsistency, namely: If so many individuals are now deemed to be mentally incompetent to judge certain matters or participate in certain activities—such as which cult to join, which drug to take, which crime to be responsible for, and so on—how can the same persons be competent to judge the politicians who determine official policy concerning these very affairs and to participate in the electoral process on which our whole society rests? Since hardly anyone today advocates completely disenfranchising mentally ill persons, the selective invocation of mental incompetence—as a justification for legal and political action—stands clearly revealed as part and parcel of the modern psychiatric apparatus of rhetorical justification and social control.

In sum, much like the idea of mental illness, the idea of mental incompetence comprises certain conceptual-cognitive characteristics (of the agent diagnosed), and certain dispositional-justificatory decisions (of the agents making the diagnosis), the latter element generally greatly outweighing the former. As a cognitive category, the idea of mental incompetence derives its force from the fact that certain diseases of the body, especially of the brain, render the patient grossly unable to care for himself. Foremost among such conditions are acute injuries and intoxications that render the person unconscious. Obviously, such a person is incompetent to decide whether he should or should not have medical care—his inability being apparent even to untrained observers. The next class of conditions, of great importance both practically and theoretically, comprises the so-called deliria and dementias: these are acute and chronic disturbances of brain function, typically caused by injury, intoxication, infection, or loss of brain cells due to as yet undetermined causes, resulting in impaired behavior without loss of consciousness. Delirium and dementia are manifestations of brain diseases that can be objectively demonstrated and diagnosed, by means of clinical tests while the patient is alive or by autopsy after he dies. The delirious or demented person, too, is likely to be unable to care for himself and may properly be treated as incompetent. It is now customary to view the person deemed incompetent because of mental illness as similar to the unconscious or demented patient. This is an extension of the analogy between mental illness and bodily illness and exhibits all of the strengths and weaknesses of that analogy. What, in fact, are the similarities and differences between these two groups of individuals?

The similarities are few and unimportant: like the demented patient, the mentally incompetent person may behave oddly and upset others. In other ways, however, the two differ: the mentally incompetent person suffers from no demonstrable disease and is usually able, indeed eager, to chart his own course in life, however harmful that may be to himself or others. Moreover, he often finds others—including lawyers and doctors—to vouch for his competence in court. I have chronicled the fate of several persons, some quite famous, who have been declared mentally incompetent to stand trial despite their protestations and despite the fact that lawyers and psychiatrists agreed that they were competent.[23] The tragic consequences of such a policy of so-called substituted judgment for the incompetent patient—a policy ostensibly aimed to help, not harm, him—are due to the fact that the person declared mentally unfit to stand trial is denied the right to trial, guaranteed by the Sixth Amendment to the Constitution, and is instead incarcerated, potentially indefinitely, in a psychiatric institution.*

---

*Prior to 1971, when, in *Jackson v. Indiana,* the Supreme Court recognized the grave abuses which this policy had spawned and placed certain limits on its applications, defendants declared mentally incompetent to stand trial often ended up spending the rest of their lives imprisoned, without trial, in hospitals for the criminally insane.[24]

NONRESPONSIBILITY AS IRRATIONALITY

A typical bodily illness, like cancer of the colon, is inferred from, and is equated with, a somatic lesion—that is, cancerous cells in the colon and perhaps elsewhere in the body. In contrast, a typical mental illness, like schizophrenia, is inferred from, and is equated with, irresponsible behavior—that is, lack of moral responsibility in the conduct of some, or most, aspects of life. Responsibility and nonresponsibility are, of course, ethical and legal concepts. In our society, not all persons are considered to be responsible; for example, the very young, the very old (senile), the mentally retarded, and certain brain-damaged persons are regarded as more or less nonresponsible. If we ask why some persons are regarded as responsible and others not, the conventional answer, given by psychiatrists as well as others, is that we can treat only rational persons as responsible and must treat those who are irrational as not responsible. Moore takes this to be self-evident. "The responsibility of the mentally ill," he asserts, "thus turns on their lack of rationality. . . . an agent's serious irrationality by itself reduces or eliminates his responsibility."[25] This is why everyone—psychiatrist, lawyer, lay person—is so quick to label others as *irrational*, intuitively realizing that this is the easiest way to deprive a person of his humanity: An individual considered to be lacking the capacity to be responsible is usually also considered—in proportion to his lack of responsibility—to be lacking the capacity to be at liberty as well.

Irrationality, the Brain, and the Person

Some persons never develop the normal use of some of their body parts and functions: for example, the congenitally blind person cannot see, and the congenitally deaf person cannot hear. Others lose the use of certain bodily functions: for example, the person suffering from muscular dystrophy has failing muscles, and the person suffering from Alzheimer's disease has a failing brain.

Although irrationality due to senile dementia is just as real as immobility due to disabling arthritis, there is an important difference between them: judgments about the mobility or immobility of a person's joint rest on a biological standard, whereas judgments about the rationality or irrationality of a person's reasoning or thinking rest on a personal or societal standard. We ascertain whether a person is rational—or correctly oriented—by determining whether he knows who he is, where he is, who the President is, and so forth. There is nothing wrong with such a standard. What is wrong is that psychiatry conflates and confuses the irrationality of dementia with the irrationality of psychosis. The former is a symptom of a malfunctioning brain, whereas the latter, as I shall presently show, is not.

Wherein lies the essential difference between the irrationality of a demented person and of a psychotic one? The demented person *displays a defect*—typically of his memory (he cannot remember the date or even who he is), and of his ability to reason (he cannot do simple arithmetical tasks that he formerly could easily do). The psychotic person, on the other hand, *asserts a false claim*—typically of his identity (he is Jesus or God), and of his reasons for engaging in acts injurious to himself or others (he is commanded by God or demons or is protecting himself from nonexisting persecutors).

If psychosis is not the symptom of a hidden—as yet undiagnosed or undiagnosable—brain disease, then what is it? The answer, I am afraid, is too simple: it is a form of behavior. Specifically, psychosis is behavior judged to be bad—injurious to the self or others. It is also a form of behavior closely connected with dishonesty: a person who is honest with himself—"true to himself," as Socrates put it—cannot, in my opinion, *be* or *become* psychotic, although he may, of course, be *called* psychotic by others.

How, then, do psychiatrists ascertain whether a particular person who has committed a violent act was or was not psychotic? The answer is: They don't. That is the wrong question to ask. The right question is: Under what circumstances do psychiatrists (and others) *ascribe* psychosis to the perpetrator of a certain act? Before answering these questions, let us briefly consider some typical instances of the assumption and ascription of responsibility and nonresponsibility.

Claiming and Disclaiming Responsibility

It is important to keep in mind that responsibility is *something* we both claim and disclaim for ourselves and attribute or refuse to attribute to others. For example, a five-year-old child is not held criminally responsible by the legal system for killing people in a house fire which he starts by playing with matches; but he is held responsible by his parents for controlling his bladder and bowels and for washing his hands before meals.

Here is an example more pertinent to our present concerns. Certain persons—called *terrorists* by those who disapprove of them, and *patriots* by those who approve of them—often claim responsibility for bombings and killings committed by unknown assailants. The terrorist killer and the insane killer both kill: the difference between them is that the former typically claims responsibility for his action, whereas the latter often disclaims responsibility for it. A similar symmetrical relationship obtains between authorities who incriminate innocent persons as guilty, and those who exculpate guilty persons as innocent: for example, French military officers claimed that Albert Dreyfus was responsible for crimes he did not commit, whereas American forensic psychiatrists claimed that John Hinckley, Jr. was not responsible for crimes he did commit. (Hinckley, it should be remembered, acknowledged his guilt.[26])

I might seem to be dwelling unduly on responsibility as a crucial parameter of psychosis. But the plain facts about this alleged illness, as against the rhetoric in which it is couched and the theories by which it is ostensibly explained, fully justify this emphasis. What are these facts? They are that a person is considered to be insane if two conditions obtain: (1) that, by conventional standards, he behaves very badly—typically, threatening to kill himself or others; (2) that he justifies his misbehavior in a conventionally unjustifiable way—typically by claiming that what he has done is good, not bad. Examples abound in the daily press.

In December 1976, Roxanne Gay killed her husband, Blenda, a defensive end on the Philadelphia Eagles professional football team, by plunging a knife into his throat while he was asleep. Witnesses at her trial testified that she "suffered from hallucinations that her husband, her family, and the police were plotting to kill her." Mrs. Gay was acquitted as not guilty by reason of insanity and was committed to the Marlboro State Psychiatric Hospital in New Jersey. On July 21, 1980, Camden (N.J.) County Judge I.V. DiMartino ordered that Mrs. Gay be released because she "has achieved that degree of mental stability where she is no longer a danger to herself, her family, or society."[27]

Actually, Mrs. Gay had advanced two claims: namely, that she was insane, and that she killed her husband because she was a "battered wife." No one nowadays is troubled by the inconsistency inherent in this combination: being a battered wife supplies a motive or reason for killing one's husband, but a motive or reason for such a deed is precisely what an insane woman is not supposed to have. According to testimony at the trial, there was no evidence that Mrs. Gay was abused by her husband. Characteristically, *The New York Times* referred to her false claims as *hallucinations.* The implication—so strong today that doubting it is to invite derision—is that a woman who hallucinates that her husband is abusing her is not responsible for killing him.

The view that mental illness renders its victim irrational and hence not responsible was stated with special clarity and force by Moore:

Since mental illness negates our assumption of rationality, we do not hold the mentally ill responsible. It is not so much that we excuse them from a prima facie case of responsibility; rather, by being unable to regard them as fully rational beings, we cannot affirm the essential condition to viewing them as moral agents to begin with. In this the mentally ill join (to a decreasing degree) infants, wild beasts, plants, and stones—none of which are responsible because of the absence of any assumption of rationality.[28]

The interpretation offered by John Hinckley Jr.'s parents for why their son shot President Reagan and three other men illustrates the same point:

"How could anybody do such a horrible thing?" The answer is schizophrenia, an overpowering mental illness that robbed John of his ability to control his thoughts and actions. . . . John . . . is *desperately* ill. . . . [T]he disease is the culprit, not the person (emphasis in the original).[29]

Life indeed imitates art. Almost 400 years ago Shakespeare used similar language to suggest the same idea, albeit only to underscore the absurdity of exculpating the doer from responsibility for his deed:

Hamlet. . . . What I have done . . .
I here proclaim was madness.
Was't Hamlet wronged Laertes? Never Hamlet.
If Hamlet from himself be ta'en away,
And when he's not himself does wrong Laertes,
Then Hamlet does it not . . .
Who does it then? His madness.[30]

But were Hamlet not responsible for avenging his father's murder, *Hamlet* would not be a tragedy. "The horrible act John committed," John's parents keep insisting, "he committed through no fault of his own. It was an act of illness. . . . [John] is a person who morally is one of the finest people you could ever meet."[31]

Cui bono? Who profits from this explanation? John Hinckley, Jr. is incarcerated in St. Elizabeth's Hospital where, I suspect, he will remain until he dies. Whereas John Hinckley, Sr. and Jo Ann Hinckley have fashioned a new career—perhaps *calling* would be more accurate—out of their son's historic deed: warning the American public about the Devil—whom they call Mental Illness.

INSANITY AND NONRESPONSIBILITY RECONSIDERED

In the past, philosophers, jurists, and lay people asked why the madman behaves irrationally, and the alienists answered: Because he is insane. Philosophers, jurists, and lay people still ask the same question, and psychiatrists still offer the same answer, now reframed in terms of mental illness. I reject this pseudoexplanation as self-serving. I believe we should turn the question around and ask: Why do philosophers, jurists, and lay people attribute irrationality and nonresponsibility to certain individuals? My answer, as I indicated earlier, is: In order to remove such persons from the category of moral agents and to justify controlling them by means of the psychiatric sanctions of the modern State. The following incident is typical.

In August 1985, several groups of ex-mental patients held their annual "International Conference for Human Rights and Against Psychiatric Oppression" at the University of Vermont, in Burlington. After demonstrators made an unlawful attempt to speak to some of the psychiatric patients at the Medical Center Hospital, one of them was not only arrested and charged with unlawful trespass, but was also ordered to undergo "psychiatric evaluation for competency and sanity."[32] I have never heard or read of a demonstrator against abortion clinics or South African racial policies engaging in similar symbolic violations of the law having been ordered to undergo a psychiatric examination to determine his competency and sanity.

Mens Rea (Guilty Mind) and the Capacity to Commit a Crime

The law recognizes insanity as a mental condition that may be *total*, abolishing the person's responsibility for what would otherwise be a criminal act, or as a condition that may be *partial*, merely diminishing or reducing it. In the former case, the defendant is not punished at all, but is almost certainly incarcerated involuntarily in a mental hospital; in the latter case, the defendant is found guilty of a lower grade of offense, receives a prison sentence commensurate with that crime, and almost certainly receives no psychiatric treatment in prison. Although legal scholars are fond of making pedantic distinctions among terms such as *partial responsibility, diminished responsibility, diminished capacity, limited capacity,* and *partial insanity,* all these phrases come to the same thing, that is, *diminished capacity* or *diminished responsibility* (the terms I shall use).

The theory of diminished capacity, as described above, is more than a century old. As a practical tactic in law and psychiatry, the defense and disposition of diminished capacity became popular in the United States only after the 1950s. In legal phraseology, the operative concept is "that if because of mental disease or defect a defendant cannot form the specific state of mind required as an essential element of a crime, he may be convicted only of a lower grade of offense not requiring that particular mental element."[33] The modern doctrine of diminished capacity was introduced with, and gained acceptance through, the rationalization that defendants so treated would receive psychiatric therapy in prison. In fact this has not happened, partly because defendants successfully pleading diminished capacity do not consider themselves mentally ill and decline treatment, and partly because no treatment is in fact made available to them. It must be noted, also, that diminished capacity is a limited defense, applicable only against crimes where specific intent is an element of the offense, such as intentional homicide or theft.

The Necessity of Mens Rea for the Criminal Law

After every sensational insanity trial that arouses the public passions and results in the defendant's acquittal as not guilty by reason of insanity—exemplified by the trial of John Hinckley, Jr.—the cry goes up for the reform or abolition of the insanity defense.* Typically mounted by politicians and psychiatrists sensitive to possibilities for self-enhancement, the resulting so-called attack on the insanity plea is an exercise in deception, self-deception, and futility. The fact is that so long as people—especially the supposed critics of the insanity defense themselves—believe in mental illness, there can be no significant change in this defense.

Attempts to abolish the insanity defense invariably founder on the following chain of logic. Anglo-American law is based on the moral principle that there can be no crime without *mens rea*, which literally means a guilty mind and is interpreted, in practice, as intent to commit a crime. Many circumstances or considerations—only one of which is psychiatric in character—may result in the legal and commonsense judgment that a person seemingly causing another person's injury or death is not legally responsible for it. Among these factors are accident, self-defense, duress—and mental illness. Since virtually everyone now believes that mental illness exists and has the effect of diminishing or annulling the subject's capacity for intentionality, an attack on the insanity defense becomes, in effect, an attack on *mens rea*, and hence an attack on the very pillar of our legal system for adjudicating guilt and

---

*Trials such as that of John Hinckley, Jr. are much more common in the United States than in other countries. So-called aberrations in the uses of the insanity defense are, in fact, a characteristic feature of the American legal system, especially as it is presently constituted.

innocence. To overcome this impasse, it would be necessary for people either to abandon their belief in mental illness, which does not seem imminent, or their belief that mental illness is synonymous with diminished or annulled mental capacity, which would be oxymoronic, since a crazy person is, by definition, viewed as someone who does not know what he is doing. Small wonder that, combining arrogance with resignation, many legal scholars have come to see the union of law and psychiatry as similar to that of a hopelessly mismatched married couple, each partner being unable to live with or without the other. No doubt, a divorce would be expensive and painful, requiring the depsychiatrization of *mens rea* and the abolition of nonpenal punishments; but, in the long run, it might prove beneficial to the man (the law), as well as the children (the body politic)—though not to the wife (psychiatry), whose economic and existential well-being depends on the marriage.

How did the law and psychiatry end up in such a parasitic relationship? To answer this question, we must briefly reconsider the differences between a person being the de facto cause of the injury or death of another human being, and that person, as moral agent, being responsible for such an outcome. The difference is obvious and all-important, as the following examples will readily convey. Suppose that Jones is driving down a highway while Smith is planning to commit suicide by throwing himself in front of a vehicle from an overpass. Smith jumps, lands in front of Jones's car, and is instantly killed. Jones is the ultimate human instrument of Smith's death, but is not responsible for, or guilty of, any crime. Self-defense and duress present similar situations. In summary, a person may be considered not responsible for his behavior in general—or for a particular act (crime) at a specific point in time—for three quite different types of reasons:

1. Because the agent is deemed to lack *mens rea* (criminal intent) for what otherwise would be an illegal act. This judgment may be based on circumstances (self-defense), or on the presence of an objectively demonstrable bodily disease (epilepsy) resulting in what is viewed as an accident rather than as an action, or on the alleged presence of an objectively nondemonstrable mental illness (schizophrenia).

2. Because the agent rejects responsibility and his doing so is viewed as the manifestation of a mental illness (schizophrenia).

3. Because, although the agent insists he is responsible, authorities coercively deprive him of responsibility against his will by declaring him to be suffering from mental illness (and therefore unable to stand trial, not guilty by reason of insanity, etc.).

I summarize the most important situations in which responsibility is considered to be diminished or annulled in Tables 8.1 and 8.2.

In the foregoing situations, in each of which one person, Jones, injures or kills another person, Smith, we consider it reasonable to *not* hold Jones responsible for a crime. It is important that we understand why. Assuredly, we do not do so because of what we learn from examining Jones's *mental state;* instead we do so because of what we learn from examining the *context of the problematic action.* That is why, in such cases, we do not examine Jones's mind—to determine whether or not it was capable of forming criminal intent; instead, we examine the situation in which the injury or death occurred—to determine the roles played in it by the various participants. The proper analogy here is not to illness or incapacity but to meaning, literal and metaphorical. Let me explain.

Examining a person's mind to determine whether or not his mental capacity is, or was, diminished is allegedly like examining his body to determine whether or not the capacity of his liver or kidneys is diminished. But since there is no such thing as a mind—since the notion of

TABLE 8.1. Responsibility Absent or Diminished

I. In the Context of Criminal Law

1. Subject injures or kills assailant in self-defense: no intent to commit a crime (no *mens rea*); no criminal responsibility; no mental illness; no punishment; no hospitalization

2. Subject injures or kills unknown person(s) when he loses control of his car during his first epileptic seizure (injury or death viewed as the result of an accident, not of an act): no intent to commit a crime (no *mens rea*); no criminal responsibility; no mental illness; no punishment; no hospitalization

3. Subject injures or kills a person as a result of an altercation during which he strikes his victim a blow, the victim falls, hits his head, dies: no intent to commit murder (*mens rea* for involuntary manslaughter only); diminished criminal responsibility (guilty of involuntary manslaughter); punishment for lesser offense; no mental illness; no mental hospitalization

4. Subject stalks and shoots a political figure or other prominent person: (seemingly) has intent to commit a crime; successfully pleads insanity; mental illness (no *mens rea*); no criminal responsibility; not guilty by reason of insanity; no punishment; hospitalization for criminal insanity

5. Subject charged with (political) crime for which he wants to stand trial and prove his innocence: declared mentally unfit to stand trial; mental illness (at the time of the trial); *mens rea* and criminal responsibility for alleged offense moot; hospitalization for criminal insanity

TABLE 8.2. Responsibility Absent or Diminished

II. In the Context of Civil (Mental Health) Law

1. Subject complains to psychiatrist of fears of killing himself or others and asks to be protected from himself: explicit rejection of responsibility for self (self-control); individual invites others to assume responsibility for him; mental illness; voluntary admission to mental hospital

2. Subject abstains from ordinary acts of self-care expected of adults in our society (e.g., does not work, speak, eat, bathe, etc.): implicit (nonverbal) rejection of responsibility for self; individual invites (coerces) others (family, physicians, the police) to assume responsibility for him; mental illness; unprotesting or involuntary admission to mental hospital

3. Subject offers no complaints and wants to be treated as a responsible person but, because of the validated complaints of others against him, is coercively deprived of responsibility; mental illness; subject declared to be mentally unfit (to be a parent, to refuse psychiatric drugs, etc.)

mind is, itself, a fiction—the idea of a *mental capacity* to form criminal intent is also fictitious; if taken literally, it is bound to lead to conclusions prefigured in the premise, as described in detail in this book. (I mean here simply that criminal intent is not something a *mind* forms or has, but something a *person* forms or has.)

In short, if we really wanted to free ourselves from the constraints imposed on us by the idea of a mental capacity to form criminal intent, and of the deceptive procedures it inexorably generates, we would have to proceed in a completely different manner in dealing with so-called crazy criminals who are now deemed to be proper subjects for diversion from the penal to the psychiatric system. How? In the way we now deal with injury or death caused by accident or self-defense, as I have just described. In such cases we do not look to experts or to esoteric procedures to solve our problem; instead we rely on commonsense methods to determine whether or not a person intended to harm another person. We proceed similarly if we want to determine whether a person uses a word literally or metaphorically: That is, we do not examine the speaker's or writer's mind psychiatrically in an effort to discover whether the word has a literal or metaphorical meaning; instead, we examine the context in which the word occurs and form our conclusion accordingly. However, because we regard mental illness as a genuine illness—as a fact or material object—we foreclose the possibility of establishing the connections between the mentally ill person's behavior and his responsibility for it in the same commonsense manner in which we approach the connections among accident, duress, self-defense, and responsibility.

Annulled or Diminished Responsibility

Because of the influence of a positivistic mental science on intellectual as well as popular thought, the law now regards mental patients as persons who possessed responsibility when they were mentally healthy but who, as a result of their mental illness, have lost it, and who, after undergoing appropriate psychiatric therapy, might regain it. This view rests on a tacit analogy between the capacity to be responsible and the capacity of certain bodily organs, especially the sense organs, to perform their functions. For example, a healthy man has sight, which he may temporarily lose because of injury or illness, and which he may regain as a result of successful treatment. Viewing responsibility on the model of eyesight, it is believed that as one type of brain lesion causes loss of vision, another type causes loss of responsibility. However appealing this notion might be, it is false: being endowed with vision is a physiological fact, but being responsible is a moral attribute. This is why we can be absolutely certain that a person is blind, but we cannot be certain that he is not responsible (unless he is unconscious).

Nevertheless, since it is believed that the mental patient is irrational and cannot make responsible decisions, others—family members, psychiatrists, courts—have to treat him as if he were a child and act on his behalf. And since often no one is willing to care for these persons (and they are often unwilling to care for themselves), society welcomes the psychiatrists' eagerness to fill that need. But there is a catch. Most people, especially at the beginning of their careers as mental patients, resist being confined in insane asylums. Hence, it is necessary to incarcerate them. The patients' irrationality and nonresponsibility justify this policy so perfectly that mental illness, irrationality, nonresponsibility, and involuntary psychiatric confinement quickly jell to form a single legal-psychiatric-social compound whose component elements can no longer be separately identified. The unity of this complex combination of psychiatric ideas, justifications, and procedures is illustrated in the following passage from the pen of Charles Mercier, a prominent turn-of-the-century British psychiatrist:

> Apart from the fact that it is desirable to cure insanity, and that in many cases a cure can only be attempted within an asylum; apart from the necessity, that often exists, of secluding a perfectly harmless lunatic in order to prevent him from squandering his means and ruining himself and his family; apart from the desirability of restraining him from performing acts which are not dangerous, but which are disgraceful, and which he himself would, on his recovery, be loudest in blaming his friends for not preventing; there remains the most important fact that the distinguishing feature of the insane

is not their dangerous aggressiveness, but their revolting indecency and obscenity. . . . probably a large majority of both men and women are or would be, if freed from restraint, more shameless and filthy in their conduct than so many monkeys. It is not merely that the public must be protected from such conduct as this. They have a right, also, to be prevented from witnessing it; and it is for this reason, more than any other, that the seclusion of the insane in asylums is necessary and right.[34]

The imagery of disease and the imagery of animality and lack of self-control—and implicitly of irrationality and nonresponsibility—are here skillfully blended into a coherent and seemingly irrefutable justification of prevailing psychiatric practices. Revealingly, except for an initial passing reference to curing the insane, there is no hint here that the insane suffer from a disease, that the problem of insanity is in any meaningful sense medical, or that the confinement of the insane is primarily for their benefit. On the contrary, what the author succeeds so well in conveying is that the insane person often presents us with a spectacle at once distressing and disgusting, justifying his segregation from the rest of society. Of course, that is a moral judgment and a recommendation for political action, with which, depending on our own moral and political values, we can agree or disagree.

Since neither rationality nor responsibility are facts of nature or measurable performances of the human body (like temperature or blood pressure), how do authorities establish whether a person is or is not rational or responsible? By recourse to the judgments of psychiatric experts who claim to be able to correlate rationality and responsibility with sanity and insanity. A nineteenth-century British alienist declared:

No mind can properly be considered to be "unsound" or "insane" which is not the subject of actual disease, the "insanity" or "unsoundness" being invariably the products—the effects or the consequences—of some deviation from the healthy condition of the brain, its vessels or investments, disordering the mental manifestations.[35]

Another psychiatrist wrote: "A monomaniac with perverted emotions and homicidal tendencies cannot, *says science*, control his conduct, and cannot therefore be held responsible for his acts" (emphasis added).[36]

Ironically, while people now regard such formulations of the nonresponsibility of the insane as exaggerated and old-fashioned, they view with enthusiasm presently popular formulations of diminished capacity—that is, the proposition that insanity reduces rather than annuls criminal responsibility. Plausible though it might seem, the idea of diminished responsibility, as ostensibly demonstrated by psychiatrists, is even more absurd than the idea of annulled responsibility, as the following reflections illustrate.

The term *diminished capacity* implies a roughly quantitative view of responsibility, consistent with our judgment that, like health or strength, a person may have more responsibility at one time than at another, and that one person may, in the same situation, have more responsibility than another. By matching different individuals against a conventional standard, we consider some to be weak or in poor health, and others to be strong and in robust health. If we viewed responsibility similarly, it would follow, as a matter of common sense and logic, that as a person's capacity to be responsible may be diminished at one time, so it may be increased at another time; and that, matched against a conventional standard, some persons may possess less, and others more, capacity for responsibility than some hypothetical mean. Indeed, if we paid more attention to the circumstances of sensational crimes, and less to the expert opinions of psychiatrists, then many such crimes—for example, that of John Hinckley, Jr.—would seem to be the acts of agents possessing increased, rather than diminished, capacity for committing criminal acts. The reason we never view crimes this way is one of the symptoms of our abject abdication of common sense in favor of psychobabble. Actually, hardly a day passes without psychiatrists examining defendants to determine their mental capacity to commit crimes. Although psychiatrists often find that a defendant *suffered from diminished capacity* to commit the crime he had committed, they never find that he *enjoyed an increased capacity* to do so. Psychiatrists seem to have an uncanny ability to find what they are paid to find. In the whole history of psychiatry, never has a psychiatrist examined a person charged with a crime and found him to have an increased mental capacity to commit a crime. This fact alone utterly unmasks the medical pretensions legitimizing psychiatric determinations of diminished responsibility.*

Increased Responsibility

If the idea of diminished responsibility (capacity) can be said to have descriptive content, so must its opposite, namely, increased responsibility. A person's responsibility for a crime is considered diminished if he acts without premeditation, under the impetus of a strong and sudden

---

*Actually neither law nor psychiatry recognizes the concept of increased mental capacity to commit a crime. Psychiatry does recognize the concept of increased intentionality, however (see Chapter 7).

impulse, for example, the man who injures or kills his wife's lover when he discovers them in the marital bed. Similarly, a person's responsibility for a crime could be considered increased if he carries out a well-rehearsed crime, for example, the man who selects his victim, stalks him, and at the right moment attacks or kills him. Typically, such a person has a clearly articulated reason for his behavior; however, normal persons are likely to regard such a person's reason as irrational or crazy, and psychiatrists are likely to interpret it as the symptoms of paranoid schizophrenia.

In 1978, then a 42-year-old chronic graduate student in mathematics at Stanford University, Theodore Streleski killed one of his teachers, Professor Karel W. deLeeuw. An exceptionally articulate and intelligent person, Streleski had what he considered to be an excellent explanation for why he killed deLeeuw. In a review of the story in *People* magazine following Streleski's sensational release from prison in September 1985, the reporter, Diana Waggoner, writes:

> He [Streleski] spent eight years contemplating grievances against Stanford and plotting a murder, systematically drawing up a short list of candidates. . . . "The essential thing was to be able to badmouth Stanford and do it with some impact," he says. "I considered other alternatives . . . I considered going to the media directly." He rejected the last option as simply impractical. "I realized that I had no leverage," he explains. "Television and the media don't cover struggling graduate students. But they do cover murderers." For Professor Karel W. deLeeuw, 48, a former Fulbright scholar and the father of three children, that dispassionate rationale was a death sentence.[37]

On August 18, 1978, Streleski packed a two-pound sledgehammer into a small flight bag and left his apartment in San Francisco for the Stanford campus. After arriving in Palo Alto, he walked to the mathematics department and waited. After deLeeuw arrived at his office and had time to settle down, Streleski stepped inside.

> "He was sitting with his back to the door," Streleski recalls without apparent emotion. "I walked directly behind him. I hit him squarely on the top of the head with the hammer and then administered two or three of what I call 'insurance blows' to the right temple. . . . He rolled back to the storage cabinet. At some point I heard what I presume was a death rattle. I covered him with a clean garbage bag like a shroud to save the feelings of the janitor who would probably find him."[38]

Streleski's surrender was equally carefully planned. After taking a train back to San Francisco, he thoughtfully called his ex-wife's family "to warn them that there might be some legal problems." He then returned to Palo Alto, had a beer and a slice of pizza, waited in a bus shelter reading a novel until 3 A.M. the next morning, then walked to a police station, turned himself in, and handed over the bloodied hammer carefully wrapped in a plastic bag.

When Streleski came to trial in 1979, a court-appointed attorney assigned to defend him wanted him to plead not guilty by reason of insanity. Streleski refused. However, he could not prevent psychiatrists from testifying that he, Streleski, was very sick, suffering from paranoid psychosis, and therefore lacked the capacity to commit murder. Perhaps because this testimony was uncontradicted, or perhaps because Streleski's behavior struck people as obviously that of a crazy person, the jury concluded that Streleski suffered from diminished capacity and found him guilty only of second degree murder. Seven years later, to the accompaniment of much media attention, Streleski was released. "'My feeling for the jury is mellow,' he says, 'because they gave me the use of the word 'murderer' at the cheapest possible cost. . . . The publicity has been used as a weapon against Stanford. I think I got out of the murder what I wanted.'" Comments Waggoner, displaying the proper deference toward our reigning mythology: "That may be so, but others take a *more rational* view" (emphasis added).[39]

The problem, however, was, and is, not Streleski's rationality, but his morality. Streleski did not lack rationality in 1978, and does not lack it now. Nor does he lack intentionality. On the contrary, his capacity to form intention is arguably superior to that of an average, normal person. What Streleski lacks is modesty, self-restraint, and respect for the lives of certain human beings whom he feels entitled to try, judge, and execute.

Here is another famous example of increased capacity officially portrayed as diminished capacity. On October 21, 1985, Dan White, a former member of the San Francisco Board of Supervisors who, in 1978, shot and killed Mayor George Moscone and Supervisor Harvey Milk, committed suicide. To virtually everyone, this confirmed the judgment that White was a victim of mental illness and thus provided further validation for the legitimacy of his successful diminished capacity defense. Certainly, if one views crime through the lenses of psychiatric excuses, then White's suicide furnishes the ultimate proof of his insanity. Revealingly, even some of Milk's supporters saw White's death in this light. "It comes as no surprise," said Supervisor Harry Britt, the gay politician who succeeded Milk on the board, "that Dan White was a very disturbed man." Added writer and gay advocate George Mendenhall: "[The suicide] points to the fact that Dan White was a mentally disturbed person."[40] Douglas Schmidt, the lawyer who secured White's courtroom victory, put it even more strongly: "Now what has happened seems to vindicate our position."[41] Martin Blinder, the San Francisco psychiatrist who achieved instant fame with his infamous "Twinkie defense," also used the suicide to support the interpretation that White had been mentally ill and that his illness caused him to commit homicide and suicide. "White killed out of a depressive despair," opined Blinder. "The suicide is entirely consistent with my diagnosis seven years ago."[42]

I found these interpretations objectionable at the time of White's trial and find them obscene now.[43] Consider the evidence. White was a morally sensitive man: He objected to homosexuality as ethically repugnant. He was a devout Catholic: He gave himself up to a priest after the shooting. If White really had diminished capacity for murder—in plain English, if he had truly *not intended* to kill Milk and Moscone—then he would have regretted the tragedy he had inadvertently caused and would not have needed to feel guilty. But evidently he did feel guilty. People who do horrible things to other people often do. Judas felt guilty and killed himself. Lady Macbeth felt guilty and killed herself. We do not interpret their suicides as evidence of their having been mentally ill, but rather as evidence of their having done evil deeds. It seems only reasonable to view White as no less human and hence no less responsible, and to interpret his suicide as evidence of his guilt for the evil he had done.

Let us reexamine White's famous diminished capacity defense in the light of his suicide. What, exactly, did it consist of? Why was there such an outrage in the San Francisco gay community against it? Thanks to the "Twinkie defense," White was convicted of voluntary manslaughter instead of murder. Who benefited from this? Clearly, White's lawyers and psychiatrists: they made money and gained fame from it. But how did White profit from this great courtroom victory? He received a shorter prison sentence than he would have if he had been convicted of murder. But perhaps a longer, more appropriate prison sentence would have enabled White to atone for his sins and, by saving his soul, might have saved his life. The liberal conscience may abolish the execution of persons who have perpetrated horrible crimes, but the conscience of the perpetrators may still demand that they pay the ultimate penalty. Like anyone not completely duped by psychiatry, White too must have felt that his defense was as phony as a three-dollar bill. He must have known—like any unprejudiced observer could infer—that his crime constituted a carefully orchestrated performance: The way he got into the building where his victims were, the way he selected his victims, the way he killed them, the way he gave himself up—every detail of this tragedy tells us something we do not, dare not, admit. What? That White's killing of Moscone and Milk showed evidence of increased, rather than diminished, mental capacity to commit a crime. (By which I mean simply that he was more capable of killing than the law's hypothetical average, ordinary person.)

Although in the past psychiatrists and priests have often bitterly disagreed, they now agree—ironically, precisely where psychiatry most decisively betrays religion and where religion betrays itself. Despite having killed himself, Dan White was given a Roman Catholic burial. "The church will not judge Dan White's soul," a spokesman for the San Francisco archdiocese told the *San Francisco Chronicle:*

> Traditionally [explained the *Chronicle*], suicide among Roman Catholics was considered a mortal sin against the laws of God, and the victim was denied the last holy rites of the church and the right to be buried in consecrated ground. "Things have changed today," said the archdiocesan spokesman. "Today it is the church's feeling that a person must be crazy to commit suicide. And we place the insane in the hands of God, for his mercy and his judgment."[44]

I cannot accept that the church feels it is its duty to judge the conduct of persons who use condoms to prevent conception, but feels it is not its duty to judge the much more important deeds of cold-blooded murder and self-determined death. Indeed, I find it hard to imagine what would constitute a more blatant evasion of a moral authority's duty to judge the issues of intentionality, moral agency, and personal responsibility than the Catholic Church's stand on suicide, exemplified by the life and death of Dan White—or what could constitute a more dramatic example and symbol of our collective flight from moral responsibility.

WHY INSANITY EQUALS NONRESPONSIBILITY (AND VICE VERSA)

In the primitive or so-called animistic world view, all the calamities that befall man are believed to be caused by human beings or agents conceived in the image of human beings (gods, spirits). It was a momentous advance of the human mind to abandon this view and accept that many undesirable things in life, such as storms or earthquakes, are not the deliberate works of enemies or evil spirits, but the consequences of natural events. By and by, people started to regard bodily diseases too as natural events, for which neither the patient nor anyone else was responsible. For example, we do not blame people for having Hodgkin's disease. However, our understanding of this sort of nonresponsibility was quickly qualified, as we learned that although a person may not be responsible for having, say, diabetes, he may be responsible for his obesity which precipitates or aggravates it. Accordingly, we now sometimes consider people to be responsible for their lifestyles which might cause them to develop certain diseases.

In general, then, while we do not consider medical patients to be responsible for being ill, we do consider them, despite their illness, to be responsible for what they do with their lives. This is especially so when the illness is chronic, in which case we typically consider the patient responsible for managing his disease. For example, although we do not regard a diabetic as responsible for having diabetes, we view him as responsible for managing his diabetes. Thus, while arteriosclerosis and AIDS, Parkinsonism and pyelitis, leukemia and lung cancer are all diseases, none makes a person so afflicted not responsible for beating his wife, robbing a bank, or killing people. In contrast, mental illness typically confers precisely this sort of total nonresponsibility on its victims. Why should this be so? Why do psychiatrists and the law not treat psychotics like physicians and the law treat diabetics—regarding them as not responsible for their disease, but responsible for their deeds? The fact that they do not reveals what, *inter alia*, the idea of mental illness really means: namely, nonresponsibility—not only for one's condition, but for virtually any aspect of one's conduct as well.*

Largely because of the effect the idea of mental illness has exercised, for more than 200 years, on the Western mind, and especially on the concept of responsibility, many people are now profoundly confused about who is, or ought to be, held responsible for certain actions and consequences. For example, some people who smoke and develop lung cancer claim that not they, but the tobacco companies that manufacture cigarettes, are responsible for their illness. Many lawyers and psychiatrists agree with them.

Similarly, most Americans now believe that people who use illegal drugs do so not because they choose to, but because they have a mysterious propensity to use certain drugs, and when they are exposed to these chemicals, have an irresistible impulse to subject themselves to their effect. This is why drug abuse is now treated as both a disease and a crime.

---

*In an article published anonymously nearly 30 years ago, a former mental patient contends—rather naively, without realizing that insanity by definition negates responsibility—that the psychotic person is responsible not only for his behavior but for his illness as well: "Simple schizophrenics, hebephrenics, and catatonics 'prove'—by words and actions which are louder than words—that they are not responsible. . . . The real truth is that the schizophrenic is responsibly guilty of some crucial misdeeds."[45]

All this points to a profound disorientation—especially in the United States—concerning the grounds for deciding whether or not a person is responsible for his behavior. One of the symptoms of this disorientation is the liability insurance crisis now plaguing the country; yet this serious socioeconomic problem is never linked (though it should be), much less attributed (as in part it well might be), to psychiatry's unrelenting war on responsibility.[46]

Responsibility Lost and Regained

Critical consideration of the connections between mental illness and responsibility thus points to a relationship of profound negation: As death negates life, insanity negates responsibility. It is not so much, as is commonly believed, that insanity diminishes or annuls the mentally ill person's capacity for responsibility; instead, it is rather that our idea of insanity itself negates our concept of responsibility. Although it appears as if nonresponsibility were a condition separate from insanity but sometimes caused by it (like anemia may sometimes be caused by cancer, each condition, nevertheless, being a distinct and separate phenomenon), in fact nonresponsibility and insanity are essentially synonymous (like poverty and lack of money, two terms for one phenomenon). This identity of meaning is epitomized by the symbolic significance of the insanity defense in modern law—namely, the view that where there is no intention to commit a crime, a crime requiring intention cannot be said to have been committed; and that, because an insane person lacks the ability to form intent, he is, ipso facto, innocent of such crimes by reason of insanity. This double presumption leads to a pat and predictable scenario which is typically presented as if it were an astounding revelation. Whenever the perpetrator of a spectacular crime is tried, what is revealed to us, time and again, is that the criminal is a victim rather than a victimizer. The story of Billy Milligan is typical.

In 1977, when he was 22 years old, William Stanley Milligan kidnapped, raped, and robbed a series of women in Columbus, Ohio, and was subsequently acquitted of all his crimes on the ground of insanity. What gave his story special journalistic appeal—he was the subject of scores of articles and of a major book—was that Milligan claimed to have anywhere from 10 to 24 *personalities*, that this claim was not seriously contested in court, and that, as a result, he was the first person in the history of American jurisprudence to have been acquitted on the ground that he suffered from a disease called *multiple personality*. Characteristically, the book on Milligan tells us very little about what he did to his victims, but tells us a lot about what others allegedly did to him. According to the dust jacket, the author presents:

> . . . [the] moving true story of Billy Milligan—a tortured man who must live with twenty-four separate personalities contained within one body. The astounded reader gets to know them all . . . forcing us to understand and sympathize with a very special human being . . . . Above all, it is the frightening and touching revelation of Billy's evolving selves that seizes the imagination and holds the reader spellbound as a victimized boy grows to fractured manhood.[47]

It seems that if something is presented as psychiatric science, the public now believes it no matter how absurd. Perhaps the more absurd, the more believable: *Credo quia absurdum.*

Mens Rea: Guilty Intent or Rational Intent?

Clearly, insofar as people want to dispose of certain troublesome persons in society by means of coercive psychiatric interventions, they will find justifications for such a policy. Accordingly, showing that insane persons who commit crimes possess no less intent—or perhaps even more intent—than do sane persons will not change the minds of the believers in insanity: they will merely fall back to what may, at present, be their strongest position, namely, the argument that the insane person is irrational and hence not a moral agent. Since this claim is a tautology, there is no way to disprove it. The most one can do is to describe it carefully and clearly.

Consider a man, like John Hinckley, Jr., who shoots the President of the United States—and three other men—and then explains that he did it to impress a young actress whom he idolized from afar. If I suggest, as well I might, that Hinckley wanted to shoot President Reagan, the believer in mental illness is likely to respond: "Well, perhaps, but if that isn't an irrational (insane) thing to do, I don't know what is." Since my imaginary interlocutor believes that shooting a bank teller while robbing a bank is rational, but shooting Ronald Reagan to impress Jody Foster is not, there is not much more we can say to each other. Moreover, since my interlocutor equates irrationality with insanity, insanity with lack of intentionality, and lack of intentionality with lack of *mens rea*—presto, John Hinckley, Jr. is not responsible for his criminal act.*

---

*In 1952, the conventional judgment of the contemporary reasonable person that a crazy deed can only be the deed of a crazy person was given the imprimatur of the United States Supreme Court, which ruled, in *Leland v. Oregon,* that while a legally insane

This is exactly the conclusion Moore reaches when he asserts that "one is a moral agent only if one is a rational agent." Moore even acknowledges the self-referential character of the idea of rationality, for he states: "Only if we can see another being as one who acts to achieve some rational end . . . will we understand him in the same fundamental way that we understand ourselves and our fellow persons in everyday life."[49] Since most people cannot, or do not want to, put themselves in Hinckley's shoes, by Moore's criteria of rationality, Hinckley is irrational. The fact remains, however, that irrationality has nothing whatever to do with diminished or absent intentionality. On the contrary, irrational persons are likely to be more stubborn—that is, more persistently intentional—than rational persons.

Actually, the so-called crazy criminal confronts us with a relatively simple choice between two ways of punishing him: namely, by depriving him of property, liberty, or life (fine, imprisonment, execution), usually called *punishment* or *criminal sanctions;* or by depriving him of his status as a moral agent (psychiatric incarceration, lobotomy, electroshock, drugging), now called *psychiatric diagnosis* and *treatment.* Because of their uncritical endorsement of the psychiatric ideology, most people—that is, leaders in psychiatry and law and their multitudinous following—do not articulate the choice this way: instead, they say it is a choice between *punishing* a person because he is an *offender,* and *not punishing* him because he is a *mental patient.* This linguistic prejudgment, as Sir James Fitzjames Stephen has remarked, precludes changing our present criminal-psychiatric system of social controls. But why, exactly, do I think this system ought to be changed? Because it punishes persons both guilty and innocent of lawbreaking, the latter often more severely than the former; and because it nominally excuses persons guilty of crimes and then punishes them under medical auspices.

Although most experts on psychiatry and the law are satisfied with the conclusion that irrational persons are insane and hence not responsible for their acts, perhaps the reader is not, and I will therefore add a few more remarks on the intentionality of the so-called insane criminal. Typically, an insane criminal is a person who kills his wife or children, allows himself to be captured without trying to elude the police, and explains his act by stating: "God told me to do it." In our day and age, that statement—in conjunction with the act—is accepted as irrefutable proof that the killer is insane. Indeed, such an act together

---

person may have the intent required for a crime, it is an "insane intent."[48] The legal literature on insanity, diminished capacity, and related matters all bear upon, and illustrate, the contention that, in a crucially important sense, mental illness in all its guises is a legal fiction (see Chapter 11).

with such an explanation is now viewed as similar to a disfiguring tumor that has eaten away a part of a person's face or body: the former person is as obviously suffering from insanity (psychosis) as the latter is from cancer (a malignant neoplasm). If insanity is defined by being so exemplified, then, of course, that is the end of the matter. But it is not the end of the matter of intentionality; on the contrary, it is its beginning, and a very interesting beginning it is.

Suppose that Jones tells Smith "Please close the door," whereupon Smith gets up from his seat, walks to the door, and closes it. Would we say that Smith did not intend to close the door? That he lacked the capacity to form an intent to close the door? Of course not. What we would say, instead, is that Smith decided to close the door and that his decision was based on Jones's request. However, when a person identified as insane offers an explanation of exactly the same type—by asserting, for example, that God told him to kill his wife—we foreclose the possibility of seeing his intentionality in such a commonsensical way. Instead we obscure the obvious by saying either that the insane actor is irrational and hence not responsible; or that his act was not based on choice, decision, or intent (as previously described), but on an irresistible impulse. Actually, long before this question became a pressing legal problem, Hobbes had struggled with it and concluded: "*Fools* and *madmen* manifestly *deliberate* no less than the wisest men, though they make not so good a *choice*" (emphasis in the original).[50] Does, then, the view that the mentally ill person is incapable of intending, planning, and controlling his antisocial actions—as formulated by psychiatrists and psychoanalysts—represent scientific progress, as it is now generally believed? Or does it represent a stubborn denial of certain obvious but painful facts of life—as I maintain—and hence a profound retrogression to prescientific thinking?

THE UNHOLY MATRIMONY OF PSYCHIATRY AND LAW

It is stating the obvious that if a bitterly unhappy marriage long endures, husband and wife must be both its victims and beneficiaries. The same goes for the unholy matrimony between psychiatry and the law: We—the American people—are both its victims and beneficiaries. By enabling us to divert certain criminals from the penal to the psychiatric system, the fiction of mental illness as destroyer of *mens rea* protects us from guilt for punishing guilty but crazy criminals; by eschewing formally punishing—and, as a result, by capriciously underrestraining and overrestraining—persons guilty of crimes, this fiction endangers the safety of our persons and property and the integrity of our political system.

The following story exemplifies the way our safety is now endangered by the policy of diverting so-called crazy criminals from the penal to the psychiatric system. A young man is committed, for the eighth time in his life, to a North Carolina State Hospital because of mental illness manifested by "violent behavior that included attacks on family members." On the day the patient is scheduled to be released, his parents meet with the psychiatrist and plead with him not to release the patient, who is still threatening to harm the family. Nevertheless, the patient is released the same day. That night he stabs his sister approximately 20 times.[51]

My long-held contention that psychiatric excuses are no less ill-founded than psychiatric incriminations, and that their consequences are perhaps even more disastrous, is illustrated almost daily by reports of crimes committed by criminals allowed to go unpunished because of psychiatrists. The following story is typical:

Fired Bay Worker Kills Ex-Boss, Dies in Gun Battle

(January 7, 1986) A one-time federal auditor ambushed and killed his former boss yesterday in a Sunnyvale office park . . . . The attacker had been fired and convicted of extortion for making threats against his bosses in the past. Court records reveal that he had been spared prison after a psychiatrist advised that he was not dangerous. . . . "In my opinion, the threats that he made were a situational response and unlikely to be repeated," psychiatrist Karen Gudiksen of Oakland wrote [in December 1984] . . . . Miller was placed on three years probation.[52]

Unfortunately, there is, literally, no end today to such stories. But one more should suffice. On October 22, 1985, a young woman, named Mary Ventura, recently released from a mental hospital, pushed another young woman, Catherine Costello, under a subway train in New York. When apprehended, Miss Ventura said, "I am sick." "Yes, Miss Ventura is sick," echoed an editorial in *The New York Times*.[53] Miss Ventura, we are to understand, is not responsible for her act. Who is? "Society has to accept the responsibility for what Mary Ventura did . . ." declares Matthew Brody, director of mental health for the Brooklyn Academy of Medicine, in a letter to the *Times*.[54] Psychiatrists insist that because mental patients *have* mental diseases, they are not responsible for their criminal actions. I maintain that because *psychiatrists* believe in mental diseases, they are responsible for causing havoc in our society.

A hundred years ago in Russia, there was not much to celebrate when it came to civil liberties, and today there is still less. We have similarly gone from bad to worse with respect to legal psychiatry. About a hundred years ago Mark Twain was moved to observe:

> Of late years it does not seem possible for a man to so conduct himself, before killing another man, as not to be manifestly insane. If he talks about the stars, he is insane. If he appears nervous and uneasy an hour before the killing, he is insane. If he weeps over a great grief, his friends shake their heads, and fear that he is "not right." If, an hour after the murder, he seems ill at ease, preoccupied, and excited, he is unquestionably insane. Really, what we want now, is not laws against crime, but a law against *insanity*. There is where the true evil lies.[55]

Mark Twain was more celebrated than heeded. Just as he was denouncing forensic psychiatry, Americans began their love affair with it.

Disjoining Rights and Responsibilities

Central to the contemporary argument favoring the general idea that insanity annuls responsibility—and in particular the idea that the insanity defense is morally desirable and practically necessary—is the denial that liberty and responsibility are two sides of the same coin. In fact, it is not possible to increase or diminish one without increasing or diminishing the other. "Liberty," said George Bernard Shaw, "means responsibility. That is why most men dread it."[56] The truth of this proposition is illustrated by the fact that Shaw's aphorism works just as well if it is turned around: "Responsibility means liberty. That is why most men dread it." This is indeed why not only many so-called mental patients, but many so-called normal persons as well, dread and reject responsibility.

Ignoring the organic connections between individual liberty and personal responsibility, the typical expert on psychiatry and the law—regardless of whether he is psychiatrist or lawyer—now advocates holding insane persons less and less responsible while giving them more and more rights. The result is an overt deprivation of responsibility and a covert deprivation of liberty, the latter masked by a deceptive rhetoric of fictitious rights.

Among these fictitious rights, the involuntary mental patient's right to treatment stands out as a monument to the hypocrisy of our Age of Madness. As I have shown elsewhere, the patient's right to treatment is, in fact, the psychiatrist's right to torture the patient in the name of treatment.[57]

Typical of the enthusiasm for *nominally* disjoining rights and responsibilities—I emphasize *nominally* because they cannot actually be disjoined any more than, say, competitive games can be disjoined from winning and losing—is Stephen J. Morse's simultaneous advocacy of the insanity defense and of a penumbra of rights for insanity acquittees (that is, persons acquitted of a criminal charge as not guilty by reason of insanity). How is it possible to assume such a self-contradictory posture? One of the things that makes it possible is using a debauched version of the English language (see Chapter 11). Thus, Morse, a professor of law at the University of Southern California, pontificates about "the actor's dangerousness and *need for incarceration*" (emphasis added),[58] as if the lawbreaker had a need to be incarcerated. But, of course, he does not; if he did, we would not need a system of law enforcement.

Nor is this all. Morse's intellectual repertoire contains such other items as the certain knowledge that "all behavior is caused. Causation is not the issue [in the insanity defense]; nonculpable lack of rationality and compulsion is."[59] By substituting culpable and nonculpable rationality for willed and caused action, Morse thinks he has offered an irrefutable justification for the insanity defense—and for psychiatrically punishing people so long as we call the punishment *treatment.*

Finally, Morse's compassion for the criminal who *needs* incarceration leads him to conclude that "We should not abolish the insanity defense unless we truly believe that every perpetrator of a criminal act deserves to be punished, no matter how crazy. If we do not believe this, and I do not see how we can, then we must retain the defense."[60] Morse may not be able to see how we can adopt such a position, but I can. And the reason I can is because if it is our intention, as it is mine, to *not disjoin* rights and responsibilities—regardless of whether a person calls himself crazy or others do so—then we must not only refrain from depriving the innocent person of liberty, but must also hold the guilty person responsible for his criminal acts.

It is important to note here that the penchant for disjoining the insane person's rights and responsibilities is a relatively recent development in psychiatry. Throughout the nineteenth century, and even as relatively recently as when I was young, psychiatrists saw the insane patient as a person similar to the infant and the idiot; accordingly, he had neither rights nor responsibilities. Such a person was then not only excused from crimes, but was also incarcerated in a mental hospital, often for life. At the same time, although such a patient had no responsibilities in the formal, legal sense of that term, he was expected to take care of himself, other patients, and the institution in which he was housed, much as a child is expected to help his parents. In short, the relationship between psychiatrist and patient was then *paternalistic* and *coercive,* but *predictable.*

The contemporary psychiatrist sees the mental patient as neither a full-fledged moral agent, nor as a completely insane person devoid of rights and responsibilities. This is why there is unceasing debate and disagreement—among psychiatrists, mental patients, lawyers, and courts—about the precise range of the patient's rights and responsibilities, which are disjoined and asymmetrical. This disjunction and asymmetry has now reached absurd and bizarre proportions, as the following examples illustrate.

On October 1, 1985, an Arizona Superior Court judge ruled on a suit brought by four former mental hospital patients asking the court to require "the state to provide comprehensive mental health services to its 7800 chronically mentally ill residents," a service estimated to cost more than 55 million dollars a year.[61] One of the plaintiffs in this case was a man, Cliff Dorsett, whose right to sue the State of Arizona was apparently not compromised by his nonresponsibility for two remarkable crimes. In 1966 Dorsett killed ("murdered," according to the newspaper story from which I quote) a woman, was acquitted as not guilty by reason of insanity, and was committed to a state hospital for treatment. The treatment was so successful that a year later he was released. Two months after being released, Dorsett killed (again "murdered," according to the newspaper story) another woman, "leaving her body in south Phoenix and her head in Glendale [a Phoenix suburb]." Eight years later Dorsett was again released. He died of emphysema in 1984, before he could enjoy his courtroom victory over the state of Arizona.[62] Evidently, when a man like Cliff Dorsett kills and kills again, American law does not regard him as a moral agent at all and does not hold him responsible for his crimes; but when he sues the state for "mental health care," the law regards him as a full-fledged moral agent and accords him the right to use the legal system to coerce the taxpayers of Arizona to provide treatment for his mental illness. Alice would never have dreamt of such a wonderland.

Here is another example of the labyrinthine disjunctions of rights and responsibilities characteristic of the present social situation of mental patients. Federal law now permanently denies former committed mental patients their Second Amendment rights to keep and bear arms. In 1985, a group called "Coalition for the FREE"* brought suit on behalf of a

---

*The participants of the Coalition are: The National Mental Health Association; Mental Patients' Liberation Front, Inc.; Share of Daytona Beach, Florida; The Mental Patients Association of New Jersey; The Mental Patients Association of Philadelphia; and The Mandala Group (of Billings, Montana). So far as I know, none of these groups has addressed the parallel issue of the mental patient's *responsibility*, namely, that if the mental patient has a right to bear arms, he must also have the duty (right) to be held responsible for any crimes he commits with them.

former mental patient, Anthony Galioto, challenging this law.[63] After the U.S. District Court for the District of New Jersey ruled in favor of the plaintiff, the case was appealed to the Supreme Court of the United States. The Coalition then filed a brief of amicus curiae arguing that the statute should be declared unconstitutional because it "irrationally discriminates" against former mental patients. The Supreme Court has agreed to hear the case. The brief is an eloquent plea for according former mental patients the same rights as are accorded other Americans:

> . . . by assuring that even convicted felons have the possibility of being rehabilitated for purposes of acquiring firearms, while totally denying such rehabilitation to former mental patients, the federal statutes are a classic example of the irrational discriminations that still exist against many former mental patients' fundamental American rights. . . . The issue of equal entitlement to licenses and privileges for former patients is clearly one aspect of this historical discrimination.[64]

Like all briefs on behalf of the rights of mental patients, this document makes no reference at all to holding mental patients, former or present, responsible for their crimes. I find it astonishing that advocates for mental patients continue to remain blind to the absurdity of ceaselessly clamoring for more rights for mental patients, but not for commensurately more responsibilities for them as well. Clearly, the reason for this is that they, too, believe in mental illness: "No one, least of all the *amici*," say the *amici*, "would urge the availability of firearms completely without reference to present mental illness."[65] In view of the definitions, meanings, and uses of mental illness, the *amici* act here like a sharpshooter who, while extolling his marksmanship, shoots himself in the foot.

Of course, some of the chickens are beginning to come home to roost—and others are sure to follow. If mental health professionals claim to be in the business of controlling their clients' behavior, and if they insist that their science tells them that mental patients are not responsible for their criminal behavior, then we should not be surprised that when a mental patient commits a crime, his therapist may be held liable for the damages. This happened in 1974 in the famous *Tarasoff* case[66] and again in 1985, in a case in Vermont.

In 1977, a 29-year-old man who had been a patient in a Counseling Center in Vermont burned down his father's barn. The circumstances, briefly, were as follows. The patient was a violent person with a long history of "impulsive assaults." A week before the incident, the patient's father asked him to falsify a Social Security document. An argument ensued in which the father called his son "mentally ill" and told him he belonged in a mental hospital. The patient told his therapist he was angry at his father and felt like burning down his barn. The therapist asked the patient to promise that he would not do so. The patient promised and then burned down the barn. The father sued and the Vermont Supreme Court found the Counseling Center liable for the damages.[67] In our secular age, this is as close as I expect to come to seeing divine punishment visited on my colleagues.

As the examples illustrate, persons denominated as *mental patients* now sometimes have more rights than responsibilities, and sometimes less. The result is that the relationship between psychiatrist and patient is today not only *paternalistic* and *coercive* but also *capricious.*

While the progenies of the unholy union of psychiatry and law may have been defective in Mark Twain's day, they are monstrous in ours. Indeed, they are like anencephalic Siamese twins: on the one side, mental patients so lacking in rationality and intentionality that they can never be held responsible for a crime; on the other, psychiatrists so grandiose and greedy that they eagerly assume the mutually incompatible responsibilities of treating the mental patient for his mental illness, and protecting everyone else from his criminal acts. Hovering anxiously over them are the members of the learned professions and the public—all doing their utmost to keep the twins alive in their parasitic embrace, lest the effort to separate them prove fatal, as if there was no fate worse than death.

PART FOUR:

THE PRACTICAL USES OF MENTAL ILLNESS

9

MENTAL ILLNESS
AS STRATEGY

You are to use the word purely as an incantation; if you like,
purely for its selling power.

—C. S. Lewis[1]

Sometimes the term *mental illness* is used as if it designated an identifiable condition like diabetes or a pattern of habitual behavior like neatness: an organic psychosis is indeed such a condition, and anorexia nervosa is indeed such a pattern of behavior. More often, however, the term refers to a strategy rather than a condition—exemplified by the Group for Advancement of Psychiatry's (GAP) definition of mental illness as "an illness which so lessens the capacity of a person to use (maintain) his judgment, discretion, and control in the conduct of his affairs and social relations as to warrant his commitment to a mental institution.[2] The GAP advances this definition as if it were *describing a disease* when, in fact, it is *prescribing a disposition.*

DEFINITIONS: DESCRIPTIVE AND DISPOSITIONAL

Every person of average intelligence and education knows that language may be used in two quite different modes: namely, to assert or describe, and to advocate or prescribe. For example, we can say, "The door is closed" or "Please close the door." Although the difference between these two modes of communication is obvious, misunderstanding or denying it lies at the heart of much of the confusion and controversy concerning psychiatric matters.

As I have noted, the phrase *mental illness* appears to refer to a condition, but typically refers to a strategy. Or, to put it differently, mental illness terms are often used as if they were descriptions of psychopathological conditions from which individuals suffer—when, in fact, they function as prescriptions for how individuals allegedly suffering from such conditions should be treated by others. I point here to a simple, but officially forbidden, truth about psychiatry—namely, that its practitioners often *first decide* what to do about a person, and *then discover* the appropriate diagnostic label with which to justify their decision. For example, if a psychiatrist wants to commit a person, he discovers that the patient is dangerously psychotic; if he wants to get him acquitted of a criminal charge by reason of insanity, he discovers that the patient was, at the precise moment of his criminal act, suffering from a mental illness that deprived him of criminal responsibility; if he wants to provide an abortion for a woman in a country where the only legal abortions are those deemed to be therapeutic, then he discovers that she suffers from a mental illness for which the indicated treatment is an abortion.

One of the advantages—or disadvantages—of focusing on the strategic meanings of mental illness terms is that it frees us from having to decide whether statements using such terms are true or false. The sentence "Please close the door" is neither true nor false. Instead, it is a command or injunction, expressing a desire and prescribing an action: we may approve or disapprove the desire, obey or disobey the order. When asked to close the door, we may reply: "Yes, sir, right away"; or "I understand you want the door closed, but I prefer that it stay open"; or "If you want the door closed, you close it." However, it would be non-sensical to say: "You are right." Let us apply these considerations to some of the confusions concerning mental illness.

Suppose someone says: "Jones suffers from schizophrenia." As a descriptive statement, we could agree or disagree and hence say something like, "Yes, you are right, he does," or "No, you have made a mistake, he does not." Both answers imply that schizophrenia exists, that Jones may or may not have it; and that even if Jones does not have it, some other people do. However, both answers are misleading and mistaken, because the sentence *Jones suffers from schizophrenia* is only seemingly descriptive, but is actually prescriptive. Its prescriptive meaning may be any of the following: "Jones should be confined in a mental hospital; should be acquitted as insane of the crimes he has committed; should not be taken seriously for the views he holds"; and so forth. Once we have translated mental illness from description to prescription, we no longer have to accept or reject the assertion about mental illness (see Chapter 11). We are now liberated, so to speak, to respond to the injunction—previously implicit but now explicit—with a clear rejoinder of our own concerning the recommended action.

Perhaps the most obvious use of the idea of mental illness occurs in the context of commitment, exemplified in my initial example of the GAP's definition of it as, in effect, committability. To see clearly why this is not a definition of a *condition*, we need to construct an analogous definition of, say, myocardial infarction. A coronary occlusion would then be defined as a disease which so lessens the competence of a person's cardiac function as to warrant his observation in a hospital's intensive care unit. Although such a statement describes what may happen to a person as a consequence of his suffering a heart attack, no cardiologist would accept it as a definition of the disease called *myocardial infarction.*

So we must go back to our starting point—the fact that the central epistemological muddle of psychiatry derives from the fact that while the term *mental illness* seemingly refers to an abnormality or illness similar to, or identical with, a bodily disease, in fact it denotes no objectively identifiable condition or phenomenon. Accordingly, in keeping with the principle that the meaning of an abstract noun such as *insanity* must be inferred from its actual use, I shall now identify, describe, and illustrate the principal uses/meanings of *mental illness*. (Since *mental illness* functions mainly as a strategic term, I have already touched on some of its such uses, and will touch on others in the chapters that follow.)

Mental Illness as Accusation or Incrimination

Descriptions of the psychoses in psychiatric textbooks are a rich source of illustrations of the accusatory uses/meanings of mental illness terms, as the following cases, culled from *Noyes' Modern Clinical Psychiatry* (7th ed.), illustrate.

The first story begins with this sentence: "P.G. was committed to a hospital for mental disease because of his peculiar religious ideas and rites, one of them being the practice of going about nude."[3] If we look at this sentence without any psychiatric prejudgments, it makes very little sense. In the first place, every religious idea is peculiar to those who do not share it. Furthermore, in free societies, holding peculiar religious ideas is considered to be an essential aspect of individual liberty and political freedom. Lastly, the meaning of *going about nude* depends on the context: in one's own home, it is a right; in a public place, it is a crime. Thus, from the very first sentence of this case history, we are confronted with a psychiatric account that purports to describe an illness (psychosis) a so-called patient has, while actually it justifies an act in which a psychiatrist engages (commitment). In this account we also get a glimpse of the collusion between patient and psychiatrist concerning the commitment:

> About this time [when he was 40 years old] he began to go to isolated spots and to walk about nude, explaining that he was taking "sun baths." Gradually he made fewer attempts to retire from sight when taking his "sun baths" . . . . Finally, after having been warned on repeated occasions by the local constable that he must not continue his exhibitionistic practices, the patient was committed to a hospital for mental disorders.[4]

The method in this madness is obvious enough. Evidently, this person wanted to drop out of the game of competitive adulthood and proceeded to do so in the manner prescribed in our society. To show that this pattern is typical rather than isolated, I shall cite two more case histories from the same textbook, illustrating similar collusions between psychotic and psychiatrist culminating in commitment.

The patient, "A.R."—diagnosed as suffering from simple schizophrenia—was first a poor student and then a poor worker. When he reached the age of 19, he gave up his job as a machine operator in a factory and showed no further interest in securing employment. When asked if he worked, he replied, "'What do I want to work for? I have a father and sister working and they are enough.' He appeared quite self-satisfied and felt that he should have a position of importance."[5] At this point, A.R. was arrested for peeping into women's bedrooms. Through the influence of his father, the charge was dropped. A year later he was again arrested but again was released on the intercession of his father. Since these strategies failed to achieve what seemed to be their intended effect, the patient escalated his symptoms:

> He came to say little unless addressed and grew antagonistic toward his father and sister. He would remain out until midnight and then come home, eat a large meal, read until 2 A.M. and sleep until noon. Finally, after his third arrest for peeping, he was committed to a hospital for mental disorders.[6]

"Such a case illustrates," comments Kolb, "how an individual is unable to complete the transition from adolescence to maturity with its adult heterosexual and social adjustments."[7] That may or may not be true. Kolb does not know, nor do I, whether this man was unable or unwilling to make this transition. In any case, I maintain that the imagery of illness and helplessness attached to such an individual functions as a justification for this particular psychiatric method of handling the problem. To be sure, in this sort of case the patient incriminates himself as a mental patient. After he does so long enough and persistently enough, his self-incrimination is given official sanction: he is diagnosed as suffering from schizophrenia and is committed.

The case history Kolb offers as typical of catatonic schizophrenia exhibits a similar pattern. The patient married when he was 20 and stopped working when he was 24. We are not told who supported him after that. What we are told is this:

> Two months before commitment the patient began to talk about how he had failed, had "spoiled" his whole life, that it was now "too late." He spoke of hearing someone say, "You must submit." One night his wife was awakened by his talking. He told her of having several visions but refused to describe them. He stated that someone was after him and trying to blame him for the death of a certain man. He had been poisoned, he said . . . . He had periods of laughing and shouting and became so noisy and unmanageable that it was necessary to commit him.[8]

Again the pattern seems clear enough. The patient produces symptoms which have the effect of coercing those about him to do something, hopefully to take care of him. Sooner or later, psychiatrists are called on to produce a diagnosis of mental illness which has the effect of counter-coercing the patient into commitment.

Some of the foregoing examples may seem dated, and indeed they are: I cite them to illustrate the paradigmatic strategic meaning/use of mental illness. At the moment it is legally and psychiatrically fashionable to commit only those persons whose mental illness renders them "dangerous to themselves or others." Accordingly, psychiatrists now manipulate the psychiatric vocabulary so as to justify forcibly ejecting chronic mental patients from state mental hospitals, a process they call *deinstitutionalization.* Not surprisingly, people now complain that psychiatrists refrain too much from committing crazy people, with the result that the patients end up in prison. The following comment in *The New York Times* is typical:

> To get someone committed the patient has to behave in a way that would get the same person arrested. Not eating, wandering the streets, refusing medical or psychiatric care are not considered legal causes for commitment . . . we criticize the Soviet Union for institutionalizing political dissidents, while we send our mentally ill to prisons.[9]

The fact that the problems to which this writer refers have nothing to do with medicine, illness, and treatment, but have everything to do with poverty, homelessness, and social deviance seems to get lost in the effort, in which nearly everyone now seems to want to participate, to manipulate the psychiatric vocabulary, and with it, both the psychiatrist and the mental patient.

Mental Illness as Excuse or Exoneration

For obvious reasons, mental illness terms are used to excuse or exculpate only in situations where a person has committed an illegal act or is accused of having committed such an act. People do not plead insanity for engaging in legal acts or meritorious deeds.

Before it was fashionable to plead insanity, it was customary to plead demonic possession. Indeed, current pleas of insanity do not differ much from old-fashioned pleas of demonic possession, as the following stories illustrate. In 1974, a 47-year-old Phoenix (Arizona) man rammed his car into the front door of St. Francis Xavier Catholic Church, then ran up the aisle and began destroying altar pieces. It took eight parishioners to restrain him. The police took him to the local psychiatric hospital where he told the officers: "I was possessed by the devil and he made me do it."[10]

The same claim made in 1981 by a young man in Connecticut charged with murder was supported not only by his relatives and friends but by his attorney as well. On February 16, 1981, Arne Cheyenne Johnson got into an argument with Alan Bono and stabbed him to death. According to *The New York Times*, the case involves

> a family that seems utterly convinced of the Devil's presence in their house and a defense attorney who intends to force evidence of that influence onto the court. "The courts have dealt with the existence of God," says Martin Minella, the attorney. "Now they're going to have to deal with the existence of the Devil."[11]

Johnson's girlfriend, Deborah Glatzel, told the lawyer and the reporters that her brother had said that "he had seen the beast [devil] go into Cheyenne's body and it was the beast who had committed the crime."[12] The reporter for the *Times* notes that this case arises at a time when there is a growing belief in the country in religion and cites a national Gallup Poll which showed that 34 percent of adults believe that "the Devil is a personal being who directs evil forces and influences people to do wrong."[13]

Of course, most of the remaining 66 percent of adults no doubt know it is mental illness that does it. In 1980, Michael Tindall, who had served as a helicopter pilot in Vietnam, was charged with taking part in smuggling hashish from Morocco to Gloucester, Massachusetts. He insisted that he did it "because of a need to relive the excitement he experienced in combat," and that this need was a symptom of his illness, the "Vietnam Syndrome." In September 1980, a federal court jury in Boston acquitted Tindall of the charges against him. "It was," reported a combined AP-UPI dispatch, "the first time the Vietnam Syndrome—an emotional malady recognized by the American Psychiatric Association and the Veterans Administration as post-traumatic stress—had been used successfully as a defense in connection with a premeditated crime."[14]

The assertion that being possessed by mental illness, rather than by the devil, excuses one from crime is stated in a more pretentious way by various legal formulas for determining the criminal responsibility of persons suspected of being insane. The Durham Rule, for example, asserts that "an accused is not criminally responsible if his unlawful act was the product of mental disease or mental defect."[15] It is important to keep in mind that all tests for the criminal responsibility of allegedly insane defendants rest on the premise that mental illnesses exist and cause people to commit illegal acts. While such a strategy of psychiatric mercy may now seem humane or even scientific to many people, it is in fact neither, as William Blackstone, the great English jurist, recognized more than 200 years ago:

> But this excuse [lunacy] ought not to be strained to the length to which our coroner's juries are apt to carry it, viz., that every act of suicide is an evidence of insanity; as if every man who acts contrary to reason had no reason at all; for the same argument would prove every other criminal *non compos*, as well as the self-murderer.[16]

Blackstone was referring, of course, to the novel strategy of evading the harsh punishments of the law against suicide by posthumously diagnosing the offender/victim as a lunatic. Perhaps because, in those cases, there was no question of psychiatrically examining the so-called patient, the strategic character of the diagnosis was clearer then than it is now.

Indeed, the evidence suggests that the strategic character of the idea of mental illness has been successfully obliterated from the consciousness of the modern intellectual. Consider by way of example the debate now raging among psychiatrists, medical ethicists, lawyers, and television commentators concerning the latest psychiatric dilemma, namely, mental illness in a death row inmate. Can a mentally ill person be executed? If not, should he receive appropriate treatment so that he may be?

This dilemma derives from the fact that, in American law, sanity is a requirement not only for executing a valid last will, but also for being validly executed. This requirement rests on two interconnected premises: One is that it is considered morally wrong to execute a person who does not understand he is about to die or the reasons for it; the other is that a seriously mentally ill person is considered to be just such a person. Obviously, this situation represents an irresistible invitation to death row inmates as well as their self-appointed benefactors for offering mental incapacity as an excuse. If the prisoner does not want to be executed, all he has to do is act crazy; if his lawyer does not want him executed, all he has to do is claim his client is crazy. In either case, officials are confronted with the question: Is the prisoner psychiatrically fit to be executed? Is he genuinely insane or only faking insanity? (See Chapter 5.) As we saw, it is not easy to tell the difference. Lay people can't do it. Lawyers can't do it. Only psychiatrists can do it. Here is a current example.

In 1974, Alvin Ford, then 24, killed a policeman while robbing a Red Lobster Restaurant in Fort Lauderdale, Florida. Tried and sentenced to death, Ford has spent the past 11 years on death row in the Florida State Prison. I do not know whether Ford prefers to be executed or imprisoned for the rest of his life. All I know is what I read in the newspapers, which say that Ford's lawyers claim he is insane and hence mentally unfit to be executed. Although lawyers and legal scholars never tire of telling us that insanity is a legal term without psychiatric significance, no sooner do they raise the question of insanity than they call for psychiatrists to verify their claim.

Ford's lawyers hired some shrinks who, not surprisingly, found Ford to be stark raving mad—a "paranoid schizophrenic." So armed, Ford's lawyers petitioned Governor Robert Graham to declare Ford unfit for execution. What could the governor do but hire his own shrinks? He got three of them. They examined Ford and, *mirabile dictu*, all three found him to be fit as a fiddle for execution. Does this mean that they found him to be sane? Not quite. No red-blooded American psychiatrist finds anyone sane, much less a murderer. Sane people don't kill. Only insane people do. Every sane person knows that. So what did these scientists of the mind find? Before answering this question, let me mention the behavior Alvin Ford is allegedly exhibiting.

Undoubtedly, by our usual standards of behavior, Ford is acting pretty crazy. The trouble is, we have no criteria for what constitutes normal behavior on death row. What would psychiatrists consider to be mentally healthy behavior on the part of a person who has seen fellow inmates executed and twice come within hours of execution himself, as Ford has? Actually, anyone familiar with Freudian ideas concerning adaptation to extreme stress by denial might say that Ford has coped quite well. He states, "I am not going to die. I'm the one who's in charge here. I make them put people in jail. I'm going to decide who gets killed." According to court records, when one of the state-appointed psychiatrists asked him, "Are you crazy?" Ford replied, "Are *you* crazy?"[17]

What, then, did the governor's psychiatrists find? Two found him to be "psychotic," but "competent for execution." The third concluded that Ford's "disorder was contrived and recently learned," in short, that he was malingering; he, too, found Ford to be mentally competent to be executed.

Ford's fate is now in the hands of America's demigods, the Justices of the United States Supreme Court: they are, of course, experts on mental illness just as they had been experts on slavery (see Chapter 11). To assist them in their deliberations, the APA lost no time filing an amicus brief on behalf of Ford. "A 30-minute interview," complained the psychoquacks," is inadequate to determine a prisoner's competency to be executed and violates his due process rights."[18] This assertion implies that a longer and differently structured interview would be adequate for determining—by *psychiatric methods*—whether or not a prisoner is mentally competent to be executed. We have been through this before. First, the psychoquacks claimed special professional competence to determine whether a defendant, at the precise moment when he committed a crime, could or could not form the intent to commit a crime; then they claimed such competence to determine whether a defendant, at the time of trial, is or is not mentally fit to be tried; now they claim such competence to determine whether a prisoner on death row is or is not mentally fit to be executed. I continue to maintain, however, that unlike the competence of the kidneys to secrete urine, competence to be executed is not the sort of thing for which a physician can examine a patient: The psychiatric examination is a charade to obscure the practical and moral problems at hand and the strategic character of the psychiatric intervention used to evade it.

The stupid mistake or stubborn strategy—the reader must decide which—of viewing insanity as a treatable illness rather than as a tactical maneuver leads to an important further step in cases such as Ford's. (Several such cases have been reported in the press during the past year.) A prisoner on death row awaiting execution presents a practical problem for the authorities—such as Governors and Justices of the

Supreme Court—who are, de facto as well de jure, in charge of his life and death. They have only two options: they must treat the prisoner either as sane and fit for execution or as insane and unfit for it. If they decide he is sane, they choose to execute a man who has been declared to be mentally ill and unfit for execution by—so some will say—conscientious, honorable, incorruptible medical professionals. On the other hand, if they decide he is insane, then—according to currently prevailing forensic-psychiatric standards and policies—they are obligated to ensure that he receives appropriate psychiatric treatment for his illness, no doubt from equally conscientious, honorable, incorruptible medical professionals. For what ultimate purpose? To make the prisoner sane enough so that he can be killed with the blessings of the rule of American law and the science of American psychiatry.

Although this dilemma clearly exposes the absurdity of the claim that mental illness is an illness (like any other); and although it clearly reveals that, under such circumstances, the *claim* of mental illness or mental health functions as a purely strategic device—all this is not only ignored, but inverted into further evidence of our need for psychiatric expertise. Indeed, the existential cannibals are already feasting on their prey. "How," ask two experts on such matters, "will the staff of a state mental hospital respond when they realize that successful treatment means the patient will die?"[19] Moreover, according to a report in *Psychiatric News*, "the patient's right to refuse treatment and the issue of informed consent further complicate such cases." But not to worry, the experts have a solution: "All inmates found incompetent to be executed should automatically be sentenced to life imprisonment. Otherwise . . . treatment of such prisoners would erode hospital morale . . . ."[20] Can the fakeries of psychiatry become any more brazen than this? I submit that instead of asking priests how many angels can dance on the head of a pin, we are now asking psychiatrists whether it is ethical for a physician to restore the sanity of an insane inmate on death row. The CAT scan, no doubt, will give us the answer.

Mental Illness as Denial of Moral Conflict and Evasion of Personal Responsibility

The acts of accusing and excusing, inculpating and exculpating, usually involve clear-cut issues and situations in which individuals are blamed or forgiven. But in certain situations involving moral conflicts and questions of personal responsibility, the lines between good and evil, right and wrong, legal and illegal are not so neatly drawn. In these situations, too, mental illness terms may be used strategically—to obscure guilt, to resolve ambivalence, to bring about a result justified by compassion, and so forth.

Long before the days of modern psychiatry, Shakespeare laid bare this tactical use of the idea of madness. Aided and abetted by his wife, Macbeth murders his way to the pinnacle of political power. His victory is spoiled, however. Lady Macbeth starts to hallucinate blood on her hands, is tormented by anguish, cannot rest or sleep. Her husband concludes that she is sick and sends for the doctor. But the doctor wants none of it. He tells Macbeth that his wife is "Not so sick, my lord / As she is troubled with thick-coming fancies, / That keep her from her rest." Macbeth is not satisfied. He presses the doctor with these immortal lines:

> Cure her of that!
> Canst thou not minister to a mind diseased,
> Pluck from the memory a rooted sorrow,
> Raze out the written troubles of the brain,
> And with some sweet oblivious antidote
> Cleanse the stuffed bosom of that perilous stuff
> Which weighs upon her heart?[21]

The doctor, however, recognizes that what ails this patient is not a disease. His famous answer is: "Therein the patient/Must minister to himself."[22] Lady Macbeth is not sick. She feels guilty for the wrong she has committed. Her husband knows this but does not want to admit it. The modern psychiatrist and the modern popular mind accept and legitimize precisely that intellectual and moral evasion which the doctor in *Macbeth* repudiates.

One of the crassest examples of the use of mental illness terms to obscure moral conflicts and avoid political decision making occurs in the relationship between psychiatrists and pregnant women. Since times immemorial, some pregnant women (and their husbands or lovers) have sought abortions. Until recently, performing abortions was medically unsafe as well as legally prohibited. In the post-World War II years, it became fashionable, in the United States as well as elsewhere, to allow pregnant women to have therapeutic abortions based not only on objectively verifiable medical criteria, such as severe renal disease with hypertension, but also on subjective and unverifiable psychiatric criteria, such as mental illness. For example, in 1968, a new abortion law was enacted in California permitting therapeutic abortions on mental health grounds. During the first six months of that year, almost 2000 women were found to require therapeutic abortions "to safeguard their mental health," while only 155 abortions were done to safeguard a woman's physical health. By the time the first nine months of 1968 had elapsed, 5000 therapeutic abortions were performed in California, virtually all of them for psychiatric reasons.[23] In the 1970s, when abortion was legalized, the psychiatric disabilities so common to pregnant women disappeared just as suddenly as they had appeared two decades earlier. Thus, whenever and wherever abortion on demand is illegal, but psychiatric therapeutic abortion is legal, the psychiatrist who prescribes an abortion follows in the footsteps of the physician who, during Prohibition, prescribed liquor.

Another arena in which mental illness terms are used to obscure moral conflict and evade personal responsibility is in connection with so-called drug abuse. The use of illegal psychoactive substances is now widespread throughout the world. Although it is obvious that no one is compelled to use such substances and that therefore, in the final analysis, people take drugs because they want to take them; and although it is also obvious that there are many complex cultural, religious, and legal reasons for the so-called drug problem—it is now fashionable to attribute the problem to the drug abusing person's mental illness. In addition, it is also fashionable to blame the drug itself and those who make it available—both the dope and the pusher being viewed as seducers infecting innocent individuals, who then succumb to the mental illness called *addiction*.[24]

Mental Illness as Denial of Human Depravity

The last strategic use/meaning of mental illness that I want to identify is its invocation to deny the depths of human depravity. We encounter this use of the term typically when a shocking crime—usually dubbed *bizarre* by the press—is committed and when the agent of that deed, though unknown, is instantly *diagnosed* as deranged or psychotic. Revealingly, the press often relapses into making use of the vocabulary of the alienists and mad-doctors in describing these alleged mental patients.

A typical story, appearing on page one of the *New York Post* on November 13, 1980, was headlined: "Angels stalk mad slasher." The subtitle added: "350-man patrol hunt for knife maniac."[25] This story concerned the search for a knife-wielding assailant who terrorized the lower East side of Manhattan and remained at large despite an intense effort to find him.

A similar story appeared in the *Syracuse Post-Standard* on October 10, 1980, a page-one headline informing the reader: "Cops hunt psycho in slaying of two in Buffalo." The first sentence of the UPI story explained further: "Several Buffalo area law enforcement agencies joined forces

Thursday in a hunt for a deranged, mentally disturbed person who killed two black cab drivers and cut their hearts from their bodies."[26] The authorities had no idea who the killer was; all they knew was that he was a *psycho.*

The New York Times uses more elegant language in reporting this sort of news. One of its typical headlines, placed discreetly on page 16, capping a story about a series of bizarre murders reads as follows: "Disturbed suspect is sought in seven ritualistic killings of Coast hikers." The report concerned the murder of seven women over a period of 15 months along the hiking trails near San Francisco. Although in this case, too, the identity of the killer or killers was an utter mystery to the authorities, the *Times* tried to tranquilize its readers with the following account:

> Although there were some dissimilarities in the cases—the two decomposing bodies were fully clothed, for example, while the latest victims were apparently forced to disrobe—Sheriff Howenstein said that the evidence pointed strongly to a single, severely disturbed killer.[27]

Note that these killings are called *ritualistic,* to insinuate the idea that the killer is insane. But it seems to me more obvious that what is ritualistic about this and similar cases is not the manner in which the crimes are committed but the manner in which they are reported—mental illness terms being used ritualistically to distract the reader from the evident depravity of the men and women who commit such crimes. I wonder, indeed, what sort of evidence Sheriff Howenstein (and other true believers in mental illness) would interpret as pointing strongly toward a *mentally healthy* mass murderer as the culprit?

Citing Sheriff Howenstein's opinion about the mental ill-health of this unknown killer was, moreover, merely the warm-up. The *Times* had an even more qualified authority on mental illness waiting in the wings to offer an opinion about the killer:

> A criminal psychologist's interpretation of evidence collected over the last year also indicated that the killer's mental state was further deteriorating . . . . The two murders Friday may have been an effort to call attention to the earlier murders in the same area.[28]

These pathetic fantasies are offered to insinuate the idea, now dear to the hearts of American madness-mongers, that every depraved act is a *cry for help* by a *victim.* But this is a truly perverse interpretation, distracting the observer's attention from the actual victims of crimes by portraying their perpetrators as themselves the victims.

Hardly a day passes without the newspapers reporting similar stories couched in such language. What should we make of them? As I see it, such accounts are simply reports of a type of behavior we colloquially call *sickening*—that is, so disgusting and upsetting that it makes *us* sick; of course, the term *sick* here is used as a metaphoric adjective, intuitively recognized as such by any competent speaker of the English language. So far probably no one will refute my interpretation. However, my next step, although equally obvious, is more likely to be rejected. I suggest that the idea that these unknown criminals engage in acts that are sickening or that they themselves are sickening has been transformed into the idea that they are *really sick.* But these persons are sick not in the sense in which persons with cancer or heart disease are sick, but only in the sense in which persons who are lovesick are sick (see Chapter 5).

MENTAL ILLNESS: STRATEGY, SELF-DECEPTION, DECEPTION

I hope I have succeeded in demonstrating that professionals as well as lay people now feel comfortable using a multiplicity of diverse criteria for determining what counts as mental illness (see Chapter 3), and then using that idea to achieve a variety of personal and social goals. Surely, one of the things we can conclude from this is that we have abandoned (assuming we had once begun) defining mental illness descriptively, and have taken, like a duck to water, to defining it strategically.

Although my thesis about mental illness as strategy may be persuasive, I realize that it suffers from a fatal flaw: it is too obvious. On the one hand, everyone now seems to believe in mental illness; on the other hand, hardly anyone acts as if he really believes in it. Consider the evidence: 60 million Americans are estimated to smoke cigarettes: they are mentally ill, suffering from Tobacco Dependence; 30 million Americans are said to use illegal drugs: they are mentally ill, suffering from drug abuse; 4 million Americans are supposed to have schizophrenia: this disease is generally acknowledged to be the number-one health problem in the United States; leaders in medicine, psychiatry, government, education, industry, and labor ceaselessly proclaim that "mental illness is like any other illness."

Nevertheless, responding to a Gallup Poll survey asking Americans, "What disease or illness do you fear the most?" the respondents placed cancer on top of the list, blindness half-way down the middle, and deafness at the bottom. Mental illness was not on the list at all.[29]

In short, the meaning of the phrase *mental illness,* like the meaning of any other ideologically loaded symbol, depends on what those who use it want it to mean. Obviously, the ritualistic use of this term means one thing to true believers in psychiatry and quite another thing to those who reject the dogma of the transubstantiation of personal problems into medical diseases.

Cui bono?

As I have noted at the beginning of this chapter, one of the crucial differences between descriptive and prescriptive statements is that while the former may be said to be true or false, the latter may only be said to be desirable or undesirable. This distinction is dramatically revealed in the history of Christianity: From its inception until the dawn of the Enlightenment, belief in God and Jesus was premised on the conviction that the Scriptures and the teachings of clerics were true; since the end of the Age of Faith to our own day, religion has been defended not so much as true but as useful.[30] Of course, long ago Plato called salutary myths *noble lies.* Nietzsche aptly renamed them *holy lies.* The psychiatric myths useful for supporting faith in the myriad pseudomedical procedures of the Therapeutic State are our noble, holy, *therapeutic lies.*

One of the most important differences between whether a statement is true or useful is that truth is typically impersonal and universal, whereas usefulness is not. If a person asserts that lead is heavier than water, it is senseless to ask the classic Roman question: *Cui bono?* (Who profits from it?) Whereas if a person asserts that alcoholism is an illness, it is very sensible, indeed, to ask: *Cui bono?* I have devoted much of this work, and especially this chapter, to showing the importance of asking—and answering—this question whenever a person or group advances a claim clothed in the mantle of mental illness.* Hobbes, whom I often cite in this book, concluded *Leviathan* by urging precisely this point of view on his readers. By substituting clinical for clerical images and words in his text, his message is as timely now as it was in 1651:

> *He that receiveth benefit by a fact, is presumed to be the author.* CICERO maketh honourable mention of one of the Cassii, a severe judge amongst the Romans,

---

Cui bono? indeed. On April 4, 1986, *The New York Times* reported:

The parents of John Hinckley, who shot President Reagan in 1981, have been honored for their efforts to educate the public about mental illness. The parents, Jack and Jo Ann Hinckley, were given the Howard Safar Memorial Award for distinguished service at the annual meeting of the National Council of Community Mental Health Centers.[31]

for a custom he had, in criminal causes, when the testimony of the witnesses was not sufficient, to ask the accusers, *cui bono;* that is to say, what profit, honour, or other contentment, the accuser obtained, or expected by the fact. For amongst presumptions, there is none that so evidently declareth the author, as doth the benefit of the action . . . . And therefore by the aforesaid rule, of *cui bono,* we may justly pronounce for the authors of all this spiritual darkness, the Pope, and Roman clergy, and all those besides that endeavour to settle in the minds of men this erroneous doctrine, that the church now on earth, is that kingdom of God mentioned in the Old and New Testament.[32]

This may sound old-fashioned but, if so, it is only because of the language. We now have our own expression for *cui bono: the bottom line.* The bottom line indeed remains: *Who profits*—in our case, from the psychiatric ideas and interventions so strenuously promoted in the modern world? Hobbes, of course, always saw the struggle for power as the hidden agenda behind clerical fraud and force disguised as benevolence, and we could do worse than heed his advice. "But *cui bono?* What profit did they [the presbytery] expect from it?" he writes in one of his typical passages. "The same which the Popes expected: to have a *sovereign* power over the people."[33] This formula is still valid: we must extend it, however, because today, in addition to psychiatrists, many others use psychiatric ideas and interventions to gain power over their adversaries—or secure other advantages for themselves.

10

MENTAL ILLNESS AS JUSTIFICATION

The liver, skin and kidneys should be stimulated to activity, and be made to assist in decarbonising the blood. The best means . . . [is] to put the patient to some hard kind of work . . . as chopping wood, splitting rails or sawing with the cross-cut or whip saw. . . . The compulsory power of the white man, by making the slothful negro take active exercise, puts into active play the lungs, through whose agency the vitalized blood is sent to the brain to give liberty to the mind.
—*Samuel A. Cartwright, M.D. (1851)*[1]

Because human life is basically social, every group possesses certain methods for ensuring the role-conformity of its members. Because human behavior is basically goal-directed, there are two fundamental methods for encouraging or enforcing role-conformity: the carrot and the stick, reward and punishment, blandishment and coercion. Although coercion is, accordingly, one of the most important facts of life, modern psychiatrists prefer to avert their eyes from it.

This was not always the case. During the infancy and childhood of psychiatry—that is, from 1650 until 1800—alienists and madhouse keepers frankly acknowledged that they controlled their patients by force. Since all insane persons were then treated as involuntary patients, those in charge of them could hardly have done otherwise. However, as psychiatry became medically more legitimate and socially more accept-able—during and since the second half of the nineteenth century—its practitioners sought increasingly to obscure, or even deny, that much of what they did, ostensibly for the patient, was imposed on him by force. In the twentieth century, the psychiatric campaign to analogize psychiatric practices vis-à-vis involuntary patients with medical practices vis-à-vis voluntary patients has been crowned by almost complete success: Since about the middle of this century the very mention of psychiatric coercion has become taboo. If the person who mentions this aspect of psychiatry is a layman, psychiatrists regard his comments as an unjust and hostile criticism of the profession; if he is himself a member of the profession, then psychiatrists regard his comments as a symptom of unforgivable disloyalty or worse.

The concept of coercion implies two closely related notions, namely, power and freedom. One person, Jones, cannot coerce another, Smith, unless he has *power* over Smith: A weaker person cannot (literally) coerce a stronger one. Conversely, Smith cannot be coerced by Jones, unless Smith has certain aspirations and desires, typically to be *free* to live, possess property, and pursue happiness: A person devoid of all wants, indifferent to whether or not he lives or how he lives, cannot be coerced. This explains why in the West people have sought to protect themselves from coercion by political means, principally by restraining the powers of the State (limited government); while in the East they have sought to protect themselves by spiritual means, principally by limiting their own desires (nirvana).

THE RELIGIOUS JUSTIFICATION OF COERCION

Since Western ideas about freedom and power derive in large part from Jewish and Christian religious traditions, let me first offer some brief remarks about these creeds. Viewed as a literary and political docu-ment, one of the striking features of the Old Testament is its preoccupa-tion with power and powerlessness: that is, with God's power—to cre-ate, destroy, and control; and with man's powerlessness—as man vis-à-vis God and as slave vis-à-vis master. It is here, at its very roots in the Judeo-Christian heritage, that an important ambivalence—or dou-ble message—about domination and submission enters the picture. One message is that God's total power and man's complete submission to Him is a good thing; the other is that man's power over his fellow man—in particular, the power of the Egyptian Pharaohs over their

Jewish slaves—is a bad thing. The story of Exodus may thus be viewed as, among other things, an expression of the fundamental aversion human beings experience when other human beings deprive them of their power of self-determination. Yet, as we know, it would be very wrong to say that the Old Testament story condemns slavery as such, that is, as a social arrangement or institution. (Exodus implies only that slavery was a wrong for the Jews at that particular time in their history.)

Coercion in Jewish and Christian History

Although the (historical) Jewish attitude toward slavery does not differ significantly from Christian or Mohammedan attitudes toward it, something else in the Jewish attitude toward the use of coercion does: namely using force to bring nonbelievers to the true faith. Although Judaism was—and in some ways still is—a proselytizing religion, its record on rejecting the use of force to convert the "heathen" is remarkable indeed. According to *The Encyclopedia of the Jewish Religion*, "The forced conversion of the Idumeans (Edomites) to Judaism by John Hyrcanus (135–105 B.C.E.) is the only such recorded case in history."[2] No other Western monotheistic religion can make such a claim. In view of the long history of Judaism, this is an especially remarkable record of nonviolence in the name of God. Perhaps it helps if God has no name.

It helps, too, that Judaism is a nonuniversalitic religion: Its doctrines do not imply, much less proclaim, that it is the right religion for everyone. In contrast, a universalistic faith—let us keep in mind here that the root meaning of Catholic is *universal*—implies that it is good for everyone. Why is this distinction—between the unlimited scope of what is Catholic, and the limited scope of what is Jewish—so important? Because, given the human propensity for domination and coercion, it is but a small step from asserting that "X is true or good for everyone," to insisting that everyone accept X as true or good—by force if necessary. This formula has justified forcible religious conversions in the past, and now justifies a broad spectrum of forcible psychiatric interventions.

Although a monotheistic God's power is necessarily total and unlimited, an earthly ruler's is not, a distinction apparently never lost on the Jews. Hence, perhaps, their simultaneous worship of both a fearsome, all-powerful God and of a Law that keeps Him in his place. Perhaps nothing illustrates more dramatically the difference between the ideological character of Christianity and Judaism than the objects of devotion upon which their worshippers are expected to gaze with awe: Christians on the icons of divinity, Jews on the divine law. Consider what each of these stands for: the figure of the crucified Christ for the Son of God who died for *all of mankind*; the Scroll, for the law God gave to Moses for the *Jews only*. It is no accident, then, that the Christian embraces the use of force in the name of God, whereas the Jew eschews not only the use of such force but the very use of God's name.

Contrast this particularistic—exclusivist, elitist—posture of the Jew and the psychoanalyst* with the universalistic—catholic, scientific—posture of the Christian and the psychiatrist. Christians believe that their ideas about religion are true not only for themselves but for everyone. Psychiatrists believe that their ideas about psychopathology and psychotherapy are true not only for themselves but for everyone. The former attitude—as we know all too well—led to the forcible spread of the Christian faith and to the glorifications of this practice. The latter attitude—though it is now generally denied, especially by psychiatrists—led to the psychiatric campaigns of forcibly imposing mental healing on unwilling subjects. Because the goods represented by Christian salvation and psychiatric cure have been considered superior to all others, their adherents have felt justified in suspending whatever value they reposed in the principle of limited power or the rule of law. To spread the benefits of Christianity and of psychiatry, no laws or limits need be observed: the end is so lofty that it justifies any means. How else can we account for Christians killing heretics with the love of Jesus on their lips? How else can we account for psychiatrists imprisoning mental patients with the love of Mental Health on their lips?†

The Patriarchal Premise

How is it that over long stretches of history and, in some parts of the world even today, religious ideas have justified the most absolute, unlimited uses of power? Although the details of the theological justifications of repression are numerous and complicated, they all come down to a single, rather simple, image: namely, to a monotheistic, male God who rules from Heaven over all mankind as a father on earth rules over his children.

---

*"The would-be Jew," Louis Finkelstein emphasizes, "must demonstrate that his desire is based on no mundane motive."[3] Similarly, the would-be psychoanalytic patient must demonstrate that he is a fit subject for analysis.

†Obviously, my foregoing analysis applies only to the Western monotheistic tradition. For example, the Hindu philosopher Radhakrishan emphasizes:

> Hinduism does not support the sophism that is often alleged that to coerce a man to have the right view is as legitimate as to save one by violence from committing suicide in a fit of delirium . . . . The worshippers of the one jealous God are egged on to aggressive wars against people of alien cults. . . . The spirit of old Israel is inherited by Christianity and Islam.[4]

A classic exposition of this religious perspective on power is Sir Robert Filmer's treatise tellingly titled *Patriarcha*.[5] Written in 1640, this work—with the arresting subtitle: "A Defence of the Natural Power of Kings Against the Unnatural Liberty of the People"—was made famous by John Locke's satirical attack on it. Locke ridiculed the author for trying to "provide Chains for all Mankind," which Filmer in fact did quite well. But what should interest us, and perhaps should have interested Locke a bit more also, was how Filmer justified the benefits—one might now say *cures*—which redounded to those enlightened enough to fasten those chains on themselves or others.

What Filmer provided in his book was nothing novel but was nevertheless very important, namely, a patriarchal—and specifically Judeo-Christian—justification of political authority. Filmer maintained that kings were entitled to absolute power over their subjects who, in turn, owed their rulers absolute obedience. Why? Because both the king's wielding of power and the subjects' yielding to it were decreed by God, the divine lawgiver. How did Filmer know this? The Bible told him so. Until God created Adam, God himself ruled. With Adam, God created a paternal authority to rule in his place. This argument, writes Gordon Schochet "implied that government—and monarchy in particular—was a natural institution and that the burden of proof was on anyone who claimed that there were justifiable, enforceable limits to political authority."[6]

A number of concepts and images come together here, such as patriarchalism, paternalism, the divine rule of kings (or other sovereigns), absolutism, slavery, and, last but not least, revealed religion (in particular Judaism and Christianity). What characterizes all of these is that each sees the political order as naturally hierarchical, familial: on the one side is the father, or Father, or Lord, or God, or his vicar on earth, king or pope; on the other side are the people seen as children, or slaves, or sinners, or a flock tended by a shepherd. Within such an image, Schochet reminds us, "Childhood was not something that was eventually outgrown; rather it was enlarged to include the whole of one's life."[7] It might be unseemly, and unnecessary, to belabor that this is the basic image of what life is and ought to be—of how power ought to be distributed in society—that informs the Jewish and Christian world views. God is our Father in heaven, the priest is called *Father*, we are His children. Just a metaphor you might say. But a master metaphor that continues to pack a powerful wallop of real, literal power. The fact is that for millennia there were no individuals. As Sir Henry Maine observed, ancient law "knows next to nothing of Individuals. It is concerned not with Individuals, but with Families, not with single human beings, but groups."[8]

The Case against the Religious Justification of Coercion

Clearly, our rhetoric justifying the use of power not only reinforces our image of it but also ultimately determines how, or whether, we try to limit it. Thus, if God is seen as all-powerful, demanding total submission to His will, and if power is wielded in the name of such a God, then not only will the wielders of power demand total submission, but those subject to authority and sharing its claim to legitimacy will also be eager to totally submit to it. To be sure, they may chafe under the yoke, but their complaints, couched in terms of misrule, will not challenge the principles legitimizing their own submission. Similar considerations apply to psychiatry and mental health as legitimizing images and principles.

It is important to emphasize, in this connection, that the great historical struggles for religious liberty, in Europe and especially in America, antedate the modern struggles for national independence. More than a hundred years before Jefferson and Madison successfully slayed clerical power in the New World, Thomas Hobbes stated the case for doing so in the Old, in terms as memorable as—though less well remembered than—those of the Founding Fathers:

> Again [he wrote in *Leviathan*], the office of Christ's ministers in this world, is to make men believe and have faith in Christ; but faith has no relation to, nor dependence at all upon compulsion or commandment . . . . Therefore the ministers of Christ in this world, have no power, by that title, to punish any man for not believing or for contradicting what they say.[9]

Sadly, but not surprisingly, liberation from oppression by the priest led, in most cases, to oppression by the politician—the interests of the State replacing the interests of God as the leading symbol for sanctioning power. I shall not be concerned here with this tragic but perhaps often inevitable metamorphosis in the grand human drama of domination and submission.* Instead, I want to comment briefly on the specifically American historical experience vis-à-vis the problem of religious oppression and religious liberty.

---

*Isaiah Berlin's observation on this theme is pertinent in this connection:

> Whatever his crudities and errors, on the central issue Hobbes, not Locke, turned out to be right: men sought neither happiness nor liberty nor justice, but, above and before all, security. Aristotle, too, was right: a great number of men were slaves by nature, and when liberated from their chains did not possess the moral and intellectual resources with which to face the prospect of responsibility, of too wide a choice between alternatives; and therefore, having lost one set of chains, inevitably searched for another or forged new chains themselves.[10]

Leaning heavily on the great thinkers of the European Enlightenment, the leaders of the American Enlightenment saw their task clearly. Simply put, it was this: for centuries, the soil of Europe was bathed in bloodshed in the name of God. Catholics persecuted Protestants, Protestants persecuted Catholics, and both persecuted the Jews. For men who worshipped liberty as well as a loving God, it was not a pretty sight to behold. Because in these persecutions the use of force was justified by appeals to gods and churches, and because the actual use of force making the persecutions possible rested on an alliance between priest and king, the mechanism for controlling this sort of violence seemed obvious enough: separate Church and State, spiritual authority and secular power. The great writings of Thomas Jefferson and James Madison are sharply focused on this one theme: taming the abuse of power justified by faith. Their words are as true and timely today as ever.

> It is error alone [wrote Jefferson] which needs the support of government. Truth can stand by itself . . . . The way to silence religious disputes, is to take no notice of them . . . . It does me no injury for my neighbor to say there are twenty gods, or no God. It neither picks my pocket nor breaks my leg . . . . Constraint . . . may fix him obstinately in his errors, but will not cure them.[11]

Madison was equally firm in repudiating clerical coercion. In 1785—then only 24 years old—he wrote:

> . . . we hold it for a fundamental and undeniable truth that . . . the Religion then of every man must be left to the conviction and conscience of every man . . . . Who does not see that the same authority which can establish Christianity, in exclusion of all other religions, may establish with the same ease any particular sect of Christians, in exclusion of all other sects?[12]

For Jefferson and Madison, and their spiritual friends and allies, religious freedom—that is, freedom from constraint or coercion of any kind enforced in the name of God—was the crux of the struggle for personal and political freedom in general. This fact is familiar enough to historians and educated persons generally. What I think is less familiar is that Jefferson and Madison also clearly recognized that so long as a people want to submit themselves to a higher authority, whether it be pope or king, church or crown, their struggle for freedom is doomed to failure by their own refusal to accept the indivisibility of rights and responsibilities across as many areas of human concern as possible.

So inspired, the founders of American freedom did two historically monumental things. First, they undermined and destroyed the idea of

God as a morally legitimate sanction for the use of force, enshrining this bold proposition in the First Amendment to the Constitution of the United States. Second, they foresaw the danger to liberty that lurks in the nation-state itself and sought to fashion protections against it, enshrining this bold vision in a constitution explicitly limiting political power. In short, the Founding Fathers rejected the religious legitimization of unlimited power by appeals to an approving deity, embracing instead the prudential principle that since, unlike God, government cannot be perfect, its power must be limited.

THE PSYCHIATRIC JUSTIFICATION OF COERCION

For millennia, men viewed theological arguments as valid, indeed lofty, justifications for coercion. Indeed, many people still share that vision: We call them *religious fanatics*, a diagnosis that makes us feel smug and superior to them. But shouldn't we judge ourselves by analogous criteria, that is, by asking: What sorts of reasoning and argument do we accept as so true, irrefutable, and lofty that its conclusions justify coercion? The answer is painfully obvious. Do we not now seek Truth in Nature and Science, much as our forebears did in God and His Will? Do we not now believe in mental illness and psychiatric treatment, much as our forebears did in diabolical possession and exorcism? But our beliefs are true, and theirs were false, might be the reader's instinctive reaction. Perhaps so. That is not the point. The point is that we use *our Truth* to justify *our coercions:* We use Mental Illness and Psychiatric Treatment as justification for pushing people around, just as our faith-intoxicated forebears used Possession and Dispossession to do so.

It is important to reemphasize in this connection that psychiatry, as we now know it, began with the practice of confining mad persons in insane asylums—a practice that, of course, needed to be justified. What justified it was the nascent idea—unknown before, say, 1600—that madness is unreason and that unreason can, in the asylum, be turned back into reason and hence sanity. The prospect of sanity tomorrow thus justified coercion and incarceration today. In the course of the next three centuries, justifying coercion by therapy became as dear to the heart of modern secular man, as justifying coercion by theology ever was to the heart of medieval man. The parallel is, indeed, arresting. In the one case, man, perpetually at risk as a sinner, is invited to rivet his gaze on a dreadful future in hell, or on a blissful one in heaven—and conduct himself accordingly; and if he does not, this vision of the future justifies his brothers, who are his keepers, to save him from perdition and put him on the road to salvation, whether he likes it or not. In the other case, man, perpetually at risk as mentally ill, is invited to rivet his gaze on a dreadful future in mental sickness, or on a blissful one in mental health—and conduct himself accordingly; and if he does not, this vision of the future justifies his brothers, who are his keepers, to save him from mental illness and put him on the road to mental health, whether he likes it or not.

Thus, the modern ideologist—in particular the communist and the psychiatrist—has wrenched the torch that lets him see the future ever so clearly from the fist of the religious zealot and holds it high himself. The eagerness with which the modern benefactors of mankind are willing to degrade, persecute, and slaughter millions of particular men, women, and children today, in order to make life better for mankind in general tomorrow, has been remarked on by many observers of our age. For example, C.S. Lewis noted wryly: "The general movement of our time [seeks to fix] men's attentions on the Future. . . . Gratitude looks to the past, and love to the present; fear, avarice, lust, and ambition look ahead. . . . We [Screwtape speaking] want the whole race perpetually in pursuit of the rainbow's end, never honest, nor kind, nor happy *now.*"[13]

Indeed, Lewis warned that this ideological passion now fuels a specifically medical-therapeutic justification for tyranny: "The new Nero will approach us with the silky manners of a doctor. . . . Even if the treatment is painful, even if it is life-long, even if it is fatal, that will be only a regrettable accident; the intention was purely therapeutic."[14]

Although Lewis was not describing the psychiatric ideologue, he might just as well have been. It is obvious that people now resort to the rhetoric of mental illness and mental treatment in countless situations and ways, but always for the same end: to justify manipulating—intimidating, incriminating, excusing, but always coercing—individuals *today* because they are mentally ill; and thus—by protecting and promoting their mental health—ensuring their liberty and happiness *tomorrow.* For a remarkable nineteenth-century illustration of this imagery, I offer the following true story.

Slavery as Psychiatric Treatment

In May 1851, Samuel A. Cartwright, M.D., a prominent Louisiana physician, published an essay entitled "Report on the diseases and physical peculiarities of the Negro race," in the then-prestigious *New Orleans Medical and Surgical Journal.*[15] Cartwright claimed to have discovered two new diseases peculiar to Negroes which, he believed, *justified* their enslavement as a *therapeutic necessity* for the slaves and as a *medical responsibility* for the masters. Here is a précis of the argument, in Cartwright's own words:

Drapetomania, or the Disease Causing Slaves to Run Away

Drapetomia is from "drapetes," a runaway slave, and "mania," mad or crazy. It is unknown to our medical authorities, although its diagnostic symptom, the absconding from service, is well known to our planters and overseers. In noticing a disease not heretofore classed among the long list of maladies that man is subject to, it was necessary to have a new term to express it. The cause, in the most of cases, that induces the negro to run away from service, is *as much a disease of the mind as any other species of mental alienation,* and much more curable, as a general rule. With the advantages of proper medical advice, strictly followed, this troublesome practice that many negroes have of running away, can be almost entirely prevented, although the slaves be located on the borders of a free State, within a stone's throw of the abolitionists . . . .

Dysaesthesia Aethiopis, or Hebetude of Mind . . . a Disease Peculiar to Negroes

Dysaesthesia Aethiopis is a disease peculiar to negroes, affecting both mind and body, in a manner as well expressed by dysaesthesia, the name I have given it, as could be by a single term. It differs from every other species of mental disease, as it is accompanied with *physical signs* or *lesions of the body,* discoverable to the medical observer, which are always present and sufficient to account for the symptoms. . . .

The complaint is easily curable, if treated on sound physiological principles. The skin is dry, thick and harsh to the touch, and the liver inactive. The liver, skin and kidneys should be stimulated to activity, and be made to assist in decarbonising the blood. The best means . . . [is] to put the patient to some hard kind of work in the open air and sunshine, that will compel him to expand his lungs, as chopping wood, splitting rails or sawing with the cross-cut or whip saw. Any kind of labor will do that will cause full and free respiration in its performance, as lifting or carrying heavy weights . . . the object being to expand the lungs by full and deep inspirations and expirations, thereby to vitalize the impure circulating blood by introducing oxygen and expelling carbon. . . . The *compulsory power of the white man,* by making the slothful negro take active exercise, puts into active play the lungs, through whose agency the vitalized blood is sent to the brain to give *liberty* to the mind (emphasis added).[16]

The justificatory rhetoric of psychiatry is here displayed in full panoply: mental diseases, physical causes, bodily lesions, and, *mirabile dictu,* effective treatments with bountiful benefits for patient and society alike. While the Report speaks for itself, I want to underscore some of its features, since the same elements continue to characterize contemporary psychiatric claims concerning mental diseases and psychiatric treatments.

1. Although *running away,* or escaping from captivity, is ordinarily thought of as a deliberate human act, Cartwright refers to it as an occurrence caused by certain antecedent events: drapetomania *"causes"* slaves to run away; the cause, moreover, is a *"disease of the mind."*

2. To prevent the full-blown development of drapetomania, exhibited by the actual running away of the slave, whipping is recommended as medical therapy; in a revealing allusion to its historical origins, the treatment is called *"whipping the devil out of them."*

3. The cure of drapetomania, and the restoration of the slave to sanity, requires that the patients be "treated like children, with *care, kindness, attention and humanity,* to prevent and cure them from running away."

4. As with drapetomania, Cartwright identifies Dysaesthesia Aethiopis specifically as a *"mental disease . . . accompanied with physical signs or lesions of the body, discoverable to the medical observer."*

5. Although Cartwright mentions not a single free Negro who has consulted him as a patient for this illness, he refers to "the *complaint* as it prevails among free negroes."

6. "Nearly all" free Negroes "that have not got some white person to direct and to take care of them" are said to be afflicted with Dysaesthesia Aethiopis.

For Cartwright, this alleged correlation was further evidence that for the black man, sanity was to be subjected, as slave, to the white man, and for the white man, sanity was to dominate, as master, the black man. Today, similar evidence makes us conclude that for the mentally ill, sanity (rationality) is to submit, as a patient, to the psychiatrist; and that for the psychiatrist, sanity (responsibility) is to dominate, as a therapist, the mental patient.

No wonder psychiatrists ignore their own history: Remembering it surely would make it more difficult to generate enthusiasm for DSM-III—or indignation over the conduct of psychiatrists in the Soviet Union. Paraphrasing Hegel, Shaw observed: "We learn from history, that we learn nothing from history." Perhaps they were right.

DEVIANCE AND CONTROL: RELIGION AND PSYCHIATRY

We are ready now to draw some parallels between religion and psychiatry, by focusing on the ideas and acts most abhorred by each of these systems of belief and social control. The core act of deviance in religion is blasphemy or heresy; in psychiatry, it is delusion or psychosis.

To appreciate the similarities between blasphemy and psychosis, we must first consider the idea of freedom of speech. Commentators on First Amendment freedoms often cite one of Justice Oliver Wendell Holmes' striking phrases to illustrate what this principle ought to mean. "The principle of the Constitution that most imperatively calls for our attachment," said Holmes "is 'not free thought for those who agree with us but freedom for the thought that we hate.'"[17]

Here, then, is a short list of some of the typical utterances that people have always hated, and still do today, and for which those who uttered them were denounced in the past as blasphemers, and are diagnosed now as psychotics.

"Jesus is the son of man, not of God."
"I should kill myself; my life is worthless."
"The government is violating my human rights."

The person who uttered the first statement was considered to be a blasphemer in medieval Catholic counties because he was said to deny the *divinity* of Jesus. The person who utters the second and third statements is considered to be psychotic in the United States or U.S.S.R., because he is said to deny *reality*—namely, that life is good and that the State is good. Because in the United States life is good, the person who wants to leave it by suicide, is, in America, ipso facto crazy; because the Soviet state is good, the person who wants to leave it by emigration is, in Russia, ipso facto crazy. The fact that everyone knows there is nothing crazy about either decision only supports the legitimacy of the authorities' use of coercion. When moral legitimacy draws its support from the masses' longing to be a happy herd, hypocrisy is a source of strength, not weakness.

The following are two more examples:

"The consecrated bread and wine of the Eucharist are the body and blood of Jesus."
"My wife is putting poison in my food and making me impotent."

The person who uttered the first statement was considered to be a heretic by certain Protestants. The person who utters the second statement is considered to be a psychotic by psychiatrists.

It is false and foolish to try to dismiss such cases as instances of religious or psychiatric *abuse*. On the contrary, they are typical examples of religious and psychiatric *persecution*—justified by blasphemy against the sacred beliefs of religious and psychiatric authorities, and made possible by people's blind adherence to the belief that such deviance amply justifies controlling the deviants. This persecutory position may be best appreciated by contrasting it with the position explicitly rejecting the use of force for the expression of opinion, as exemplified in one of Thomas Jefferson's letters to his grandson, written in 1808:

> When I hear another express an opinion which is not mine, I say to myself, he has a right to his opinion, as I to mine, why should I question it? His error does me no injury, and shall I become a Don Quixote, to bring all men by force of argument to one opinion? If a fact be misstated, it is probable that he is gratified by a belief of it, and I have no right to deprive him of the gratification. If he wants information, he will ask it, and then I will give it in measured terms; but if he still believes his own story, and shows a desire to dispute the facts with me, I hear him and say nothing. It is his affair, not mine, if he prefers error.[18]

Consider, in this connection, that but one century before Jefferson—only a little more than 300 years ago (in 1648, to be exact)—the Parliament of England enacted "An Ordinance for the punishing of Blasphemies and Heresies," the punishment, in each instance, being death. What were the acts to be punished? They were such things as asserting:

> that there is no God . . . that the Son is not God, or that the Holy Ghost is not God . . . or that Christ is not God equal with the Father . . . or that the Holy Scripture is not the word of God . . . or that the Bodies of men shall not rise again after they are dead.[19]

Some of these utterances are, of course, still offensive to many people. Suffice it to add here that the long history of persecution for blasphemy was based on the biblical injunction, "You shall not revile God" (Exodus 22:28). Since the writers of Exodus did not say which God, this phrase was equally useful for Catholics and Protestants. Jefferson, who did not mince words when it came to denouncing religious bigotry, spoke contemptuously of "the incomprehensible jargon of the Trinitarian arithmetic, that three are one, and one is three."[20]

Enough, then, of religious blasphemies, that is, of the thoughts that the devoutly religious hate. What about psychiatric blasphemies, the thoughts that the devoutly rational hate? Psychiatrists have long had their *Index of Prohibited Behaviors,* called psychiatric diagnoses. In 1982, the American Psychiatric Association published its current catalog of blasphemies, punishable with involuntarily imposed or otherwise unwanted psychiatric interventions and a broad range of other social sanctions, especially when associated with the additional offense of *dangerousness to self or others.* A few examples of these offenses must suffice here:

Elective mutism, [a blasphemy usually displayed by children, manifested by] continuous refusal to speak in almost all situations, including at school.[21]

Anorexia nervosa, [manifested by an] intense fear of becoming obese . . . [and] refusal to maintain minimal body weight.[22]

Tobacco dependence, [a blasphemy, we are warned, that is] obviously widespread.[23]

Pathological gambling. [Uneducated persons may confuse this with bad luck or losing, just as they may confuse *kleptomania* with theft.][24]

Transsexualism, [manifested by] a persistent wish to be rid of one's genitals and to live as a member of the other sex.[25]

Atypical gender identity disorders or paraphilias, [manifested by the subject's reports of] unusual or bizarre imagery or acts necessary for sexual excitement. [These psychiatric blasphemies are especially odious because] frequently these individuals assert that the behavior causes them no distress and that their only problem is the reaction of others to their behavior.[26]

Why do we need this master list of contemporary blasphemies and heresies? The compilers of DSM-III are eager to tell us. We need it to help the sinners repent: "Making a DSM-III diagnosis represents an initial step in a comprehensive evaluation leading to the formulation of a treatment plan."[27] There are three important ideas implicit in this smug claim: first, that every disorder classified by the compilers is a bona fide illness; second, that every such illness is remediable by means of a bona fide treatment; and third, that the treatment to be applied to the blasphemer ought to be chosen by the psychiatrist, not the patient. But surely, if a man has a right to declare that there are three gods, or 13, or that there is no God, then he must also have the right to declare that he has three personalities, or 13, or that he belongs in the body of a person of the opposite sex, or that he is God, or any other idea that we may deem to be true or false, religion or heresy, reality or delusion.

But we cannot simply leave it at that. We know that human beings rarely form even small groups—much less large, complex societies—without resorting to the use of some force. Thus, the practical question before us comes down to choosing those uses of force we approve, and rejecting those we disapprove. For the reasons I have stated, I reject the psychiatric use of force. On the other hand, for those who believe that mental health is more important than freedom, coerced psychiatric practices will be justified by their therapeutic rationale, just as for those who believe that redemption is more important than freedom, coerced religious practices are justified by their theological rationale.

On Guarding the Guardians

Unfortunately Dostoevski was only half-right when he observed that "If there is no God, everything is permitted." As all history shows, everything is permitted even if there is a God, since the perpetrators of evil have never failed to secure His blessings.

The human condition is precarious indeed. Because it is our fate not only to act but also to have to account for our actions—to ourselves as well as to others—we have an imperative need to justify our behavior. To satisfy it, mankind has evolved a short, but apparently serviceable, shopping list of standardized justificatory images and slogans: God, patriotism, compassion, and, of course, Science and Treatment. The havoc wreaked by men and women heaven-sent or therapy-bent on helping others, especially those who want nothing to do with them, is banal. I mention it only because the notion of *psychiatric help* is such a widely accepted justification for coercion today, especially in the United States. What lessons, then, can the history of power justified by the absolute authority of God teach us about the problems of power justified by the absolute authority of Science (or pseudoscience)?

The Reformation was fueled in large part by the dissatisfactions of Catholics, some of them priests, with the abuses of the then prevailing religious practices. Protestantism is thus intimately connected with the development of fresh ideas about both limited government and religious freedom. The battle over blasphemy now entered a new phase. Some of Martin Luther's views are especially pertinent in this connection.

Early in his career as a critic of clerical "abuses," Luther advocated complete religious liberty—in effect, a separation of Church and State. "Every man," he wrote in 1523, "should be allowed to believe as he will and can, and no one should be constrained [for religion]."[28] He was fierce in his opposition to the Inquisition, declaring that "one could not be a Catholic without being a murderer," adding proudly that "We do not kill, banish, or persecute anybody who teaches other than we do. We fight with the Word of God alone."[29] However, as Luther's power grew, he changed his tune, ending his life urging that Jewish synagogues and prayerbooks be burned, that rabbis be forbidden to teach, and that the Jews be forcibly converted to Christianity. He also insisted that the Catholic Mass was blasphemous and urged its suppression by the government.[30]

Interestingly, a number of elements in the Protestant-Catholic relationship, and especially in Luther's criticisms of the Roman Church, have reemerged, in different terms, in the relationship between contemporary critics of psychiatry and conventional psychiatrists. To begin with there were two distinct aspects to the Reformation protest against Catholicism. One had to do with the nature of God: Was he a single God or a Trinity? The other had to do with the power of the Church: Should religious deviance be punished by means of secular power or should religious differences be tolerated? The original Protestant position on the first question was to reaffirm the monotheistic definition of God given in the Old Testament. This is how, in the sixteenth century, the term *antitrinitarians* came to be applied to some Protestants. Protestants might have responded by asserting that they were not antitrinitarians but only *unitarians*—that is monotheists.

Because I don't accept the expanded (multitarian) definition of disease, I have been accused of denying the reality of mental illness and called an antipsychiatrist. Actually, like the Protestants who reembraced the strict, unitarian-monotheistic definition of God, I have simply reemphasized the strict, unitarian-materialistic definition of disease. It is important to note in this connection that people did not find it very interesting that the Jews had always rejected the doctrine of the Trinity. But people began to find it very interesting indeed when Christians—even Catholic priests—began to reject this idea and reembraced an earlier and stricter definition of a nontrinitarian deity.

It is no secret that most physicians—that is real doctors, not psychiatrists—have always maintained, and still maintain, that mental patients are not really ill, that mental illnesses are not real illnesses, and that psychiatrists are not real doctors. To be sure, real doctors say such things only derisively, in jest; still, much of what I have written about mental illness and psychiatry is similar to what, say, surgeons have long maintained. But when I—a professor of psychiatry in a medical school—reject the idea that there exist illnesses of the mind or psyche—not to mention the terrible mental illnesses that affect whole nations, societies, cultures, or mankind itself—and reemphasize the definition of disease as a bodily, material phenomenon, people find it very interesting indeed. In short, my claim that mental illness is an oxymoronic fiction is similar to the claim that a monotheistic trinitarian God is an oxymoronic fiction.

The second parallel between the antitrinitarians and my criticism of psychiatry is equally striking. What animated the critics and criticisms of the early Protestants? The fraud and force, the deceptions and coercions, that had come to pervade the practices of the Catholic clergy and the Roman Church. In other words, the Protestants—the name is important—protested against two things: Indulgences and the Inquisition. The former symbolized fraud, the latter symbolized persecution—both practiced, of course, in the name of God. The Reformers insisted that buying indulgences does not ensure salvation and that the Word of God cannot and must not be spread by force. What has animated me and my criticisms of psychiatry? The fraud and force, the deceptions and coercions, that pervade psychiatric practices. I insist that a decent and honorable life cannot be achieved by buying (or otherwise receiving) psychiatric treatments—because problems in living are not diseases that can be cured, whether by drugs, electricity, or any other treatment for mental illness. And I maintain that involuntary psychiatric interventions are not cures but coercions and urge that psychiatrists reject such methods.[31] However, although I condemn the therapeutic rape of the patient by the psychiatrist, I defend the legitimacy of psychiatric practices between consenting adults—not because psychiatric help or psychotherapy is necessarily beneficial for its recipient (though it may be), but because infringing on people's freedom to give or receive such help, like infringing on the freedom to give or receive religious help, constitutes a crass violation of inalienable human rights.

These parallels between religion and psychiatry, between the use of fraud and force in the name of God and in the name of Mental Health, bring us full circle to the problem of unlimited power and the mechanism for limiting it. The unlimited power of the Church rested on two pillars: God, the grand legitimizer, spiritually justified the use of any means in His name; and the State, the ultimate repository of power, actually possessed the means for controlling deviants. When these two forces were allied, the result was total power wielded irresistibly by a totalitarian system. Similar considerations obtain for Mental Health, the grand legitimizer of our present age, and its alliance with the State. Thanks to this historical parallel, we need not invent a new mechanism for limiting the power of this new alliance between Psychiatry and the State.

Today, the psychiatrist is empowered not only to provide services to those who want them but also to persecute, in the name of Mental

Health, those who do not want them. Faced with this situation, we have three basic options: We can take away the psychiatrist's power (to incarcerate the innocent or exculpate the guilty), we can take away his tools (lobotomy, electroshock, or neuroleptic drugs), or we can leave things as they are. Taking away the psychiatrist's power would be like the Founding Fathers' abolishing priestly power: Psychiatric help, like religious help, could be given to anyone who wants it; but it would no longer justify the use of force. Taking away the psychiatrist's tools would be like the communists' abolishing various religious practices: People would be protected from psychiatric abuses (as defined by the State), albeit paternalistically, by being treated like children who need the State's protection from their wicked exploiters and their weak selves. Leaving things as they are would be like continuing to support a status quo of forcing help on people in the name of God: We would continue to prattle about the rights of mental patients, as if heretics could have rights in a theocratic society; and we would congratulate ourselves on our humanitarian laws guaranteeing the *mental patient's right to treatment*, as if inquisitors had ever wanted to deprive heretics of their right to worship the God of their persecutors.

Indeed, Jefferson never tired of trying to separate the priest from his power, an effort that was then widely interpreted as hostility to religion itself. In a letter to John Adams written on June 15, 1813, Jefferson refers to an earlier communication "on the subject of religion . . . [which] by its publication will gratify the priesthood with new occasion of repeating their comminations against me. They wish it to be believed that he can have no religion who advocates its freedom."[32] This is precisely the position of organized psychiatry today vis-à-vis the handful of psychiatrists who eschew coercion. To paraphrase Jefferson, the psychiatrists wish it to be believed that he can have no psychiatry who advocates its freedom. I think the psychiatrists are right, and that Jefferson protested too much. When the United States was in its infancy, the clergy throughout the world were so closely allied with coercion that the two were, for all practical purposes, inseparable. The same is now true for psychiatry. Without coercion, psychiatry would be so unlike what we now call *psychiatry*, that my colleagues are right in believing that by opposing psychiatric coercion I oppose psychiatry itself.

By separating Church and State, religion was deprived of its power to abuse the individual, and the State was deprived of one of its major justifications for the use of force. The upshot was a quantum leap toward greater individual liberty such as the world had never seen. By separating Psychiatry and the State, we would do the same for our age: At one fell swoop psychiatry would be deprived of its power to abuse the individual, and the State would be deprived of one of its major justifications for the use of force. The result would be another major advance for individual liberty—or, perhaps, the advent of another system of justificatory rhetoric and persecutory practice, replacing both the religious and psychiatric systems.

PSYCHIATRIC POWER RECONSIDERED

Like the power of the priest in the past, so the power of the psychiatrist at present is a fact or social reality. We may look upon such a fact as a solution or as a problem. Obviously, so long as we view it as a solution, we try to perfect it, not to abolish it. On the other hand, as soon as we begin to view the use of power by a person as problematic, and if at the same time we also question the high-minded pretext with which he justifies his power, there is hope of our being able to limit or even abolish his power by questioning and perhaps successfully undermining his justification for using it. Acting as the agents of the dominant social institution, men always claim to be using force *to do good*. The justificatory image and idiom for doing good thus typically covers both consensual and coerced actions. Therein lies a gigantic logical error and ethical mischief that we must expose and reject. In a free society, acts between consenting adults are permissible (in a sense, good) because they betoken the freedom of the actors, not because the contents or consequences of the acts are necessarily beneficial. We can sell cars, vacations, and stocks regardless of whether buying them benefits the purchaser. Nor do benefits justify coercion: You cannot force a person to buy stocks or bonds, even if you can prove that he will make a profit on the purchase.

The Psychiatric Premise

The logic and ethics of psychiatric paternalism entail altogether different premises, rules, and standards. Thus, in his dealings with the voluntary patient, the psychiatrist typically deemphasizes the issue of whether his client wants, or has a good reason for wanting, his services, dwelling instead on the beneficial effects of the therapy; similarly, in his dealings with the involuntary patient, the psychiatrist justifies his coercions, especially nowadays, by insisting on the therapeutic—indeed, life-saving—powers of his practices. This perspective has been dubbed the *thank-you theory* on the ground that the recovered mental patient's gratitude for getting involuntary electroshock or neuroleptics is adequate justification for psychiatric coercions.* The result is the psychiatrist's passionately held conviction that what justifies psychiatric interventions—voluntary or involuntary—is not consent but the presence of mental illness and the promise of its cure. "No matter what the law does, we'll always treat all the patients we want," declares Loren Roth, a professor of psychiatry at the University of Pittsburgh and a leading authority on psychiatry and the law.[33] By patients, Roth, of course, does not mean persons who would like to avail themselves of a treatment they cannot afford; he means persons who look to the law to protect them from psychiatric coercion justified as treatment. The point is that psychiatrists love to be despots, and, like all despots, revel in being both coercive and compassionate, oppressive and merciful.

Because of the reasons reviewed above, I believe that our efforts to bring about psychiatric *reforms* in the past have been, and our preoccupation with psychiatric *abuses* (especially in other countries) today are, completely misconceived and misdirected. We stubbornly combine and confuse two different problems and questions: One is, What are the proper or improper uses of psychiatry? The other is, Should psychiatric practice be based on the principle of coercive paternalism or on the principle of free contract? Or should there perhaps be—as I have suggested many years ago—two radically different and distinct kinds of psychiatry, one based on coercion, and another on contract?

Psychiatrists who like to debate the problem of psychiatric abuses— especially American psychiatrists who glory in righteously condemning Soviet psychiatrists—are, without exception, psychiatric paternalists: The premise behind their posture is that if psychiatry is practiced *properly*—that is, if it is not politically abused—then psychiatric paternalism is a valid guiding principle for the profession and there is no need to limit the powers of psychiatrists. But this is a tragically false and futile position. To begin with, it is impossible to know, or establish in a morally and politically unbiased way, what is or is not psychiatric abuse. As all history teaches us, oppressors tend to view their use of power as good, whereas the oppressed tend to view their coerced conditions as bad. Thus, American psychiatrists calling Russian psychiatric practices *abuses* is but a feeble and ironic echo of American mental patients calling psychiatric practices in the United States *abuses.*

In addition, we know, as Lord Acton emphasized, that power tends to corrupt and that absolute power tends to corrupt even more. We also know, as Thomas Jefferson pointed out, that if men were angels there

---

*For the ingratitude of such patients, see "The Psychiatrist's Love Affair with Coercion" in Chapter 4.

would be no need for limited government, or for any kind of government. My point is that the currently fashionable effort to combat psychiatric abuses is either a stupid and misdirected enterprise, or a ploy to preserve unlimited psychiatric power, or both. The only way to limit psychiatric abuses is by limiting psychiatric power. And that puts the problem of psychiatric power back where it squarely belongs, in the realm of religion, morals, and law—in a word, in the realm of politics.

Losing Liberty through Psychiatry

Lest I seem obsessed with opposing coercion, whether justified on clerical or clinical grounds, I should like to say that I am no more obsessed with this theme than were the men who drafted the Virginia statute for establishing religious freedom and the First Amendment to the U.S. Constitution.

While George Washington would have been content to have all Christian churches equally established, Jefferson, Madison, and their allies wanted much more. The result was the passage, in January 1786, of the statute for establishing religious freedom in Virginia, whose opening words are perhaps even more relevant to our present psychiatric situation than they were to the religious situation Americans faced 200 years ago:

> Well aware that Almighty God hath created the mind free; that all attempts to influence it by temporal punishments or burdens, or by civil incapacitations, tend only to beget habits of hypocrisy and meanness, and are a departure from the plans of the Holy Author of our religion, who being Lord both of body and mind, yet *chose not to propagate it by coercion* on either, as was his almighty power to do (emphasis added).[34]

Surely, this is a remarkable rejection of nearly 1500 years of persecution carried out in the name of the Christian God. Viewed against this backdrop, then, is it not a spiritual regression for us to embrace coercion in the name of our modern, secular God—Mental Health?

Although these reflections might seem far-ranging, they basically come down to reinforcing the old adage, that the pen is mightier than the sword. After all, power is force that people wield over other people. Since those who wield power are always fewer in number than those over whom power is wielded, no person could rule, much less govern, without his power being credibly legitimized by certain ideas. It is these ideas that sanction some to use power and require others to submit to it. In the end, the whole structure of power—religious, political, psychiatric—rests on certain ideas packaged in the master metaphors of our language. As psychiatrists, psychologists, and professionals in the allied disciplines, it behooves us, then, to scrutinize our own ideas—particularly the *idea* of mental illness—which we must judge, of course, by its uses and consequences. I, for one, find it wanting not only as a conceptual aid but, most importantly, as a justification for violence against those who act or think differently than we do.

Ideas, as Richard Weaver never tired of emphasizing, are important because they have consequences. If the consequences are powerful, as they sometime are, then the ideas that generate them are also powerful. The divine right of kings was such an idea: it justified the absolute rule of monarchs. The subhumanity of the Negro was such an idea: it justified American slavery. Mental illness is such an idea: it justifies institutional psychiatry.

Moreover, if we accept that, because they know God's will, priests are justified in coercing sinners, we can expect that the contours of their coercions will vary—but their justifications will have no trouble keeping pace with their practices. The same goes for our accepting that, because they are experts on mental illness, psychiatrists are justified in coercing the mentally sick. My own experience as a psychiatrist bears this out.

When I was a young psychiatrist, psychotics were hospitalized for a long time, often for life. Psychiatrists then claimed they always hospitalized mental patients for exactly the right length of time—but most people believed the patients were confined too long.

Now that I am an old psychiatrist, psychotics are hospitalized for a short time, often only a few days. Psychiatrists still claim they always hospitalize mental patients for exactly the right length of time—but most people now believe the patients are confined too briefly.

The rationalizations for the duration of the confinement have kept pace with these changes. Four decades ago, psychotics were considered to be chronically ill and dangerous; since their illness was not considered to be responsive to specific treatment, protracted custodial care was regarded as the most humane and scientific method of treating them. Now psychotics are considered to have acute episodes and to be nondangerous; since their illness is considered to be responsive to specific pharmacological treatment, brief periods of hospitalization combined with intensive chemotherapy are regarded as the most humane and scientific method for treating them.

These are all fables, of course. The will to believe in mental illness and the need to do something ostensibly for—but, in fact, to—mental patients forms an irresistible mixture of justifications and motives that, in our Age of Madness, can make virtually any mental health policy seem both humane and scientific.

11

MENTAL ILLNESS
AS LEGAL FICTION

We know insanity is a mysterious disease, that it may exist without physical indications, is often cunningly concealed so as almost altogether to baffle detection even by a specialist, or may be so occult as to cause the most eminent alienists to clash as to its existence in an instance.

—*Warner v. Packer* (1910)[1]

Because the idea of insanity, unlike the idea of illness, originates from a legal (or quasi-legal) context, it is impossible to understand it without paying proper attention to this context. My aim in this chapter is to examine a specific legal aspect of insanity, namely, its role as a legal fiction. According to *Black's Law Dictionary* (4th ed.), a legal fiction is:

> An assumption or supposition of law that something which is or may be false is true, or that a state of facts exists which has never really taken place . . . A rule of law which assumes as true, and will not allow to be disproved, something which is false, but not impossible.[2]

In the American historical-legal experience, the classic example of a legal fiction is the status of the Negro slave as part-person or property. No less lofty a legal document than the Constitution of the United States defines enslaved blacks this way. The institution of American chattel slavery rested, as I shall discuss in a moment, on the legal fiction that slaves were not persons but *personalty* (that is, possessions or chattel).

The idea that some individuals who *seem* to be adult men and women, with appropriate rights and responsibilities are *in law* (de jure)—and hence also *in fact* (de facto)—not really persons because they are *insane*—is, in my opinion, also a legal fiction. I would venture to say that just as the view of the Negro slave as property was the grand American racial-legal fiction before the Civil War, so the view of the disturbed and disturbing person as mentally ill has been the grand American medical-legal fiction since then. Indeed, the idea of insanity illustrated in the opinion in *Warner v. Packer*, cited as the epigraph at the beginning of this chapter, is as apt an illustration of this Santa Claus function of insanity as one could wish for.

A fiction is an untruth we believe to be the truth because we want to believe it. No one denies that this phenomenon exists, especially among children. No one denies that it exists among adults too, especially among those professing a religion different from ours. No one denies that it exists even among scientists, especially if they support a theory whose validity one rejects. But the masses of people, especially the masses of modern intellectuals, reject the idea that their favorite facts may also be fictions. "It has become too easy to see," warned Herbert J. Muller, "that the luckless men of the past lived by mistaken, even absurd beliefs; so we may fail in a decent respect for them, and forget that the historians of the future will point out that we too lived by myths."[3]

So the problem remains: How do we recognize our own fictional beliefs? The trouble is that this question is phrased incorrectly: The person who believes that *his* idea—which *we* may think is a fiction—is true, experiences his belief as a solution, not as a problem. In that sense, there is no problem. There is only the human intellect at work—showing ourselves, and each other, different images of the world around and within us. And there are only different religious and political—and now also psychiatric—systems, allowing us to pick the images we want, and reject those we do not want.

INSANITY AS A LEGAL FICTION

What does it mean to assert that we should try to understand a particular concept as a legal fiction? Lon L. Fuller, a distinguished legal scholar, offers this answer:

To obtain an understanding of any particular [legal] fiction we must first inquire: What premise does it assume? With what proposition is it seeking to reconcile the decision at hand? In most cases the answer is easily discovered.[4]

Much of what I say in this book constitutes precisely such a functional analysis of the meanings and uses of mental illness. Of course, Fuller is right when he observes that the function of a legal fiction is easily discovered. "What premise does it (mental illness) assume?" It assumes that the idea of illness is applicable to the mind (or whatever we mean by the mind). "With what proposition is it seeking to reconcile the decision at hand (psychiatric coercions and excuses)?" It seeks to reconcile the decision to deprive innocent persons of liberty, and to exonerate guilty persons of responsibility, with the proposition that insanity is an illness which annuls free will and responsibility, and with the claim that so treating certain persons does not violate our commitment to a political philosophy of individual freedom and responsibility under the rule of law.

Legal Fiction as Literalized Metaphor

Legal authorities, no less than psychiatric ones, insist that mental illness is a fact, and, more specifically, that it is a disease like any other.

Mental disease . . . is a medical problem (Edwin Keedy).

Mental illnesses . . . are the subject matter of medical science (Carter v. U.S.).

We do not insist on a legal formula in diagnosing other diseases; why in this instance? (Simon Sobeloff).[5]

How can insanity be a fiction when so many thoughtful and educated persons consider it to be a fact? The answer is simple. Observers of the human condition, even the most brilliant ones, have time and again missed or misunderstood the fundamentally metaphoric nature of language. For example, Thomas Hobbes (1588–1679) defined "Words used metaphorically" as employed "to deceive others."[6] Similarly, John Locke (1632–1704) believed that "The artificial and figurative application of words . . . [is] for nothing else but to insinuate wrong ideas, move the passions, and thereby mislead the judgment."[7] Such observations miss the point that language, in any of its forms, can be used equally easily and well to inform or misinform. Distinguishing truth from falsehood requires not purging our language of metaphors, but taming our passions to control and dominate others. In reality the relationship between language and the passions is a reciprocal one, language inflaming and deforming the passions, and the passions inflaming and distorting language, both spoken and heard.

Not surprisingly, the hostility exhibited by Hobbes and Locke towards metaphors reemerges in the attitudes of some philosophers and jurists towards legal fictions. Jeremy Bentham (1748–1832) reviled legal fiction as "a syphilis which runs in every vein [of English law] and carries into every part of the system the principle of rottenness."[8] Standing as they did at the threshold of the Enlightenment, we can forgive Locke, Hobbes, and Bentham for their positivistic protests against metaphors as mischief-making devices. Their *tropophobia,** however, is alive and well in the writings of modern positivistic legal philosophers, such as Felix S. Cohen, who calls legal concepts "supernatural entities," and fulminates against "jurisprudence . . . [as] a special branch of the science of transcendental nonsense."[10] Cohen's view reflects the modern prejudice that anything that is not science is nonsense and leads to the nonsense of classifying economics and psychology as "positive sciences."[11]

On the other hand, already in the eighteenth century, William Blackstone (1723–1780) recognized that the law cannot do without fictions, some of which may be "highly beneficial and useful."[12] At the same time, he was keenly aware of the strategic character of legal fictions, remarking that, ". . . while we may applaud the end, we cannot admire the means."[13]

Insanity as a legal fiction is precisely such an unadmirable means to an end many people now applaud, namely, caring for insane persons. That there are grave dangers in the pursuit of ostensibly noble ends with palpably ignoble means I need not dwell on. Suffice it here to add that contemporary activist lawyers and judges, intent on promoting what I call *therapy by the judiciary,* have eagerly embraced as truths not only the fictions of the law but the fictions of psychiatry as well. For them, expert opinions rendered in court by psychiatrists have the logical status of scientific facts and the moral force of divine commandments.

LEGAL FICTION AS A MASK

In his important work titled *Persons and Masks of the Law,* John T. Noonan, Jr. makes two very important points: one is that legal fictions are necessary for maintaining a social order based on a dominant ideology;

---

*The fear of tropes or metaphors, a term suggested by Donald Hall.[9]

the other is that such fictions often conflict with our intuitive sense of justice and thus generate dangerous divisions in society.[14]

Noonan starts with an observation about law that applies equally well to psychiatry. "The definition of law," he writes, "depends on the purpose of the definer."[15] However, instead of acknowledging this premise, "many of those who write about jurisprudential matters analyze rules abstractly, without reference to their aim, and argue about each other's definitions."[16] The same situation prevails with respect to definitions of mental illness and other key psychiatric concepts. Thus, we have mental diseases like oppositional behavior, ego-dystonic homosexuality, and tobacco dependence, and arguments about whether these conditions should or should not be classified as mental diseases. While officially the classifier's motives are concealed behind the absurd contention that psychiatric nosology is a collection of facts, in practice, those engaged in creating new mental diseases advance various reasons for their decisions. Some say that we ought to classify X (whatever the behavior may be) as an illness because only then can we conduct neurobiological *research* into its causes and cures; others say that we should do so because the patients need *treatment* and cannot ask for it themselves; still others say that we should do so because the victims cannot be held *responsible* for their criminal acts.

Concealing the Person behind Rules and Roles

Classifying persons as mental patients and creating legal fictions involving human beings lead to the same result: The person, concealed behind a mask, is rendered less than fully human or even completely nonhuman. "Rules," observes Noonan, "not persons, are the ordinary subject matter of legal study."[17] Similarly, psychopathological processes, not troubled or troubling persons, are the subject matter of psychiatry.

I have remarked earlier on how attaching a medical diagnosis to a person makes him, in his role as *patient,* similar to—and exchangeable or fungible with—other patients similarly diagnosed (see Chapter 4). The fungibility of the patient role is especially important in psychiatry because the persons we call *mental patients* have *personal* problems. Since the person as an individual is the very paradigm of the nonfungible, viewing him as a mental patient represents the profoundest possible change in perspective.

Classified as depressives, phobics, and schizophrenics, mental patients are considered to be more alike than unlike: they can be counted as similar and treated similarly. Such similar treatment of similar things is, of course, a hallmark of scientific medicine, pitting psychiatry squarely against itself: Is psychiatry a medical enterprise concerned with treating diseases, or a humanistic enterprise concerned with helping persons with their personal problems? Psychiatry could be one or the other, but it cannot—despite the pretensions and protestations of psychiatrists—be both.

It is worth noting here that even Harry Stack Sullivan, generally regarded as one of the most humanistic modern psychiatrists, succumbed to the lure of an *impersonal* psychiatric science:

> Let me say that insofar as you are interested in your unique individuality, . . . you are interested in the really private mode in which you live—in which I have no interest whatever. The fact is that for any scientific inquiry, in the sense that psychiatry should be, we cannot be concerned with that which is inviolably private.[18]

Evidently it did not occur to Sullivan that if this is the price of being scientific, it might be better not to pay it than to betray the patient and forfeit being scientific (in the sense of being truthful) in the bargain.

The Roads to Chattel Slavery and Psychiatric Slavery

Noonan uses the American experience with slavery to illustrate how legal fictions may serve the purpose of dehumanizing persons and how lawyers and legal scholars may act as agents, rather than as critical analysts, of the resulting system. "Indifference to persons in legal history and legal study," he writes, "is dramatically illustrated by their [prominent legal scholars'] unconcern for a major function of Anglo-American law for three centuries, the creation and maintenance of a system in which human beings were regularly sold, bred, and distributed like beasts."[19] Noonan demonstrates how legislators, lawyers, and judges suppressed the commonsense perception that Negro slaves were human beings and "said not a word on how the legal system made a person a non-person."[20]

"How could a lawyer," Noonan asks, "look upon persons as kitchen utensils?" How can a doctor, we might ask, look upon persons as the carriers of diseased brains or as bundles of unconscious impulses? "The split between the ideals of the American Revolution and the maintenance of slavery," adds Noonan, "was evident to contemporaries."[21] The split between our ideals of individual liberty and responsibility and the maintenance of institutional psychiatry is no less evident to many people today. But cultural contradictions have plagued most civilizations and more than impassioned impatience is needed to resolve them. Consider the problem that confronted Americans on the eve of the birth of their new nation:

> At least half of the property cases before the Chancellor [in colonial Virginia] involved the disposition of slaves. He could not have compassion for each of them as a person and still be a judge. His role in a slave system necessitated the use of masks . . . . Legal education has often been education in the making and unmaking of persons.[22]

Who knows how many cases coming before judges today involve questions concerning the mental health of defendants or litigants? How can judges and psychiatrists have compassion for every single so-called mental patient as a person and still be judges and psychiatrists? They cannot. Thus, combining their efforts and talents, doctors and lawyers, using the mask of mental illness, have created and maintained a system of medical-legal fictions to transform citizens into mental patients— that is, free and responsible adults into unfree and nonresponsible quasi-children.

SLAVERY AND PSYCHIATRY

Since mask and role are similar but not identical, and since both are useful for our analysis of mental illness, a brief remark about the differences between them is in order here. Like clothes, roles may hide individuality, but can also accentuate and define it; whereas masks conceal, falsify, even obliterate individuality. Unlike a role, a mask, says Noonan, signifies "a legal construct suppressing the humanity of a participant in the process. . . . 'Property,' applied to a person, is a perfect mask. No trace of human identity remains."[23] Just so have the various semantic masks used by alienists and psychiatrists—from moral insanity and masturbatory madness to schizophrenia and bipolar illness— suppressed the humanity of the mental patient.

". . . Three Fifths of All Other Persons"

In order to illustrate what is a legal mask or fiction—specifically the mask that hid the face of the American slave until 1865, and the mask that hides the face of the American mental patient today—I want to present some information with which every educated person is familiar.

Few people would deny that the Framers of the Constitution of the United States of America comprised some of the finest minds and loftiest spirits that ever graced Western civilization. However, because of the existence of the institution of slavery, they felt it reasonable and indeed necessary—in the Constitution itself—to define black slaves (without so calling them) as three-fifths human. Thus was a remarkable legal fiction created to legitimize a peculiar human institution—a fiction, let us remember—that Americans found themselves unable to reject without a bloody civil war. Although this painful history is familiar enough, it might be worth quoting the text of the Constitution here, as a sobering reminder not only of the difference between legal fiction and truth but also of the social imperatives energizing such fictions.

The Preamble to the Constitution declares that its purpose, among other things, is to "secure the Blessings of Liberty to ourselves and our Posterity." Then, in Article I, Section 2, this revered document states:

> Representatives and direct Taxes shall be apportioned among the several States . . . according to their respective Numbers, which shall be determined by adding to the whole Number of free Persons, including those bound to Service for a Term of Years, and, excluding Indians not taxed, three fifths of all other Persons.

Moreover, the Constitution—and this is perhaps less often remarked on in discussions concerning the constitutionality of this or that policy—not only legitimizes slavery but makes any interference with it explicitly unconstitutional:

> No person held to Service or Labour in one State, under the laws thereof, escaping into another, shall, in consequence of any Law or Regulation therein, be discharged from such Service or Labour, but shall be delivered up on Claim of the Party to whom such Service or Labour may be due. (Article IV).

In short, the Constitution, ratified less than 200 years ago, specifically denied the notion that the black slave had a claim to liberty and that those assisting him to escape from slavery were engaging in a legally legitimate enterprise. We might try to remember this when psychiatrists and lawyers righteously tell us that it would be unconstitutional to interfere with the policies of civil commitment and the insanity defense—the legal interventions by which the idea of insanity is legitimized as true and valid.

It is sobering to reflect that only a little more than a century ago human beings were sold and bought in the United States as well as in Russia. Here slavery was justified by the blackness of the slave. How was it justified in Russia? A brief digression on this seemingly unrelated topic may be rewarding here.

The Trade in Souls

Unlike his American counterpart, the Russian slave—usually called *serf*—was white. Hence, blackness could not be used to obscure his humanity. Yet his humanity was effectively obscured by a language game that reveals the profound significance of Christianity for the Russian mind: the serf was called a *soul*. Nor was this a mere euphemism: While there is a Russian word for *serf*, in the official Russian census serfs were called *souls*. (The masters had to pay a tax on each serf, hence the need for an official census.) Thus, in America the humanity of the slave was obscured by the legal fiction that he was *three fifths of a person*, which degraded him into property; in Russia, the humanity of the slave was obscured by the legal fiction that he was a *soul*, which, while seemingly exalting him as an immortal spirit permitted degrading him as a person. Nikolai Gogol's famous satire, *Dead Souls* (1842), is based on this metaphoric disguise of the serf.[24]

Self-contradiction is, of course, inherent in every master metaphor: How can bread be the body of a God? How can a human being be three fifths of a person? How can an immortal soul be dead and how can a living person called a *soul* be traded like cattle—and, most ironically, why would anyone want to buy a *dead soul*?

The protagonist of *Dead Souls*, the immortal Pavel Ivanovich Chichikov, decides to go into the business of buying dead souls because souls could be used as collateral for a government loan, and because, legally, serfs existed and were taxed until formally taken off the rolls by a government census-taker. Hence the ultimate legal fiction of the dead soul—the serf that has died between one census and the next and was therefore de facto dead but de jure alive. The following dialogue, at the beginning of the story, takes place between Chichikov and a woman from whom he wants to buy some dead souls:

"... Well then, Natasia Petrovna, will you sell them to me?"

"Sell what to you?"

"Why, all those serfs who died."

"How can I sell them to you? ... what do you want them for?" the old woman asked, her eyes popping.

"Now that's my business."

"But since they are dead."

"And who is trying to maintain that they are alive? . . ."

"I really don't know. I've never traded in dead people before. . . . really, my friend, this has never happened to me before—to sell folks who've passed away. When it comes to live ones, I've sold some."[25]

Gogol's aim, of course, was to denounce the system of serfdom, which was then accepted as the natural order of things. At the end of the novel, he addresses the reader directly.

. . . Isn't there anyone among you who has enough Christian humility to ask himself—oh, not in public, of course, but in private, searching his soul— a question along these lines: "Am I not, even slightly, somewhat of a Chichikov?" . . . And you, Russia—aren't you racing headlong like the fastest troika imaginable? . . . And where do you fly to, Russia? Answer me! . . . She doesn't answer.[26]

Jefferson expressed the same sentiment when he wrote: "I tremble for my country when I reflect that God is just."[27] We should all tremble, for all of humanity.

The Case for Psychiatric Slavery

As the Constitution affirmed the truth of Negro inferiority and the rightness of chattel slavery, so the Supreme Court now affirms the truth of mental illness and the rightness of psychiatric slavery. In the classic case of *Robinson v. California*, decided in 1962, the Supreme Court asserted the medical reality of mental illness and the legal validity of psychiatric coercions committed in its name.[28] Ruling that it is unconstitutional to punish "any person addicted to the use of narcotics" because such a condition is a mental disease and hence its punishment would be "cruel and unusual," the Court declared:

It is unlikely that any State at this moment in history would attempt to make it a criminal offense for a person to be mentally ill . . . . In the light of contemporary human knowledge, a law which made a criminal offense of such a disease . . . [would be unconstitutional].[29]

The Court's references to "at this moment in history" and "contemporary human knowledge" are revealing: they imply that we now know something about the human propensity to take drugs that, say, Jefferson did not know.

Indeed, the entire Robinson case, and especially Justice William O.

Douglas' concurring opinion, reads as a contemporary defense of the reality of mental illness and the rightness of psychiatric slavery:

> The addict [asserts Douglas] is a sick person. He may, of course, be confined for treatment or for the protection of society. Cruel and unusual punishment results not from confinement, but from convicting the addict of a crime. . . . If addicts can be punished for their addiction then the insane can also be punished for their insanity. Each has a disease and each must be treated as a sick person.[30]

What the Court could not look straight in the face in 1962 is similar to what the Framers could not look straight in the face in 1787: namely, *their own indenture* to their own dominant institutions. Once the United States became a separate nation, it was necessary to count the persons in it: This then raised the problem of who should be counted as a person. If the Negro slave was so counted, he could no longer, in good conscience, be enslaved. Similarly, once the federal government outlawed the possession and use of certain substances—the possession and use of which were perfectly legal in 1776 and, indeed, as recently as 1913—it then became necessary to do something with or to the persons who violated that prohibition: This now raises the problem of whether to define and control such persons as criminals or mental patients or both. For the Framers, it was unthinkable to regard the Negro slave as a person. For the Justices of the Supreme Court today, it is equally unthinkable to regard antidrug laws as unconstitutional. "The addict," Justice Douglas asserted, "is a sick person. He may, of course, be confined for treatment . . . ."[31] But the addict *is* no more sick than the Negro *is* a slave.

Any society can tolerate only so much freedom: as liberty is enlarged in one area, it is constricted in another. I believe the contemporary criminalization of possessing and using certain chemicals will seem as bizarre to future generations as the justification of slavery seems to the present one. During the last years of his life, Thomas Jefferson suffered from headache, insomnia, and chronic diarrhea, problems he managed by medicating himself with Laudanum (tincture of opium).[32] Although every American president now has the right, under certain circumstances, to launch nuclear missiles, under no circumstances does he now have the right to medicate himself with opium.

The Case against Slavery: Chattel and Psychiatric

The face that man can conceal by means of legal masks he can, of course, reveal by means of historical analysis and rational criticism. It does not diminish Noonan's achievement to observe that it is no longer difficult to do what he has done so ably, namely, to reconstruct the semantic and legal processes by which the Negro slave was dehumanized. The modern mind unhesitatingly rejects the view that a black human being is property rather than person. Today the difficult task is to criticize the contention that the madman is a person rather than an insane patient.* This is a daunting task now, just as it was a daunting task to defend the humanity of the Negro slave before the Civil War: linguistic and legal habit served then, and serve now, to validate a dehumanized and infantilizing slave/ insane image of the victim and a superhumanized and paternalistic mas-ter/doctor image of the victimizer. From the beginning of the slave trade in the American colonies, writes Noonan, "'slave' and 'Negro' were terms . . . indicating a special legal status. . . . Africans in Virginia, having arrived by means of purchase, were viewed as *property.*"[34]

Similarly, since the beginning of psychiatry, with the construction of insane asylums in the seventeenth and eighteenth centuries, *mad* and *insane* became terms indicating a special legal status. Madmen in mad-houses, having been transported to the asylum against their will, were viewed as nonpersons.[†] As the semantics of slavery supported the slave trade and the institution of slavery, so the semantics of psychiatry support the trade in lunacy and the institution of psychiatry. In colonial Virginia, legislators and courts "presented a doctrine on the morality of slavery"[36]; in contemporary America, legislators and courts present a doctrine on the morality of psychiatry. The former taught that slavery was good, identifying slaves with soil and property:

> As long as the teaching of the lawgivers was accepted, slavery could not be criticized without aspersion on the goodness of wealth itself. In the Virginia

---

*In this connection, the following passage from C.S. Lewis is an apt reminder: "[O]ne passes to the realization that our own age is also a 'period,' and certainly has, like all periods, its own characteristic illusions. They are likeliest to lurk in those widespread assumptions which are so ingrained in the age that no one dares to attack or feels it necessary to defend them."[33]

†"Infants, idiots, and the insane" were never intended to be included by the Enlightenment humanists and philosophers among *persons* possessing inalienable rights to life, liberty, and property. Thus, in his *Two Treatises on Government,* John Locke states: "Lunaticks and Ideots are never set free from the Government of their Parents. . . . Madmen, which for the present cannot possibly have the use of right Reason to guide themselves, have for their Guide, the Reason that guideth other Men which are Tutors over them, to seek and procure their good for them."[35] In the past, the principle of paternalism justified the domination of women by men, of blacks by whites, and of colonial people by Europeans; today, it contin-ues to justify the domination of the insane by the sane. Even contemporary libertarian political philosophers and theorists cannot countenance the idea that individuals whom psychiatrists call *insane* or *psychotic* are persons and should be treated as such.

colony, a 1705 statute defined plantation slaves as real estate and merchant's slaves as personalty. The care and consideration lavished by lawmakers on all forms of property proclaimed to the dullest intellect that ownership was desirable. . . . Property was the most comprehensive and most necessary of social categories.[37]

Mutatis mutandis, lawgivers now teach that involuntary psychiatry is good, identifying insanity with ill health and psychiatry with treatment.[38] Thus, as long as the teaching of lawgivers is accepted, psychiatry cannot be criticized without casting aspersions on the goodness of health and treatment. Accordingly, compulsorily (civilly or criminally) hospitalized mental patients are now defined as childlike quasi-persons—unable to care for themselves and/or unable to control their illegal behavior. In the Virginia colony, property was the supreme category; in America today, health is. For who, *in his right mind,* can be against health? No one. Our language and laws thus render reasoned opposition to psychiatry all but impossible. Effective legal criticism of slavery awaited the development of a successful refutation of the idea that persons called *slaves* are not persons. I long maintained that effective legal criticism of psychiatry requires a similarly successful refutation of the idea that persons called *mental patients* are not persons. In two books, published in 1961 and 1963, I tried to formulate such a refutation.[39] Since my critique is similar to the classic critique of slavery, let me briefly recapitulate the latter, as outlined by Noonan.

The moral and legal foundation for the opposition to slavery lay in an extremely influential book, published a dozen years before the American Revolution. In his *Commentaries on the Laws of England,* William Blackstone, the first professor of the Laws of England at Oxford and one of the most celebrated English jurists of all time, maintained that "English law consisted in the rights of persons and the rights of things."[40] But who were to be counted as persons? Blackstone answered: "Natural persons [are] such as the God of nature formed us."[41] While accepting the possibility of expanding the category of persons by creating "artificial persons," such as corporations, Blackstone rejected the possibility that the category could be artificially contracted. The purpose of man-made law, he insisted, "was to protect persons in the enjoyment of those absolute rights, which are vested in them by the immutable laws of nature."[42] This reasoning led him to an unqualified rejection of slavery: Since it is self-evident that, regardless of skin color, human beings are persons, slavery is opposed to natural law. My claim that, regardless of psychiatric diagnosis, mental patients are persons, is a similar contention. Asserting such a claim, however, runs head on into

the apparently universal passion of human beings to exploit and dominate other human beings, preferably under the guise of some paternalistic ideal. Opposition to slavery was slow in gaining ground because it
ran head on into the defense of slavery as a defense of private property,
as well as into its defense as an integral part of Christian compassion
and morality.

Writing several decades before Blackstone, Montesquieu satirized
this obstacle as follows:

> It is impossible that we should suppose those people [Negro slaves] to be
> men, because if we should suppose them to be men, we would begin to
> believe that we ourselves are not Christians.[43]

While some people still believe they are good because they are Christians, even more people now believe they are good because they profess
to help sick people and are willing to support such efforts in the face of
any obstacle, be it financial, legal, or scientific. Psychiatrists and their
followers are now in the forefront of those claiming to want to help such
persons. Since they can do so only if certain individuals are denominated
as mentally ill and treated as nonpersons, it is impossible for psychiatrists—paraphrasing Montesquieu—to suppose that mental patients are
persons, because if they supposed them to be persons, then psychiatrists
might begin to believe that they themselves were not Therapists.

The question of when a human being is not a person—or, to put it
differently, which human being is *in fact* not a person—has perplexed
humanists, philosophers, psychiatrists, and legislators for a long time,
with no end in sight. Montesquieu tried to solve the problem by appealing to our "intuition of personhood"[44], an attractive idea but an untrust-
worthy criterion. The intuition of personhood held by the American
Founding Fathers—surely not a group of evil men—was not wide
enough to protect blacks in their personhood. The intuition of personhood held by legislators and psychiatrists today is similarly not wide
enough to protect persons called mental patients in their personhood,
as the following—now acutely relevant—example illustrates.

In January 1986, *Newsweek* magazine published a feature essay on
the "homeless mentally ill," which prompted a former beneficiary of
mental health services to write to the Editor: "Many of us so-called
'homeless mentally ill' have preferred the chill of the night air to the
cold reality of psychiatric treatment . . . and the damage of involuntary treatment and incarceration . . . . I am thankful for those who
have fought for my constitutional rights to be free from dehumanizing,
intrusive 'treatments.'"[45]

This plea is evidently too simple to be taken seriously in our sophisticated age when we coerce in the name of compassion. Nor do we pay attention to the lesson dumb animals—to whom madmen used to be compared—teach us. After all, do we not provide more food, more comfort, and better health care to the inmates of zoos than they could possibly provide for themselves? Why, then, do we have to cage them? Because they would rather perish in freedom than live in captivity. Just so many mental patients would rather die from psychiatric abandonment than live with psychiatric attention. Have we sunk so low that we actually believe that animals value freedom more highly than human beings? I can think of few instances where the American press and television have failed us more miserably than in their portrayal of the mentally ill. We are now confronted daily with thousands upon thousands of persons who, having experienced the bountiful benefits of the American mental health system, say with actions that speak louder than words that they do not want psychiatric help. How do the men and women of our *free* press interpret this phenomenon? By telling the freedom-loving American people one thing only, namely, that the homeless mentally ill are so crippled in mind that they do not even know how to come in from the rain. I think that is a horribly dangerous misinterpretation.

As I see it, we (normal people) have families, jobs, property—which we are all too ready to trade for a little, or even a lot of, loss of liberty. Homeless mentally ill persons have none of these things. So why should they not cling to liberty, the only thing they have left that can still give them some dignity, with the same desperation with which a drowning man clings to a piece of wood? Why should they not value liberty more, not less, than we do? So long as we refuse to so interpret the predicament of the homeless mentally ill, we will be unable to do anything *for* them, and will only feel tempted to escalate our violence *against* them.

Of course many Americans recognized that chattel slavery was not as good for the Negro as its defenders claimed it was, and many now recognize that psychiatric slavery is not as good for the mental patient as its defenders claim it is. But unable to let go of either form of domination, our Founders engaged in, as do we, endless and futile efforts at *reform.*

Noonan emphasizes the agonizing moral discomfort that slavery—a well-established institution in 1776—created in the minds of the Founders. We know that. And we also know that since they nevertheless wanted to recognize slavery as a legally valid institution, they tried to reform it. After founding a new nation, Jefferson and his fellow lawmakers created:

new legislation for Virginia, that parodied the revolutionaries' statement of the inalienable liberty of human beings. "Be it enacted by the General Assembly that no person shall henceforth be slaves within the commonwealth, except such as were so on the first day of this present session of the Assembly, and the descendants of the females of them."[46]

The bill also banned the importation of slaves, thus providing an added incentive for breeding them. Keenly aware of the historical situation in which Jefferson and his fellow creators of the new America found themselves, Noonan asks: "Can they be blamed for not attempting the impossible [the abolition of slavery]?" "Obviously not," he answers.[47] But Noonan does not stop there:

> By not attempting the impossible, they reinstituted slavery by law. For that decision they were responsible—that is, it must be recognized that they as human beings performed the acts by which slavery was continued as a legal institution. They chose to participate in the system. With their own hands they put on the masks of the law and imposed them on others.[48]

Noonan rightly observes that Jefferson, Madison, and their fellow lawyers bore a heavy burden of responsibility for perpetuating slavery: "Without their [the lawyers'] professional craftsmanship, without their management of the metaphor, without their loyalty to the system, the *enslavement by words more comprehensive than any shackles could not have been formed*" (emphasis added).[49] Similarly, the shackles formed by psychiatric words, reinforced by judicial power and sanctions, now support an intricate web of psychiatric coercions and excuses known as the mental health system. A society in which a subsystem such as slavery or psychiatry is an integral part of a larger social-political system leaves little room for neutrality on the part of the citizen: He either supports the subsystem or he opposes it. If he supports the subsystem in the present, he may, in the future, be considered to have been disloyal to the higher values embodied in the larger system. I recognize that the historical situation today is not compatible with any person or group succeeding in abolishing institutional psychiatry. But is it not better to try to abolish psychiatric slavery and fail, than to support it and succeed?

MENTAL ILLNESS AS CANON LAW FICTION

When people think of psychiatry today, they associate it with medicine, science, and the law; and when they associate it with the law, they connect it with the codes of civil and criminal jurisprudence of modern, secular societies. It is important to keep in mind, however, that modern psychiatry is also highly respected—and fully recognized as a medical science—by Western religious bodies, especially the Roman Catholic Church.

Although the Church does not formally recognize modern developments in the natural sciences—for example, the bearing of geological knowledge on the age of the earth, or of genetics on evolution—it warmly embraces what it calls "developments" in the science of psychiatry. A moment's reflection will show us why this should be so.

Like civil law, criminal law, and psychiatry, Canon Law is concerned with issues such as free will, intent, consent, guilt, responsibility, and punishability. Moreover, as a codified system of sanctions, it, too, needs excuses. In its approach to all of these matters, modern Canon Law makes extensive use of the legal fiction of mental illness. Recognizing insanity as a bona fide illness, Canon Law distinguishes between two kinds of insanity: absolute or complete, and relative or partial. Absolute insanity is

> a mental disease or disorder that renders a baptized person over 7 years of age habitually incapable of any human acts . . . . Such a condition . . . creates a general legal disability regarding the personal exercise of rights, the incurrence of criminal liability, and subjection to ecclesiastical laws. A person absolutely insane . . . assumes the legal status of an infant.[50]

Mental illness thus has a somewhat different meaning and function in Canon Law than in American civil or criminal law. For example, Canon Law speaks of the rights and responsibilities of children over seven years old; under secular law, children of that age have few rights and even fewer responsibilities, regardless of their mental state. As to relative insanity, Canon Law defines it as follows:

> A mentally ill person who is not absolutely insane, however, might be insane with regard to a given act. . . . [Thus] a person might be legally "sane" for one thing, e.g., voting validly in an ecclesiastical election, and yet be legally "insane" for another, e.g., making a religious vow.[51]

Canon Law also recognizes "the doctrine of diminished responsibility . . . temporary mental disturbance, e.g., from drunkenness or passion, might remove or diminish imputability . . . ."[52] Here, the excuses provided by Canon Law and forensic psychiatry converge.

Moreover, since concepts such as action, intent, and will play a crucial role in religion, we find psychiatric considerations popping up all over *The Code of Canon Law* (drafted by the Canon Law Society of America).

For example, for a marriage to be a valid contract in the eyes of the Church, the parties must have "consensual capacity"—which, *mirabile dictu*, is impaired by a wide range of mental disorders. After genuflecting before "contemporary advances in medical science," the Canon Law Society of America declares that "One may be incapable of a human act at the time of consent for various reasons. The first broad category is mental illness."[53] Considering the scope of DSM-III, this suggests that there may not be many valid Catholic marriages in America today.

Sadly, the theologians who have drafted this document view the mentally ill as not fully human: "The person suffering from a permanent [mental] disorder is presumed to be habitually incapable of an internal will act."[54] Since theologians cannot and do not diagnose mental illness, this amounts to ceding a great deal of territory to their psychiatric competitors. To make matters worse still, the priests are particularly impressed by psychiatric advances in sexology: "An advance was made in 1957 with a decision which held that although a nymphomaniac was capable of eliciting a will act, she was nevertheless incapable of fulfilling the essential obligations of fidelity and, therefore, her consent [to marriage] was invalid."[55] Since the priests fail to mention that men suffering from the dread disease of satyriasis—the male analogue of nymphomania—are similarly incapable of consenting to a valid Catholic marriage, it seems that they pick and choose from the rich wares of the psychiatric taxonomist only those items that suit their own purposes or prejudices. This impression is supported by their silence concerning elective abortions which, psychiatrists maintain, are one of their most effective prophylactic measures against the mental illness caused by unwanted pregnancy. In fairness it should be said, however, that the Church no longer considers homosexuality a sin. Now that the psychiatrists no longer consider it an illness the priests at least do: it is an illness, they say, that renders a man—but apparently not a woman—"incapable of fulfilling the marital obligations . . . ."[56] But would it not be more accurate to say that such a person is unwilling, rather than unable, to fulfill his marital-sexual obligation? It gets worse. For example, the priests are positively overawed about the scientific advances psychiatrists have made in understanding the nature and effects of personality disorders: "The classification and nomenclature used for the different disorders vary; yet the essential conclusions remain the same: a person gravely afflicted has a severely weakened or nonexistent freedom of choice . . . ."[57]

I cite all this not so much to criticize the churchmen for making what I regard as grave mistakes in moral philosophy, but rather to show the wide-ranging uncritical acceptance of psychiatry in our day: no important institution—secular or clerical, legal, medical or scientific—is judiciously skeptical of psychiatric ideas and interventions. The Church's all but complete capitulation to psychiatry is illustrated by phrases such as the following recurring throughout the whole text of *The Code of the Canon Law*: "The clinical diagnosis of a mental disorder, even a tentative one, is a clinical and not a juridical issue."[58] The theologians evidently feel it would be sacrilegious to doubt or disagree with a psychiatrist's *clinical diagnosis*, even if it is only tentative. One shudders to think what they must think when they are face to face with a definitive psychiatric diagnosis—such as psychohistorians like to make, for example, of Jesus. But inconsistencies have never impaired a fiction, legal or psychiatric. Clearly the difference between the forensic psychiatry of our secular society and the psychiatric Canon Law of the Church is like the difference between a glass half-full and one half-empty.

VARIETIES OF FICTIONS: RELIGIOUS, LEGAL, SCIENTIFIC, AND PSYCHIATRIC

My aim in this chapter has been to analyze the idea of mental illness as a legal fiction, much as some years ago, in *The Myth of Mental Illness*, I analyzed it as scientific fiction. Actually fictions, or myths, have always been, and always will be, with us. What changes through the ages is not the existence of fictions in society but their content and consequences. That, indeed, is what we really mean when we speak of social change. Thus, when faith ruled the world, people accepted the fictions of religious mythology legitimized as theological truths. As recently as a few hundred years ago, common folk and leading intellectuals alike believed that saints and demons existed in the same sense that human beings exist. Accordingly certain abnormal behaviors, now called mental illness, were then viewed as manifestations of possession with good or evil spirits; and the madman, accordingly, was regarded either as a saintly soul obeying divine commandments, or as a dangerous maniac possessed by demons. From the seventeenth century onward, the religious concept of insanity metamorphosed into a medical concept: Ceasing to be a divine inspiration or devilish possession, insanity became an illness. Thus did the Age of Faith become the Age of Reason, and thus did insanity become a legal and scientific fiction. It may be useful, at this point, to review the main differences between these two kind of fictions.

The Fiction of Mental Illness: The Usefulness of Untruth

Scientific fictions, usually called *hypotheses* or *theories*, are attempts to articulate empirically verifiable or falsifiable observations. That the earth is a flat disc or that space is filled with a colorless and weightless substance called *ether* are examples of scientific fictions destroyed by having been proven false. On the other hand, legal fictions, or the fictions of ideologies and religions, are either patently false or not subject to disproof (for example, the existence of gods).* In addition, there is an important difference between the way scientific and legal fictions affect ordinary people: The concept of ether, a leading fiction of nineteenth-century physics, had no *direct* effect on the everyday lives of the American people, whereas the concept of mental illness has a profound, *direct* effect on the everyday lives of the American people today.

Legal fictions, as I have noted, are not attempts to articulate empirically verifiable observations. *Black's Law Dictionary* identifies a legal fiction not only as an untruth, but specifically as one that the rules of the legal game "will not allow to be disproved."[59] The point is that a legal fiction need not be true—it is enough that it be useful. Similarly, the idea of insanity (or any other psychiatric concept) need not be true—it is enough that it be useful. Indeed, the idea of mental illness is now viewed as so indispensable that even sophisticated ethicists and philosophers are unable to see through its fictional character. The following excerpt—from an essay by the philosopher Edmund Byrne—is illustrative:

> The concept of mental illness has long played an important and, for the most part, constructive role in human affairs. And for this reason, if no other, it should not be discarded lightly or without good reason. It is, therefore, not surprising that in spite of some well reasoned attacks on this concept as being unduly identified with a "medical model" and as reifying a "myth," the statutes of almost every jurisdiction in the United States, including some of those most recently revised, persist in relying upon it as the basis upon which to articulate rules for confining those who, though not at fault, seem unable to behave or function "normally." That there are such persons in ours as in every society is beyond dispute. The focus of definitional controversy is elsewhere, namely, on the question of who not only fits into the designated

---

*There is a pervasive distrust in our society about the possibility of examining religious ideas without being either too critical or too uncritical. Probably for this reason, writers on legal fiction avoid drawing a connection between legal and religious fictions, which is a pity. Religious fictions are prototypical of legal and other social science fictions. Indeed, such fictions can be said to exist only for nonbelievers. For believers, religious fictions are religious truths, or, at least, religious mysteries. Viewing religious fictions as untruths, indeed as conscious and deliberate falsehoods, is rightly regarded as a symptom of religious disbelief or heresy. In short, fictions—legal, religious, or psychiatric—are bandages that cover deep existential wounds: they cannot be removed, or even disturbed, without causing great pain to the collective psyche.

category but fits *so manifestly as to require intervention on the part of the state* . . . . That such intervention has come to be exercised primarily upon a finding of mental illness is largely a historical accident—one which, however, is readily understandable if one bears in mind the *science-centered ethos of modern Western civilization* (emphasis added).[60]

Unlike psychiatrists, Byrne acknowledges that the cutting edge of the concept of mental illness is "the question of who not only fits into the designated category [of mental patient], but fits so manifestly as to require intervention on the part of the state . . . ." This language—falsely implying that the so-called mental patient requires intervention when, in fact, it is those who impose such intervention on him who require it—exemplifies the use of the idea of insanity as a legal fiction. Assuredly, the controversy about mental illness is not merely or abstractly about definitions of illness. It is about power and State intervention. And so it was in the case of slavery too.

Byrne's final assertion—that State intervention "has come to be exercised primarily upon a finding of mental illness is largely a *historical accident*" (emphasis added)—is absurd. Was it a historical accident that State intervention supportive of slavery was exercised primarily upon a finding of blackness? In fact, nothing but blackness could justify slavery to Americans in the past, and nothing but mental illness can justify psychiatry to Americans today.

Insanity as Fiction, Ideology as Reality

Especially when they want to appear candid, legal scholars and philosophers of psychiatry love to mouth, as if it were a kind of epistemological mantra, the assertion that "Insanity is a legal term . . . not a medical one, and refers to a legal disability . . . rather than a medical or psychiatric condition."[61] But if that is what insanity is, why are lawyers so eager to have psychiatrists diagnose it, testify about it in court, and confine those who suffer from it?

In Chapters 1 and 3, I have shown that pathologists do not consider the term *mental illness* to refer to a disease in the medical sense of the word. Legal scholars, as we have seen, often say that insanity is a legal term, but in fact treat it as if it were a medical concept; moreover, they also often explicitly repudiate the view that insanity is a legal term and insist that it is a medical concept. Consider the following contradictions:

Norval Morris, a professor of law at the University of Chicago, flatly asserts that insanity is *not a legal concept*: "The layman often asks:

'What is the legal definition of insanity?' There is, of course, no such definition."[62]

Herbert Fingarette, whom I have cited earlier, asserts just as flatly that insanity is *not a medical concept*: "Insanity, mental illness, mental disease—these are not medical concepts."[63]

Shakespeare may have had the right idea when he suggested: "The first thing we do, let's kill all the lawyers."[64]

The more carefully one reads the literature on the legal uses of insanity, the more clearly one sees how brazenly hypocritical the legal scholar's attitude is toward it. For example, Morris's disclaimer notwithstanding, Fingarette offers a legal definition of insanity: "It is in connection with responsibility-impairment that I think such notions as 'mental disorder,' 'mental disease,' 'mental illness,' 'insanity,' 'neurosis,' et al. have their root significance."[65] In short, Fingarette wants to remove the element of illness from insanity and to replace it with irrationality. However, as an apologist for psychiatry who approves of coercive mental health measures, he brings mental illness and the psychiatrist back through a side door. "Rationality," he urges, "especially in association with mental disease, still suggests, as it ought, that testimony from medical men [in insanity trials] can be both relevant and important."[66]

Stephen J. Morse's writings exhibit the same inconsistency. He states that "mental health experts have no expertise whatsoever about the ultimate issue of legal insanity precisely because it is a . . . legal issue."[67] But then he too reintroduces the psychiatrist into the picture: "Experts [psychiatrists] should be limited to offering both full clinical descriptions of thoughts, feelings, and actions and relevant data based on sound, scientific studies."[68] But why, in trying a person accused of a crime, is a clinical description of his thoughts (whatever that might be) preferable to an ordinary description of them? It is obvious why: To justify his psychiatric incarceration:

> We should be clear that it is unjust to *punish* someone who is not responsible. . . . A fixed hospital term . . . is also improper for the same reason: hospital commitment should be related to continuing disorder.[69]

Thus, we come back again to the realization that involuntary mental hospitalization is the tail that wags not only the psychiatric dog, but the legal superstructure that is its master—and the society they both serve.

These alternating and self-contradictory claims regarding insanity illustrate and support my contention that insanity is a legal fiction. To be sure, it is a legal fiction of a particular sort—one that makes use of psychiatric rather than, say, economic or political concepts and rhetoric. In this respect, too, the idea of insanity resembles the idea of slavery. Legal scholars made inconsistent claims regarding slavery also—defining the status called *slave* legally, while ostensibly determining who qualifies for it hematologically, by asking: "How much Negro blood does he have?" Although lawyers define the status called (involuntary) *mental patient* legally, ostensibly they determine who qualifies for it psychiatrically by asking: "How crazy is he?" Of course, in the age of chattel slavery what really mattered was not only how much Negro blood a person had in him, but where he was, who he was, and who wanted to make him a slave. Similarly, in the modern age of psychiatric slavery, what really matters is not only how crazy a person is, but where he is, who he is, and who wants to make him a mental patient. This is why, in the final analysis, lawyers *use* expert psychiatric testimony, psychiatric rhetoric, and the psychiatric disposition of the targeted person *as they see fit*. Unlike illness, which in a sense *belongs* to doctors, insanity *belongs* to lawyers.

Realization of the thoroughly fictional character of the idea of insanity brings us back to square one, namely, to the fact that, as human beings, we differ from other animals in being thoroughly symbolic beings. Thus, when we find death unbearable, as most people did until modern times, we make believe that, instead of being the end of life, death is its true beginning. Similarly, when we find life unbearable, as many people now do, we make believe that life truly begins only after we attain mental health. In short, with religion we falsify our death, with psychiatry our life. No wonder that M. Scott Peck—a born-again Christian psychiatrist—is now the most widely-read mental health guru in the United States.[70]

Finally, whatever people mean by insanity, they—professionals and lay people alike—perceive it as an *alien power* ever ready to enslave and oppress them.[71] This is why I have long maintained that mental illness is an ideological idea that fuels psychiatry as an ideological theory and movement of liberation (promising to liberate the mental patient from his illness). The fact that mental illness is a fiction, and that those posturing as the mental patients' liberators are the problem rather than the solution, has, of course, not in the least impaired the credibility of the mental health movement. The human dread of disorder and the craving for order through dependency as a remedy for it are so powerful that they obliterate, in each generation, the memory of what ideological liberators have wrought throughout history.

12

MENTAL ILLNESS AS EXPLANATION

The worst affliction of all is, and continues to be, that one does not know whether one's suffering is an illness of the mind or a sin.
—Soren Kierkegaard[1]

My aim in this, the final, chapter is to briefly review how and why the idea of mental illness has proven to be such a useful explanatory concept. Although the term *mental illness* is useful mainly because it is considered to be the name of a type of illness, its reference to the mind requires some critical attention also. Accordingly, I shall begin by offering some remarks on the first half of this key term, namely, on what is *mental* or *mind*.

IS MENTAL ILLNESS "MENTAL"?

There is endless talk today about mental illness without people giving much thought to what they mean by qualifying this alleged disorder as mental. I believe it is safe to assert that most people use the adjective *mental* to indicate that the illness in question is not bodily—as in the humorous assurance: "Don't worry, it's all in your mind."

The question, What is mind? has puzzled philosophers and psychologists for millennia and I am not about to review the billions of words they have said on this subject. Let me suggest only that we distinguish among three concepts, namely, brain, behavior, and mind. The first two are not particularly problematic. Brain is a bodily organ, like heart or lung, differing from other organs only in having different functions. As to behavior, while it is not the name of a material object or bodily organ, its referent is equally clear: by behavior we mean the person's "mode of conducting himself" or his "deportment" (*Webster's*). In other words, behavior is the name we attach to a living being's conduct in the daily pursuit of life—that is, the way he eats, mates, fights, and so forth; it is important to emphasize that bodily movements that are the products of neurophysiological discharges or reflexes are not behavior. For example, a lion's hunting a prey is behavior; but the constriction and dilation of its pupils in response to light or darkness is not. The point is that behavior implies action, and action implies conduct pursued by an agent seeking to attain a goal.

Transcending the Riddle of the Mind

Because psychiatrists have always claimed that mental illness is like any other illness, I began this book by examining what the experts on diseases—the pathologists—say about this assertion. We thus discovered that these experts recognize no such entity or thing as mental illness. They view the phenomena called mental illness as diseases only insofar as they are diseases of the brain, in which case the term *mental illness* is redundant and misleading.

In addition to interpreting the term *mental illness* as referring to a species of bodily illness, we might also interpret it as referring to mental diseases, that is, a disease of the *mind*. But the mind, as we saw, is an abstract noun that cannot, except metaphorically, be said to be sick. So much then for the *illness* part of mental illness. What about the mental part?

Since the middle of the last century, the term *mind* has ceased to be a part of the vocabulary of scientists and has, instead, become a part of the vocabulary of philosophers. This may explain why philosophers write at length about the mind without mentioning mental illness, and why psychiatrists write at length about mental illness without mentioning the mind. As everyone knows, the modern professionals who claim mental illness as their territory are psychiatrists, psychologists, and neuroscientists who, as their names imply, study brains and behaviors. This is why scientific psychiatry and psychology have, in effect, got rid of the mind, and why Colin Wilson is so excited to discover that "It is one of the absurd paradoxes of psychology that it has taken three centuries to reach the conclusion that men actually possess a mind."[2] Unfortunately, in saying this, Wilson demonstrates that his heart is in the right place, but his mind—pardon that word again—is not. Why should Wilson or anyone think that psychologists and psychiatrists study the mind? They study, and control, human beings and their behavior. So I agree with Morse Peckham that we would do better to recognize the term *mind* for what it is:

> For twenty-five hundred years the struggle has been going on to decide whether or not the mind is an entity. . . . [But] there are a good many words, of which "mind" appears to be an excellent example, for which there is no something. It is an illusion that there is something. The something that the word allegedly names does not exist.[3]

What, then, does *mind* mean? It does not mean anything. Instead, like mental illness itself, the word *mind* is a tool we use for certain purposes—especially for the purpose of explaining behavior:

> . . . human behavior [Peckham continues] is both predictable and unpredictable. I do not think that such a notion will surprise anyone, but what has been made of it is quite astonishing, for one of the most important uses of the word "mind" is simply to explain this predictability and this unpredictability by subsuming both under that word.[4]

This brings us back neatly to the subject of this chapter, namely, to the idea of mental illness as an explanation of behavior. Since our ideas about explaining insane behavior are inextricably intertwined with our ideas about explaining sane behavior, it is now necessary to relate both the idea of insanity and my critique of it to conventional contemporary psychiatric and philosophical explanations of mentally healthy and mentally sick behavior.

MENTAL ILLNESS AS BRAIN DISEASE

Many people—in and outside of the mental health professions—now assume that insanity is a brain disease and thus take it for granted that its explanation must be sought in neurobiological terms. In this way, the presumption that behavior denominated as mental illness is the manifestation of disordered brain function determines—prejudges perhaps is more accurate—not only what counts as *understanding* such behavior but also what counts as *trying to understand it.* This is why my criticisms of the neuropathological and psychopharmacological fakeries of psychiatry are often misinterpreted as opposition to "research about how the brain works"—an absurd contention. My objections to the claims of organic psychiatrists lie elsewhere, in what I consider to be two fundamental misconceptions: one is a misunderstanding of the differences between the literal and metaphorical meanings of words; the other is a misunderstanding of the relationship between chemical processes in the body and human experiences or so-called mental states.

Empirical Discovery Cannot Change the Metaphorical into the Literal

We understand the difference between the literal and metaphorical uses of the word *father.* Suppose, however, that a person did not know this or chose to ignore it, and focused instead only on the fact that the priest is called *Father.* Suppose, further, that impressed by the literal meaning of the term *father,* he set out to investigate the private lives of priests in an effort to prove that they are literal fathers. Such a researcher might indeed discover that some priests are real (biological, literal) fathers. But what would that prove? Only that some priests have children—who might call them not only *father* but also *daddy* or *papa.* The origin and functions of the clerical-legal term *Father* would remain what they had been: The discovery that some—or even all—metaphorical fathers are also literal fathers would have no bearing at all on the idea of the priest as Father.

The situation with respect to bodily illness and mental illness is similar. As the designations *literal father* and *metaphorical father* come into being in completely different ways and serve completely different functions, so the designations *literal disease* and *metaphorical disease* also come into being in different ways and serve different functions. Suppose, then, that someone were to ignore these differences and focus instead on the fact that mentally ill persons are (said to be) ill and went looking for brain lesions in their heads. Suppose, further, that he found that some of them had brain lesions. What would he have discovered? Only that these particular persons had brain diseases and were therefore neurologically ill. The origin and functions of the medicolegal term *mental illness* would remain what they had been: The discovery that some metaphorically ill persons are also literally ill would have no bearing at all on the idea of insanity as an illness.

The expectation that chemical processes (abnormalities) will explain mental states (illnesses) rests partly on the foregoing confusion of literal with metaphorical diseases and partly on a similar confusion of the relationship between brain and behavior. The latter confusion is perhaps best clarified by reference to what we now know about the relationship between bodily chemistry and personal experience. We know, for example, that adrenalin mediates anger and that lactic acid accumulates in muscles during exercise. This makes us realize only more clearly that adrenalin does not cause anger, nor lactic acid fatigue. Thus, even if a chemical substance were found in the brain associated with behavior we now call *schizophrenic*, such a discovery would no more establish the chemical etiology of schizophrenia than did the discovery of adrenalin establish the chemical etiology of anger.*

The Moral Unneutrality of the Idea that Mental Illness Is Brain Disease

In addition to the considerations just set forth, I object to the claims of biological psychiatrists because I maintain that it makes no sense to select patients on moral or legal grounds, and then study them as if they were medically ill. No sooner does a wicked person, like John Hinckley, Jr., show up on the evening news, then there is speculation—by newscasters, psychiatrists, and the public alike—about what kind of mental illness he suffers from. However, when a virtuous person shows up on the news—like the man who, at the cost of his own life, saved several people from a plane crash in the Potomac—there is no such speculation. Ours would be a strange brain indeed if it would regularly cause horrible behavior but could never cause heroic behavior.

I also object to the posture of (self-proclaimed) scientists who claim a purely scientific interest in advancing brain research because, in the context of contemporary debates about mental illness, such a claim is an exercise in hypocrisy. Interest in brain research, as I have indicated earlier, appears to be scientific and praiseworthy, and so it might be in principle; but it is neither scientific nor praiseworthy in practice, when it is used, as it is typically in psychiatry, to justify coercive mental health interventions. To my knowledge, no one publicly identified for

---

*As I have discussed earlier (see Chapter 3), the model of neurosyphilis has no bearing on alleged diseases such as manic-depression and schizophrenia. The treponema pallidum, the microorganism responsible for syphilis, together with the human host's response to it, cause destruction of cells and tissues: Paresis is a progressive disease of the brain which, if untreated, results in death. There is not the slightest evidence for progressive destruction of brain cells and tissues in patients diagnosed as manic-depressive or schizophrenic. There is evidence, of course, that the somatic treatments of these unreal diseases cause real destruction of brain cells and tissues, but that is another story.

his interest in investigating the biological basis of mental illness condemns psychiatric coercions and excuses. I know of no mental health researcher who would be willing to say (approximately): "I believe that mental diseases are brain diseases and that we must concentrate our efforts on discovering their precise nature and cure. In the meantime, however, we must stop using the diagnosis of mental illness to justify incarcerating innocent persons and excusing guilty ones." Because of the absence of anything remotely resembling such an expression of opinion by a person interested in organic psychiatry, I conclude that claims about the organic etiology of mental illness and the need for brain research are tactics to conceal psychiatry's (not so) hidden agendas—namely, denial of free will and responsibility and justification of coercion.

Finally, physicians and scientists who claim that mental diseases will yield their secrets to medical research and then stand revealed as brain diseases act as if such a discovery would automatically obliterate the stubborn moral and legal problems which the behavior of so-called mental patients pose. This is simply not true. Actually, there is nothing unusual about discovering a new disease. Legionnaire's disease and AIDS were unknown 25 years ago. The discovery of AIDS—even though it is an infectious disease with a fatal outcome—has not resulted in the use of that diagnosis as justification for depriving AIDS victims innocent of lawbreaking of their liberty, or for excusing them of punishment for crimes they have committed. How or why, then, would the discovery that schizophrenia is a brain disease justify the continued use of that diagnosis for civil commitment, involuntary treatment, and the insanity defense? The discovery that schizophrenia is a neurophysiological disorder—say, like epilepsy or multiple sclerosis— would strengthen rather than weaken my argument about the problem of free will and personal responsibility associated with the idea of insanity. The epileptic is, of course, not responsible for his epilepsy: that is, he is not responsible for having a seizure threshold lower than that of normal persons. But the epileptic is responsible for his social conduct. Accordingly, epilepsy is not a justification for depriving a person of his liberty or for excusing his criminal conduct. The discovery that a brain lesion renders its victim prone to schizophrenic behavior would make such a person resemble the epileptic. He would not be responsible for his tendency to schizophrenia, but would be responsible for his behavior, even when under the influence of his illness. The diagnosis of schizophrenia would thus become just as irrelevant to civil commitment and the insanity defense as the diagnosis of epilepsy is today. The schizophrenic patient, his family, and society would thus continue to face the same problems they face now—except that they would be deprived of the option of managing their problems by having recourse to civil commitment, involuntary treatment, and the insanity defense. In short, viewing mental illness as not an illness and viewing it as being "like any other illness" converge in a most important consequence—namely, in undermining the rationale for psychiatric coercions and excuses.

Finally, the posture—whether held sincerely or hypocritically—of being interested in psychiatry *qua* brain research may simply be a symptom of naive scientism. I say this because if our aim is to understand human behavior—especially the sort of dramatic and destructive behavior that typically provokes contentions of mental illness—then why should we consider it more important to investigate how the brain is put together and works than to investigate how a particular person is put together and works? Why should trying to understand the molecular biology of nerve fibers be considered more important and relevant than trying to understand the experience of worthlessness, the desire for attention, boredom, envy, fear, greed, and the many other mental states that make human beings persons? My point is that viewing mental illness as brain disease prejudices our criteria of what counts as a scientific fact: Statements about dopamine receptors—which lay people cannot understand—become facts, while statements about hatred and revenge—which lay people can understand but may not want to—become nonfacts. Thus, in a recent highly acclaimed popularization of the discoveries of modern psychiatric science, the reader was offered the following *facts:*

> "The brain is an organ; it produces thoughts about the same way the kidney produces urine." This fact was supplied by an anonymous neuroanatomist.[5]

> "Aggression is like any other disease." This fact was discovered by Paul Mandel, a neuroscientist at the Center for Neurochemistry in Strasbourg, France.[6]

> "People who act crazy are acting that way because they have too much or too little of some chemicals in their brains. It's just a physical illness!" This fact was uncovered by Candace Pert, a researcher at the National Institute of Mental Health in Bethesda, Maryland.[7]

> "Schizophrenia, the most expensive and devastating of all the common mental illnesses, has been revealed as a physical ailment involving a malfunction in the dopamine system at the base of the brain." This fact was told to John Franklin, the Pulitzer Prize winning author of

The Mind Fixers, by all of the neuroscientists he interviewed for his series of articles on mental illness.[8]

Not surprisingly, the result of all this research on mind fixing is the bizarre distortion of reality that has long characterized psychiatry. For example, it is now accepted as a fact that John Hinckley, Jr. suffers from schizophrenia and that schizophrenia is a brain disease; but it is not accepted as a fact that he shot President Reagan because he wanted to and that he is now being punished, rather than treated, in a mental hospital.

FREE WILL AND DETERMINISM

Undergirding the controversy concerning mental illness—in other words, concerning what constitutes the correct explanation of certain abnormal, bizarre, deviant, despicable, destructive, or self-destructive behaviors—lies the age-old controversy about free will and determinism. As everyone knows, the explanation of human behavior most deeply rooted in Western thought accounts for personal conduct in terms of free will—that is, by attributing the actor's behavior to his choice of a particular aim and the means he selects for attaining it. A person acts in a certain way because he wants to bring about a certain consequence, for example, gratifying his desire for food or sex, money or power. An act here is seen as a consequence of personal choice.

The other explanation makes use of a diametrically opposite principle. Instead of accounting for personal conduct in terms of aims or goals, it accounts for it in terms of causes or compulsions, such as poverty or mental illness. In contrast to teleological or motivational explanations of human behavior, deterministic explanations are causal, based on the assumption that personal conduct results from certain anterior events. Thus, a person acts in a particular way because demons, poverty, genes, or mental illness compel him to so behave. Personal choice has nothing to do with the matter.*

The roots of this dichotomy lie in the fact that the most important characteristic distinguishing human beings from animals, plants, and

---

*For a characteristic articulation of this view, consider the following passage, penned by one of the leading British psychoanalysts of the post-World War II years: "The analyst must above all be an analyst. That is to say he must *know positively* that all human emotional reactions, all human judgments, and even reason itself, are but the tools of the unconscious; and that such seemingly acute convictions which an intelligent person like this possesses are but the *inevitable effects of causes* which lie buried in the unconscious levels of his psyche" (emphasis added).[9]

nonliving things is that we possess a highly developed capacity to use symbols. This capacity is manifested by creating, sending, receiving, and interpreting messages ranging from simple gestures and grunts to incredibly complex verbal, mathematical, musical, and other notations. It is these specifically human characteristics that account for culture and for two important cultural phenomena. One is the primitive, animistic (mis)interpretation of all signs as of the same kind, regardless of whether they are *given off passively,* like the signs of an impending storm by a darkening sky, or are *given actively,* like the signs formed by human speech. The other is the modern, materialistic (mis)interpretation of all signs, again as of the same kind, regardless of whether they are *given off,* like the electrocardiographic signs of a myocardial infarction, or are *given,* like the linguistic signs of delusions.

The animistic interpretation of nature, as the term implies, entails viewing all signs as portents issued by imaginary agents fashioned after the model of human beings. Rain, drought, earthquake, disease, death—everything that happens in the world—is thus interpreted as an expression of the sentiments, desires, or wills of gods, ghosts, or spirits. In such a world, nothing happens; everything is willed by (quasi-human) agents.

The materialistic interpretation of nature, as the term implies, entails viewing all signs as the manifestations of physicochemical processes, such as human beings observe when they look at nature. Joy and sadness, fear and elation, anger, greed—all human aspirations and passions—are thus interpreted as the manifestations of unintentional, amoral, biochemical and biophysical processes. In such a world, nothing is willed; everything happens.*

Accordingly, while the *animistic* savage interprets *natural deaths*—for example, deaths due to injury or disease—as murder, the *scientific* psychiatrist interprets *unnatural deaths*—for example, deaths due to suicide or murder—as happenings instead of actions. Ironically, the psychiatric explanation of mentally ill behavior suffers from the same sort of error as does the animistic explanation of natural events: While the psychiatrist views human actions as the consequences of natural events, the primitive views natural events as the consequences of choice

---

*The contemporary, perhaps especially American, aversion to frankly acknowledging intentionality is revealed by the colloquialism *make it happen.* This phrase is a favorite of radio and television personalities engaged in giving what used to be called *advice to the lovelorn:* Instead of suggesting that the person who calls in *decide* or *do* something, they invariably tell him to *make it happen* (*it* referring to whatever either the caller wants to do or the media therapist wants him to do). This, of course, is an oxymoronic use of the term *happen,* which implies precisely that it is something not under our control.

by (quasi-) human agents. As the primitive had spiritualized nature, so the psychiatrist now animalizes man. It seems that when we try to explain the human condition, we—human beings—have a hard time finding a happy medium between making too much or too little of intentionality: When we are culturally underdeveloped, we treat objects as agents; when we are culturally developed, we treat agents as objects. Thus, the primitive tries to understand nature in terms of human nature, while the psychiatrist tries to understand human nature in terms of nature. In our roles as modern scientists, we have corrected the savage's mistake. Who will correct the psychiatrist's mistake, and ours for supporting it?

The Search for Causes in Psychiatric Explanations

Psychiatrists and other behavioral scientists continue to pour out an uninterrupted stream of articles and books allegedly demonstrating that man has no free will. By debunking free will and responsibility, professionals in the mental health discipline seek to legitimize themselves as bona fide scientists; at the same time, they also try to endear themselves to the politicians and the public by promising to control crime, which they call *excessive violence*. Typical of this trend—and much loved by the press and the public alike—is the claim that medical science has finally proved that violence is caused by brain disease and that medical specialists can, on the basis of objective evidence, predict future violence. In a major story on the Fourth World Congress of Biological Psychiatry in the "Science" section of *The New York Times*, the reporter quotes Alan Gruber, director of neuropsychobiology at the Center for Memory Impairment and Neurobehavioral Disorders in Boston, stating: "I would submit to you that we can predict human aggressive behavior 90% of the time."[10] Another speaker, Frank Elliot, a neurosurgeon, "described exhaustive studies of 321 excessively violent individuals [of whom] . . . more than 90 percent showed evidence of brain dysfunction and neurological defects." Added Elliot: "We have been looking at abnormal brains for a generation and calling them normal."[11] Needless to say, the scientists who make such claims do not bother to define what constitutes aggressive behavior or excessive violence. Is a professional boxer or bullfighter engaged in violent behavior? Or a member of the French military forces blowing up an unarmed ship in a New Zealand port?

Attributing violent behavior to brain mechanisms is, of course, only the bio-neuro-psycho-scientist's foot in the door of free will. After removing the idea of responsibility from our explanations of so-called criminal or violent behavior, he moves on to complete the determinist's dream, the destruction, once and for all, of the idea of free will.

"Is free will a fraud?" asks Richard Restak, a well-known physician-writer on brain-mind problems, in the title of an essay published in *Science Digest*. In the subtitle he answers his question: "Do we make our own choices? Plot our destinies? Are we truly conscious? New research indicates that the answer to all of these questions may be no." What evidence does Restak have to support his contention? None. "Where in the brain does this [free] will reside?" he asks. His answer speaks for itself: "There is not a center in the human brain involved in the exercise of will any more than there is a center in the brain of the swan responsible for the beauty and complexity of its flight."[12] It is such research and such reasoning that now pass for behavioral research and behavioral science.

The Case against Psychiatric Determinism

Whether the idea of insanity explains or explains away, whether it solves or creates a problem, comes down to a simple question: Do we want two types of accounts of human behavior—one to explain the conduct of sane or mentally healthy persons, and another to explain the conduct of insane or mentally ill persons? I maintain that we do not need, and should not try, to account for normal behavior one way (motivationally), and for abnormal behavior another way (causally). Specifically, I suggest that the principle, "Actions speak louder than words," can be used to explain the conduct of mentally ill persons just as well as it can the behavior of mentally healthy persons. Consider, by way of illustration, the following typical cases of insanity reported in the press:

> Willie Robinson, 42, was placed under "police protection" at the Wesson Unit of Bay State Medical Center [in Springfield, Mass.] yesterday [June 23, 1980], a short time after he allegedly went berserk with a long-bladed kitchen knife in the crowded waiting room of the hospital's Springfield Unit. . . . [At the hospital], Robinson assaulted the guard and several women and allegedly pinned a [six-year-old] boy to the ground near an ambulance entrance and stabbed him repeatedly, screaming, "I'm the king! I'm the king! Now I've done it. I'm done." [The boy died.][13]

> A Roxdale [Ontario] woman signed her husband out of a psychiatric ward against medical advice days before he stabbed her 58 times in front of their three children, an Ontario Supreme Court jury heard yesterday. . . . William Szeman, 41, pleaded not guilty yesterday [June 26, 1980] to second degree murder by reason of insanity. Lawyers on both sides of the case . . . agreed that Mr. Szeman should be found insane. The insanity finding needed only the jury's official approval and that took less than 15 minutes . . . . The jury was

told that Mr. Szeman, an auto body worker who came to Canada from Hungary in 1957, was admitted to the psychiatric ward of Etobicoke General Hospital last April 18, three days before the murder. Metro Police Sergeant Donald Sampson testified that . . . Mr. Szeman told him he worked with Germans, Hungarians, and Poles who hated him because he had fought against them during the last world war. Mr. Szeman would have been 7 when the war ended . . . . Mr. William Peacock [a neighbor] said that Mr. Szeman, walking by him after his arrest, said: "She was trying to poison me." There was no evidence that was true.[14]

The pattern obvious in the behavior of these and other like-minded persons, yet systematically neglected in psychiatric theorizing about them, has several significant features:

1. The (so-called) patient engages in dramatically destructive acts, injuring or killing people.
2. The patient makes false claims about himself: that he is a king or that he fought in the Second World War and was being poisoned by his wife.
3. The patient justifies what he has done: as a right (as king or god), or as self-defense (against being poisoned).
4. The patient feels relieved by his act and exults in it. In the first case, the killer exclaimed, "Now I've done it. I'm done." In the second, he was found "prancing and dancing near the body of his wife, which lay on the pavement in the driveway."

The standard psychiatric explanation—which attributes such berserk acts to an acute, overwhelming disorder of the brain rendering the patient irrational and violent—does not and cannot account for any of these features. In particular, it cannot account for why the patient feels proud rather than ashamed of what he has done. In the language of the McNaghten Rule, the oldest Anglo-American test of criminal insanity, such malefactors are said not to know right from wrong. But this is patently not true: in fact, they insistently assert their judgments of right and wrong. The evidence thus points not to *their inability* to judge right from wrong, but to their *inversion* of our judgments of right and wrong. Stripped of psychiatric rhetoric, a person is typically diagnosed as psychotic when two conditions obtain: first, that by conventional standards he behaves very badly—often threatening to kill himself or others; second, that he justifies his misbehavior in a conventionally unjustifiable way—often by claiming that what he had done is good, not bad.

The attempt to explain psychosis psychiatrically faces another serious difficulty which can be summed up in the following question: Why do certain (hypothesized) brain diseases causing psychoses invariably manifest themselves in dramatically bad behavior rather than in dramatically good behavior? Somatic disease processes manifest themselves in bodily changes in both directions: for example, a person may have too few red cells in his blood or too many; his blood pressure may be too low or too high; his heart may beat too slowly or too fast; he may be underweight or overweight; he may be shorter and weaker than the average or taller and stronger. Revealingly, the disease we call *psychosis* never works that way: the psychotic patient attacks and kills people, but never assists and helps them. Why are we—psychiatrists as well as lay people—so eager to attribute wicked behavior to psychosis, and why do we never attribute virtuous behavior to it? The answer is obvious: because good deeds do not disturb and threaten us; hence, good deeds do not generate a desire to explain them away by attributing them to insanity, nor do the doers of good deeds make us feel that we must protect ourselves from them by diagnosing them as mentally ill and depriving them of liberty.

Of course, like all human behavior, so-called insane behavior has a variety of motivations. Many such acts—for example, those illustrated by the stories I have cited—are inspired by an intense craving for attention and fame in a person who can achieve that goal in no other way than through a dramatic act of violence. Such an act and its aftermath also satisfy the actor's intense craving for being distracted from his own insignificance, from the drudgery and ordinariness of his everyday existence and its frustrations, in short, from the bleakness and futility of his life. Insanity, then, has this in common with war: each provides a surpassingly successful distraction from everyday problems—insanity for the individual, war for society.

MENTAL HEALTH AS ACTION, MENTAL ILLNESS AS EVENT

Psychiatrists are not the only persons professionally concerned with human behavior and the predicaments of the human condition. Among others concerned with this subject, the most important ones are philosophers, ethicists, and jurists. Without their support, the views now generally regarded as psychiatric (and to which I usually so refer) could not have come into being and could not have become as dominant as they have. It is a curious and exceedingly interesting fact—the details of which cannot detain us here—that all great modern philosophers and students of human behavior—John Locke, David Hume, John Stuart

Mill, even Ludwig von Mises—have taken for granted that while most human behaviors can be attributed to motives and make sense, some behaviors have no motives and are *bizarre* or *senseless*. In short, rational behavior is the behavior of sane persons, irrational behavior, the behavior of insane persons. The philosopher Peter Winch puts it this way:

> It is important to notice that, in the sense in which I am speaking of rules, it is just as true to speak of the anarchist as following rules in what he does as it is to say the same thing of the monk. The difference between these two kinds of men is not that the one follows rules and the other does not; it lies in the diverse *kinds* of rules which each respectively follows. . . . The anarchist's way of life is thus a *way of life*. It is to be distinguished, for instance, from the pointless behavior of a berserk lunatic.[15]

This statement is a remarkable example of the hold the psychiatric perspective has even on the best of minds. Yet, this view of the lunatic's behavior—albeit now shared by scientist, philosopher, and layman alike—is not only odd, it is also false. I call this view odd because the point of the berserk lunatic's behavior is perfectly obvious, often painfully so: its sense lies, and may be inferred from, its aim or consequence, in exactly the same way as we ascertain the sense of a normal person's behavior. For example, a berserk lunatic may claim to be Jesus or kill his wife. The point of such a person's behavior, I dare say, is to be revered like Jesus or be rid of his wife. (Why a person chooses such ends and means is another question, the answer to which is often easily obtained by asking him.) Moreover, since people, including philosophers, often do not know whether a person is or is not a lunatic until psychiatrists identify him as such, it is not true that such a person's behavior is, *prima facie*, pointless. On the contrary, the fact is that when we find a certain behavior exceptionally disturbing, we say that the actor is a lunatic or psychotic and that his behavior is senseless or pointless. We used to say that such a person was a witch or was possessed by demons. Whether we realize it or not, when we call a person a lunatic or psychotic or mentally not responsible we are engaged in giving things names which, as Thomas Carlyle wisely observed,

> are but . . . custom-woven, wonder-hiding Garments. Witchcraft, and all manner of Specterwork, and Demonology, we have now renamed Madness, and Diseases of the Nerves. Seldom reflecting that still the new question comes upon us: What is Madness, What are Nerves?[16]

The imagery of insanity—of senseless mentally sick actors performing bizarre acts—is a fiction that psychiatrists have labored long and hard to foist upon us, and themselves, as facts. Because of their efforts—and more particularly because of the efforts of post-Enlightenment men and women to deny the existential and moral depths to which human beings may sink—it is now generally accepted that insane persons are irrational and not responsible for their conduct. Because this belief performs indispensable services in modern societies, it is accepted as true.

Mental Illness: *Cui Bono?*

Because of the reasons previously discussed, virtually every educated person now believes that some human behaviors are actions, the consequences of personal choice, while others are events, the consequences of mental illness. The fact that this dichotomy, and the premises built into it, lies at the heart of all contemporary attempts to explain insanity cannot be exaggerated. The typical first step in explaining the behavior of a mentally ill person is thus to view it as a nonaction. Michael Moore states it clearly when he writes:

> The bodily motions of epileptics during a grand mal seizure or perhaps the word salads of schizophrenics would seem to be nonrational activities . . . . This kind of pattern of action is the primary symptom of the mental incapacities we label mental illness . . . . Being mentally ill means being incapacitated from acting rationally in this fundamental sense.[17]

I have discussed the error—or advantage—of this strategy before (see Chapter 7): the bodily motions of an epileptic during a grand mal seizure are not irrational or nonrational acts, because they are *not acts* at all. Surely, it would be more honest to admit that we regard the acts of insane persons as irrational because they are—or because we believe they are—false or wicked; in short, because they contradict the facts and violate the rules of life as we, and others in our society, see them.

But that is not what we do. If it were, there would be no mental illness to write about. What we do—consistent with the belief that sane persons act (responsibly), and that insane persons are the victims of an illness (for which they are not responsible and which makes them not responsible)—is that we let psychiatrists and philosophers construct a special set of explanations to account for the behavior of persons said to be mentally ill, and let lawmakers attach a special set of excuses to behaviors categorized as mental symptoms, and a special set of justifications to behaviors categorized as mental treatments. For example, psychiatrists and others accept that the mentally healthy person who sets his house afire to collect the insurance does so to accomplish his particular aims and call him an *arsonist;* but they insist that the mentally ill person who sets his house afire does so because his illness compels him to do it and call him a *pyromaniac.* In the same way, psychiatrists distinguish between the thief and the kleptomaniac, the responsible murderer and the nonresponsible schizophrenic, and so forth, maintaining that mentally healthy persons commit crimes because they choose to, and mentally sick persons because they are compelled to.

Conventional psychiatrists and I agree about why the arsonist, thief, or other mentally healthy person commits a crime. We disagree about why the mentally ill person does so: I believe we can extend the type of explanation we use to account for the behavior of the mentally healthy person to account for the behavior of the mentally ill person as well. To be sure, there may be dramatic differences in the goals each pursues: for example, one may set a fire to make money while another may do so to gain attention or get room and board in a publicly financed institution. The point is that both types of persons can, given the appropriate incentive or punishment, refrain from setting fires.

The psychiatrist posits the existence in nature of two different types of human beings: the mentally healthy and the mentally ill, the rational and the irrational. The actions of the former, he claims, are properly explained teleologically, in terms of goals; those of the latter, however, must be explained causally, in terms of mental diseases and irrational impulses. Against this view, I maintain that we do not deal here with two different classes of *human beings,* but with two different types of *explanations of human action.* The proof of this pudding lies in the fact that the psychiatrist has no objective way of ascertaining which person belongs in which category. How, then, does he make the distinction? By means of what he calls *clinical judgment,* a euphemism concealing moral judgments behind pseudoscientific diagnoses, and social strategies behind pseudotherapeutic dispositions.

In short, I contend that the idea of insanity need not be true or valid; it is enough that it be useful. Thus, the real question before us remains: How is the idea of mental illness useful? I hope that in the preceding chapters I have succeeded in answering this question. Since not a day passes without newspapers reporting a story illustrating the utility of mental illness explanations, I want to add here a recent—wonderfully revealing—example of it.

Everyone knows that some white persons dislike black persons, and vice versa. However, discrimination based on skin color, especially in publicly financed jobs, is now against the law. Differential treatment based on mental health considerations is another matter, as the following news item illustrates:

Louisville, KY, June 7 (1985) (AP)—This city may have to find an all-white job setting for a city employee because he says he has a mental problem that makes him fear working with blacks. The Kentucky Workers' Compensation Board ordered a search for a job with all-white co-workers for Gary Pearl, a 39-year-old former street cleaning supervisor, ... Mr. Pearl was granted a disability benefit of $231.47 a week until he returned to work. The board, in a unanimous ruling April 29, ordered that Mr. Pearl "undergo therapy and that exhaustive efforts be made [to find a job for him] in an all-white setting if necessary for his employability."[18]

Clearly, the idea of insanity is not merely useful, it is indispensable—in much the same way religious ideas were indispensable until recently. "Who is there who does not see," wrote Thomas Hobbes in *Leviathan*, "to whose benefit it conduceth, to have it believed, that a king has not his authority from Christ, unless a bishop crown him?"[19] Actually, in Catholic countries many did not see that because they did not want to see it, much as most people today, because they do not want to see it, do not see the ritual-political character of psychiatry's paradigmatic procedures.

If Mental Illness Did Not Exist . . .

As I have noted earlier, mental hospitals—or madhouses, as they were originally called—came first, and mental illness second: in other words, the social system of confining lunatics preceded the idea that the persons so confined were ill. Why do I think this is so important? Because the idea of mental illness as an illness conceals the simple fact that the primary function of the public mental hospital has always been, and still is, to provide room and board for society's *misérables*—the homeless, the unskilled, the unemployed, those unable or unwilling to care for themselves and for whom no one else is willing to care. Once in a great while even psychiatrists acknowledge this, as does C.H. Hardin Branch, professor of psychiatry at the University of Utah, when he remarks that "We are left with the tired, the poor, the unwanted, the disengaged, the unproductive, the people who are neither physically ill nor morally evil."[20]

This caretaking function—previously provided by the churches or the keepers of poor houses, if provided at all—had to be, and has to be, rationalized and justified. Why should able-bodied, healthy people be given free room and board—that is, room and board at the taxpayer's expense? And why should physicians—medical doctors—provide this service? Because, so goes the answer, the persons served are the mentally *ill* and it is this *illness* that renders them unable to care for themselves. But if they are ill and hospitalized, why are they confined like prisoners, unable to leave, forbidden to reject the care so solicitously given them? Because, so goes the answer, mental illness deprives the mentally ill of their ability to determine and pursue their own best interests; hence, they must be cared for compulsorily, like children. In addition, madmen and madwomen were, and still are, considered to be dangerous or potentially dangerous to themselves or others. Thus, confining the insane was, and still is, justified on the dual grounds of *parens patriae* and the police power: the mental patient must be protected from himself, and the community must be protected from the mental patient.

Similar considerations apply to the other paradigmatic psychiatric procedure, the insanity defense. As civil commitment rests on, and enshrines, the belief that there are two kinds of *innocent persons* in the world, sane and insane—so the insanity defense rests on, and enshrines, the belief that there are two kinds of *guilty persons* in the world, sane and insane. Sane persons possess the rights and responsibilities accorded to them by law; insane persons, because of mental illness, possess no such rights and responsibilities. *Ergo*, members of the latter group may rightly be incarcerated even if they do not break the law; and if they do, then they ought to be treated, not punished. This explains why incarcerating innocent persons in mental hospitals and freeing guilty persons from prisons have always been, and continue to be, the psychiatrist's two most important social functions. Clearly, if mental illness did not exist, it would be necessary to invent it.*

CONFRONTING THE HUMAN PREDICAMENT

Although modern man has rejected the revelatory tales of the Bible, he has replaced them with the apocalyptic pseudoexplanations of psychiatry and psychoanalysis. The view that the human condition is so mysterious that it is past ordinary human understanding—that some special knowledge or skill is needed to peer into its depths—has thus remained essentially unchanged. In Biblical times, people turned to prophets to unravel the mystery of life—and prophets there were aplenty. During the better part of two millennia in the Christian West, people turned to the Scriptures to unravel it—and priests there were aplenty. Nowadays they turn to psychiatrists, psychologists, social

---

*I here paraphrase Voltaire's famous remark: "If God did not exist, it would be necessary to invent him." ("Si Dieu n'existait pas, il faudrait l'inventer.") Voltaire was extraordinarily proud of this aphorism. "Though I am seldom satisfied with my lines," he wrote to Frederick the Great, "I must confess that I feel for this one the tenderness of a father."[21]

workers, and other experts on mental health—and such experts there are aplenty.

Moreover, as in homeopathic medicine where poisons cure what they cause, in psychiatry mystery explains mystery—hence the apocalyptic character of psychiatric theories. But the idea that our life is a dark mystery; that our personal problems cannot be understood by common sense, intelligent inquiry, and some earnest effort; that the secrets of our inner life or unconscious mind can be penetrated and unravelled only by a few select adepts—all this is false. Understanding why people act the way they do—what they value and what gives their lives meaning—is far easier than understanding the atomic structure of matter or the chemical composition of stars millions of light-years from the earth.

Throughout this book I have tried to show that while people ostensibly believe that mental illness exists and look to psychiatrists to explain what it is, in fact people use the idea of mental illness to explain certain human predicaments and to justify certain social policies. In its explanatory (or pseudoexplanatory) function, psychiatry thus resembles, and is a replacement for, religion. I shall briefly sketch the parallels between them.

Psychiatric and Religious Explanations of Behavior

Although the resemblance between religious and psychiatric explanations of behavior has been noted by some students of the human condition, few have seen it as clearly as Morse Peckham. Human beings, Peckham emphasizes, cannot live without constantly manufacturing explanations of their own behavior and of the behavior of others:

> We cannot manage others without explanation, nor can we manage ourselves. We justify our actions and our plans by explaining their importance—their value—both to ourselves and to others. Social interaction without explanation is inconceivable: it may be the very condition of human existence.[22]

Man's passion for explanation, however, is both his glory and shame, or, as Peckham puts it: "It is man's cross that the constructive power of explanation is equaled by its destructive force."[23] The reason for this—according to Peckham, with whose interpretation I agree—is that the human mind is too easily satisfied: "Inexplicability is satisfied by an explanation, and everybody is satisfied by any explanation some of the time."[24] In support of this seemingly self-evident but important observation, Peckham offers the following comments:

They [inexplicable phenomena] must be caused and caused, moreover, by unobservable (not, note, unobserved) forces. The unobservable force-producing entity for which a word exists is the mind. Therefore, if the responder judges himself to be culturally modern, he asserts that such phenomena are mentally produced. If he is willing to be judged more old-fashioned . . . he uses another word which is said to refer to an unobservable force-producing entity, God.[25]

What Peckham suggests is that psychiatric (mental) explanations of behavior are, in fact, merely restatements of religious (divine) explanations of it. He thus sees the entire "economic institution of psychiatry" as satisfying our need for explanations of behavior. Psychoanalysis, he adds, has been a great gift precisely because:

It makes rich explanations of absolutely any behavioral dissolution quite easy, and it provides an extraordinary and by now nearly random range of such explanations. Its trouble, as has been said often enough, is not that it explains but that it explains entirely too much.[26]

Being in possession of a system that explains too much, together with the conviction that one is so right and others so wrong that one is justified, in the name of one's beliefs, to coerce others are the twin threads that run through the entire fabric of religion, psychiatry, and psychosis and point to certain crucial characteristics they share. I summarize these characteristics, by epitomizing the explanations they typically offer, as follows:

The *religious person's* (fanatic's) explanations of behavior are *God-centered*, reflecting his overabsorption with his deity and its demands. The typical form of such an explanation is: "Those who love God and submit to his laws are pure and will be saved; all others are corrupt and terrible punishment awaits them."

The *psychiatrist's* (psychoanalyst's) explanations are *mental illness-centered*, reflecting his overabsorption with psychopathological entities and their consequences. The typical form of such an explanation is: "The patient is mentally ill, bent on harming others or himself; I, his psychiatrist, and his family are mentally healthy and all our efforts are devoted to helping the patient get well."

The *psychotic's* (schizophrenic's) explanations are *self-centered*, reflecting his overabsorption with his own self, his desires and frustrations. The typical form of his explanation is: "I am a harmless person, innocent of malicious thoughts or deeds; I am persecuted and tortured by misguided relatives and destructive psychiatrists."

In short, the crucial similarities among religious, psychiatric, and psychotic explanations—and among the persons who deeply believe in them—are: (1) Each of these systems of ideas—that is, religion, psychiatry, psychosis—is capable of explaining everything. (2) The true believer of each is willing and, indeed, eager to explain everything; saying "I don't know" or "It is none of my business" is alien to his thinking and to what he regards as his duty. (3) Because each of these actors feels strongly that he is right and that those who disagree with him are wrong, and is also convinced that his being in possession of the truth imposes special responsibilities on him, each feels deeply justified in using fraud and force to impose his views and will on others.

The result is utter cognitive chaos about what is mental illness, what causes it, and what cures it. To underscore the present impossibility of intelligently discussing the nature or causes of mental illness, I have listed its principal meanings, discussed throughout this book, in Table 12.1. Clearly, if this is the way the term *mental illness* is used, it is folly to try to ascertain what *it is*, what causes *it*, or how to cure *it*.

TABLE 12.1. The Meanings of "Mental Illness"

A. Mental illness as abnormal condition:
  1. Proven disease of the brain
  2. Putative disease of the brain
  3. Deviant behavior
B. Mental illness as patient role:
  1. Voluntary mental patient: person assumes the role of mentally ill patient
  2. Involuntary mental patient: person is cast into the role of mentally ill patient
C. Mental illness as strategy:
  1. To accuse or incriminate
  2. To excuse or exonerate
  3. To avoid or evade moral conflict
  4. To deny human depravity
D. Mental illness as legal fiction:
  1. To justify involuntary mental hospitalization and treatment (cf. B.2, C.1, and C.2 above)
  2. To justify the insanity defense and other psychiatric diversions (cf. B.2, C.2, C.3, and C.4 above)
  3. To justify coercions and excuses incompatible with our moral and legal principles and thus legitimize disjoining rights and responsibilities (cf. C.1 and C.2 above)

Mental Illness as a Barrier to Understanding

If this analysis of the explanatory function of the idea of mental illness is correct, then it follows that instead of explaining anything, mental illness is actually like a stone wall or a smokescreen that keeps us from approaching or seeing what ostensibly interests us and what we want to explain. Thus, the most formidable barrier against progress in psychiatry lies in the fundamental political-philosophical premise that the psychiatrist's account of the psychotic's behavior constitutes an explanation, but that the schizophrenic's account of his own behavior does not: accordingly, the psychiatrist feels justified in dismissing the latter as the *senseless symptoms* of a *psychotic patient*. Actually, understanding the nature of this disqualification of the ideas of insane persons is crucial for our understanding of the revisioning of mental illness and psychiatry I am proposing.

Once madness became an accepted category in Western thought, insane persons were demarcated from sane persons by the different ways their behavior was *interpreted* and hence *seen*. Initially, the mad person was viewed as had been the person possessed by demons, that is, as *not a person* at all (or as *not himself* because he had been dispossessed of himself by demons or the disease that possessed him). By the beginning of the nineteenth century, the insane person's thought, speech, and behavior were authoritatively regarded as meaningless. Imitating the modern physician's viewing bloody urine as a pathological product of diseased kidneys, the asylum physician insisted that the madman's utterances were the pathological products of his *fevered brain*: another metaphor, to be sure, but one that was also interpreted literally. Herein lay the first and most fundamental disqualification of the insane person's self-explanation.

The next disqualification, which did not displace the first but rather coexisted with it, consisted of viewing the insane person's utterances and behavior as *irrational*. This led to the interpretation that although the psychotic's speech and behavior were speech and behavior, they made *no sense*: psychiatric terms such as *word salad* and *thought disorder* betoken this view of granting the psychotic's productions *the sense of being nonsense*.

This was the scene upon which Freud entered. Before him stood a stage upon which mad men and mad women performed—spoke and acted—and whose performances were officially deemed to make no sense. It was a setting ready and waiting for someone—he had to be a physician, of course!—to decipher the meaning of madness. It does not belittle Freud's achievement to point out that since everyone then believed that what crazy people said made no sense, it was relatively easy to show that this was not so: *all one had to do was listen to what the patient had to say and recast it in one's own authoritative voice.* Presto, thanks to a novel *medical* theory, the insane person's speech and behavior made sense and could be understood. In my view, here is where Freud betrayed the patient and the truth: Instead of validating the mental patient as a bona fide moral agent, he invalidated him once more and in the subtlest of all ways—as a person who does not understand himself and hence can give no valid account of his own behavior. Only the psychoanalyst (psychiatrist) can do that. As a result, while in the nineteenth century only the psychotic person's behavior was viewed as senseless, under Freud's influence this perspective was extended to the so-called neurotic person's—and, indeed to everyone's—behavior as well: all of us are in the grip of unconscious drives and impulses; hence, none of us knows himself.

Freud's enthusiasm for viewing all human behavior as irrational is perhaps the clearest manifestation of the fact that notwithstanding certain humanistic and ennobling elements in his doctrine, his fundamental attitude toward men and women was antihumanistic and degrading. With the Freudian premise that everyone is irrational until proven otherwise, we have indeed come a long way from the days when Thomas Jefferson wrote indignantly that "It is an insult to our citizens to question whether they are rational beings or not . . ."[27] In our day it is the mark of the compassionate and informed citizen—especially if he is a mental health professional, policeman, prosecutor, or judge—that at the very first sign of a difference or disagreement between himself and another person, he ought to question whether the other is rational, assume that he is not and that his irrationality is a symptom of insanity, and treat him as such to ensure the proper cure of his underlying craziness.

The upshot of this profound ideological transformation is that the meaning of the *mental patient's self-history* is thrice invalidated—first, as the pathological secretion of a diseased brain; then, as the irrational ravings of an insane person; and finally, as the symptomatic derivative of unconscious mental processes (to which only the psychoanalyst has access).

The reluctance to grant explanatory status to the mental patient's self-explanation is, of course, an integral part of the modern deification of science as the only key to (correct) explanation. We have somehow forgotten that granting an account the status of an explanation is not the same as agreeing with it as true or valid. After all, we grant such a status to religious and mythological explanations, without necessarily agreeing that they represent reality correctly. If we bear this distinction in mind, it is obvious that the verbal behavior of the psychotic—that is, the cognitive content of his psychosis—constitutes a bona fide explanation of behavior. This is especially clear in the case of the paranoid schizophrenic, whose explanations are especially elaborate and dramatic. Of course, we, normal persons, do not, and need not, agree with or accept his explanation. However, what makes it particularly difficult for people to adopt such a view is that the psychotic's explanations are intolerably offensive, typically for his family, for psychiatrists, and for anyone obsessed with rationality. This is why normal persons prefer to view such accounts as not explanations at all—a posture sadly at odds with Samuel Johnson's dictum that "Every man has the right to utter what he thinks is truth, and every other man has the right to knock him down for it."[28]

CLOTHES, BUT NO EMPEROR . . .

Inventing metaphors and then mistaking them for the names of material objects is an inevitable part of the human condition. In the past, this enterprise characterized religion; today, it characterizes the so-called sciences of man—that is, sociology, psychology, and especially psychiatry. Thus, psychiatrists now believe in the reality of delusions and psychoses, and psychoanalysts in the reality of the libido and the unconscious with the same fervor with which theologians believed in the reality of demons and witches and the high temperature and humidity that prevailed in hell. Exploding such myths is often compared to the discovery that the legendary emperor, whose finely woven clothes anyone but a fool could see, is naked. Although this is true, turning the story around makes it even truer. After all, one of the most striking things about modern psychiatry is that it is a veritable cornucopia of theories and therapies of mental illness. Textbooks of psychiatry often exceed in size textbooks of medicine. Explanations of mental illness advanced in this century alone—from masturbatory madness to dopamine deficiency—run into the hundreds if not thousands. Methods of curing mental illnesses are equally numerous. Thus, seeing through the riddle of mental illness is not so much like seeing that the emperor is naked, but rather more like realizing that the emperor's wardrobe is rich and dazzling beyond the dreams even of emperors—but that there is no emperor.

REFERENCES

Complete references for books are listed in the Bibliography.

EPIGRAPH

1. Peirce, C. S. "How to make our ideas clear" (1878), in Wiener, P. P., ed., *Values in a Universe of Chance,* 123.

PREFACE TO THE ORIGINAL EDITION

1. Weaver, R. *Ideas Have Consequences.*
2. Selden, J. Quoted in Thomas, K., *Religion and the Decline of Magic,* 435.

INTRODUCTION

1. Stephen, J. F. *Liberty, Equality, Fraternity,* 176.
2. See Szasz, T. S., ed. *The Age of Madness.*
3. Wiener, P. P., ed. *Dictionary of the History of Ideas.*
4. American Psychiatric Association. *Diagnostic and Statistical Manual of Mental Disorders,* 3rd ed., 6. (Hereafter cited as *DSM-III.*)
5. Ibid.
6. Landers, A. "Dear Ann Landers," *Syracuse Herald-Journal,* June 24, 1970, 50.
7. Jefferson, T. "Letter to John Tyler" (1804), in Stevenson, B., ed., *The Macmillan Book of Proverbs,* 1016.
8. Twain, M. *Pudd'nhead Wilson,* 113.

CHAPTER 1: DEFINING ILLNESS

1. Robbins, S. L. *Pathologic Basis of Disease,* 1st ed., 1.
2. Minogue, K. *Alien Powers,* 38.

3. Hern, W. Quoted in Scholberg, A. "The abortionists meet: 1979 and 1980." *Primum Non Nocere* 1 (December 1980): 5.

4. Kolata, G. "Obesity declared a disease." *Science* (March 1, 1985): 1019.

5. Franks, L. "A new attack on alcoholism." *New York Times Magazine*, October 20, 1985, 48.

6. Koop, E. Quoted in Hoffer, W. "Public health strategies eyed to curb homicides." *American Medical News* (October 25, 1985): 21–22, 21.

7. Ibid.

8. Bowker, J. *Problems of Suffering in Religions of the World*, 2.

9. Ibid., 21.

10. Ibid., 74.

11. Ibid., 94.

12. See Szasz, T. S. *The Manufacture of Madness*.

13. Minogue, K. *The Liberal Mind*, 7.

14. Ibid., 8.

15. See Caroll, J. B., ed. *Language, Thought, and Reality*, especially 207–219.

16. Yellin, S. "Daughter disowned after marrying gentile." *Syracuse Herald-Journal*, February 23, 1985, A-6.

17. "Ethiopia wants Israel to return Falashas." *San Francisco Chronicle*, March 25, 1985, 9.

18. "Rich man swaps matrimony for priesthood." Ibid., 3.

19. Carrell, S. "Pharmacist's role in lethal injections debated." *American Medical News*, March 8, 1985, 16.

20. Taylor, S., Jr. "Fed loses 'non-bank' bank case." *New York Times*, January 23, 1986, D-1.

21. Rosecan, J. S. "Drug use is different from drug addictions." (Letters), *New York Times*, January 9, 1986, A-22.

22. Guze, S. B. "Nature of psychiatric illness: Why psychiatry is a branch of medicine." *Comprehensive Psychiatry* 19 (1978): 295–307, 296.

23. Cartwright, S. A. "Report on the diseases and physical peculiarities of the negro race." *New Orleans Medical and Surgical Journal* 7 (1851): 691–715; also, Szasz, T. S. "The sane slave." *American Journal of Psychotherapy* 25 (April 1971): 228–239.

24. *Stedman's Medical Dictionary*, 21st ed., 456.

25. Robbins, S. L. *Pathologic Basis of Disease*, 1st ed., 1.

26. Robbins, S. L. et al. *Pathologic Basis of Disease*, 3rd ed., 1.

CHAPTER 2: BEING A PATIENT

1. *Nathanson v. Kline*, 186 Kan. 393, 406–407, 350 P.2d. 1093, 1104 (1960) (dictum), cited with approval in *Woods v. Brumlop*, 71 N.M. 221, 227, 377 P.2d. 520, 524 (1962) (dictum).

2. Roberts, S. "Judge overrules Health Department on jurisdiction in Gross case." *New York Times,* December 2, 1985, B-1.

3. *In re Estate of Brooks,* cited in Lappé, M. "Dying while living: A critique of allowing-to-die legislation." *Journal of Medical Ethics* 4 (1978): 195–199.

4. Burger, W. In *Application of President and Director of Georgetown College,* 331 F.2d., 1010 (D.C. Cir. 1964).

5. Bryn, R. M. "Compulsory lifesaving treatment for the competent adult." *Fordham Law Review* 44 (1975): 1–36, 33.

6. See Szasz, T. S. "The psychiatric will: A new mechanism for protecting persons against 'psychosis' and psychiatry." *American Psychologist* 37 (July 1982): 762–770.

7. See Szasz, T. S. *The Myth of Psychotherapy.*

8. Rahman, F. "Medicare makes a wrong diagnosis." (Op-ed), *New York Times,* January 23, 1986, A-27.

9. Szasz, T. S. *Ideology and Insanity,* 235–236.

CHAPTER 3: DEFINING MENTAL ILLNESS

1. Kraepelin, E. *Lectures on Clinical Psychiatry,* 1; *Einführung in Die Psychiatrische Klinik,* 1.

2. Hamilton, M. *Fish's Clinical Psychopathology,* 14.

3. Pert, C. Quoted in Franklin, J. "The mind fixers." *The Evening Sun* [Baltimore], July 23–31, 1984; special reprint, 1–23.

4. Goodrich, M. M. "Worn and boring." (Letters), *Washington Post,* October 5, 1985, A-17.

5. Quoted in, Evey, J. "Dated notions." (Letters), *Philadelphia Inquirer,* January 14, 1986, 10-A.

6. Goodwin, F. Quoted in ibid.

7. See Bleuler, E. *Dementia Praecox or the Group of Schizophrenias.*

8. Wise, P. M. "Presidential address." *American Journal of Insanity* 58 (July 1901): 79–98, 80.

9. Pauling, L. "Academic address," in Rinkel, M. *Biological Treatment of Mental Illness,* 31–32.

10. See Mackay, C. *Extraordinary Popular Delusions and the Madness of Crowds.*

11. Chodoff, P. "DSM-III and psychotherapy." *American Journal of Psychiatry,* 142 (February 1986): 201–203, 201.

12. Kety, S. "The syndrome of schizophrenia," in Kerr, A. and P. Snaith, eds. *Contemporary Issues in Schizophrenia,* 33.

13. Ibid., 37.

14. Guze, S. B. "Mental disease classification." *Hospital Practice* (August 1980): 77–81, 77.

15. Spitzer, R. L. and J. Endicott. "Medical and mental disorder," in Spitzer, R. L. and D. F. Klein, eds. *Critical Issues in Psychiatric Diagnosis,* 18.

16. Ibid.
17. Twain, M. Quoted in Zimmerman, J. "Management issues in information management." *Information Management* 18 (February 1984) 16–19, 17; I have been unable to locate the original source.
18. Spitzer, R. L. and J. Endicott. "Medical and mental disorder," 18.
19. Klein, D. F. "A proposed definition of mental illness," in Spitzer, R. L. and D. F. Klein, eds. *Critical Issues in Psychiatric Diagnosis*, 52.
20. Lipton, M. "Discussion," ibid., 324.
21. Torrey, E. F., et al. *Washington's Grate Society*. Public Citizen Health Research Group, Document #1010, April 23, 1985; 10.
22. Brown, T. Quoted in Slovenko, R. "The meaning of mental illness in criminal responsibility." *Journal of Legal Medicine* 5 (March 1984): 1–61, 7.
23. Jung, C. G. *Memories, Dreams, Reflection*, 128.
24. Spitzer, R. L. and J. Endicott. "Medical and mental disorder," 23.
25. Ibid.
26. Ibid.
27. Ibid.
28. De Assis, M. "The psychiatrist" (1881–1882), in De Assis, M. *The Psychiatrist and Other Stories*, 1–45.
29. Freud, S. *Introductory Lectures on Psychoanalysis* (1915–1916), in Freud, S. *The Standard Edition of the Complete Psychological Works of Sigmund Freud*, 15: 457. (Hereafter cited as *SE*.)
30. See Szasz, T. S. *Karl Kraus and the Soul-Doctors*, 19–42.
31. Minogue, K. *Alien Powers*, 51.
32. Abrams, S. "The psychoanalytic normalities." *Journal of the American Psychoanalytic Association*, 27 (1979): 821–835, 828.
33. Jahoda, M. *Current Concepts of Positive Mental Health*, 13.
34. Menninger, K. *The Vital Balance*, 32–33.
35. Katz, J. In *U.S. v. Torniero*, 570 F.Supp. 721 (D.C. Conn, 1983); quoted in Slovenko, R. "The meaning of mental illness in criminal responsibility." *Journal of Legal Medicine*, 5 (March 1984): 1–61.
36. Menninger. *The Vital Balance*, 77.
37. Klein, D. F. "A proposed definition," 58.
38. Ibid.
39. Group for the Advancement of Psychiatry. *Criminal Responsibility and Psychiatric Expert Testimony*, Report #26, May 1954, 8.
40. "Fake invalid misled friends for 4 1/2 years." *Syracuse Herald-Journal*, September 13, 1985, A-3.
41. Greshin, B. "Liability insurance coverage for a lunatic's assault." *New York State Bar Journal* (November 1984): 14–17.
42. Van Buren, A. "Alcoholism is a disease, not lack of resolve." *Syracuse Post-Standard*, November 4, 1985, B-4.

43. Ibid.

44. Fingarette, H. "Insanity and responsibility." *Inquiry* 15 (1972): 6–29, 7.

45. Ibid., 10.

46. Ibid., 11, 6.

47. Ibid., 20.

48. Moore, M. S. *Law and Psychiatry*, 196–197.

49. Ibid., 245.

50. Ibid., 244.

51. *Durham v. United States* 214 F.2d 862 (D.C. Cir.), 1954; see also Szasz, T. S. *Ideology and Insanity*, 98–112.

52. Marshall, J. *Intention in Law and Society*, 101.

53. Edelson, M. *The Idea of Mental Illness*, 68.

54. Hobbes, T. *Leviathan*, 62.

55. Marmor, J. "Systems thinking in psychiatry." *American Journal of Psychiatry*, 140 (July 1983): 833–838, 837.

56. Marshall, J. *Intention in Law and Society*, 120.

57. Spitzer, R. L. and J. Endicott. "Medical and mental disorder," 34.

58. Kolb, L. C. *Noyes' Modern Clinical Psychiatry*, 7th ed., 80–81.

59. *DSM-III*. 5–6.

60. Wilson, C. *New Pathways in Psychology*, 224.

61. Ibid., 247.

62. Chesen, E. S. *Religion May Be Hazardous To Your Health*, 37, 46.

63. Yao, R. Quoted in "Fundamentalists Anonymous set up to counter 'mental disease.'" *Battle Cry*, January/February 1986, 1.

64. Peck, M. S. Quoted in Bartlett, K. "Diabolic dealings: Psychiatrist tells of meeting Satan during exorcisms." *Arizona Republic*, December 15, 1985, AA-12, 13.

65. Peck, M. S., Quoted in Roiphe, A. "Gunfight at the I'm OK corral: M. Scott Peck duels with the devil." *New York Times Book Review*, January 19, 1986, 22.

66. Alexander, F. *The Medical Value of Psychoanalysis*.

67. Hanley, J. "How to offset psychiatry's disappearance." *American Medical News*, June 7, 1985, 18.

68. Hoffer, A. and H. Osmond. *What You Should Know About Schizophrenia*, 1.

69. See Robbins, S. L. et al. *Pathologic Basis of Disease*, 3rd ed.

70. See Kissane, J. M. ed. *Anderson's Pathology*.

71. See Sodeman, W. M., Jr. and T. M. Sodeman. *Sodeman's Pathologic Physiology*.

72. Torrey, E. F. "It is a disease." (Letters), *Philadelphia Inquirer*, January 14, 1986, 10-A.

73. Adams, R. K. and M. Victor. "Derangements of intellect, mood, and behavior, including schizophrenia and manic depressive states," in Isselbacher, K. J., et al., *Harrison's Principles of Internal Medicine*, 9th ed., 150.

74. Hackett, T. P. and E. M. Hackett. "Schizophrenia," in Petersdorf, R. G., et al., eds. *Harrison's Principles of Internal Medicine,* 10th ed., 2211.

75. Hackett, T. P. and E. M. Hackett. "Affective disorders," in ibid., 2206.

76. McHugh, P. "Neurologic and behavioral diseases," in Wyngaarden, J. B. and L. H. Smith, eds. *Cecil's Textbook of Medicine,* 17th ed., 2: 2002, 2006.

77. Lehman, H. E. "Schizophrenia: Clinical features," in, Kaplan, H. I. et al., eds. *Comprehensive Textbook of Psychiatry/III,* 3rd ed., 2: 1153. (Hereafter cited as Kaplan, *CTP-III.*)

78. Guze, S. B. "Mental disease classification." *Hospital Practice* (August 1980): 77.

79. Ibid.

80. Rose, I. "To view schizophrenia without stigma." (Letters), *New York Times,* March 26, 1986, A-22.

81. Ahmann, S. "Conversation with the experts: Long-term psychotherapy held useful in treating schizophrenia." *Clinical Psychiatry News* 14 (March 1986): 8–9.

82. Arieti, S. *Understanding and Helping the Schizophrenic,* 6.

83. Ibid., 7.

84. Ibid., 6, 8.

85. Berlin, I. *Four Essays on Liberty,* 23.

86. Ibid.

87. Dubovsky, S. L. and M. P. Weissberg. *Clinical Psychiatry in Primary Care,* 164.

88. Leo, J. "Battling over masochism." *Time,* December 2, 1985, 76.

89. "Board takes action on DSM-III-R diagnoses." *Psychiatric News,* January 3, 1986, 1, 24.

90. Spitzer, R. L. Quoted in Goleman, D. "New psychiatric syndromes spur protest." *New York Times,* November 19, 1985, C-1, 16.

91. Leo, T. "Battling over masochism."

92. Ibid.

93. Nadelson, C. "Psychiatry as medicine." (Letters), *The Baltimore Sun,* February 9, 1986, 6-E.

94. Suarez, L. and E. Barrett-Connor. "Is an educated wife hazardous to your health?" *American Journal of Epidemiology* 119 (1984): 244–249, 244.

95. Dunham, B. *Man Against Myth,* 95–96.

96. See "Soviets consider rejoining World Psychiatric Association." *Psychiatric Times,* December 1985, 1.

97. Bleuler, E. *Dementia Praecox,* 279.

98. See Szasz, T. S. *Schizophrenia.*

99. Sedler, M. J. "The legacy of Ewald Hecker: A new translation of 'Die Hebephrenie.'" *American Journal of Psychiatry* 142 (November 1985): 1265–1271, 1265.

100. Ibid.
101. Ibid., 1267.
102. Ibid., 1266.
103. Ibid.
104. Ross, E. D. and A. J. Rush. "Diagnosis and neuroanatomical correlates of depression in brain-damaged patients." *Archives of General Psychiatry* 38 (December 1981): 1344–1354, 1344.
105. Ibid.
106. Ibid., 1353.
107. *DSM-III*, 7.
108. Ibid., 6.
109. See Bayer, R. *Homosexuality and American Psychiatry.*
110. Beethoven, L. von. *Beethoven: Letters, etc.,* 194.
111. See Szasz, T. S. *The Myth of Mental Illness; Heresies; The Theology of Medicine; The Myth of Psychotherapy; Sex By Prescription.*
112. Turner, J. *Without God,* 9.

CHAPTER 4: BEING A MENTAL PATIENT

1. Jaspers, K. *General Psychopathology,* 8.
2. Ewalt, J. and D. Farnsworth. *Textbook of Psychiatry,* 12.
3. Aristotle. "Nichomachean Ethics," in McKeon, R., ed., *Introduction to Aristotle,* 460.
4. See Moran, R. "The origin of insanity as a special verdict: The trial for treason of James Hadfield." *Law and Society Review* 19 (1985): 487–519.
5. See Szasz, T. S. *Law, Liberty, and Psychiatry,* and *The Therapeutic State.*
6. Fowler, N. Quoted in "Schizophrenia: The minister acts." *The Times* (London), February 17, 1986, 8.
7. Ibid.
8. Jonsen, A. R. and B. Eichelman. "Ethical issues in psychopharmacological treatment," in Gallant, D. M. and R. Force, eds. *Legal and Ethical Issues in Human Research and Treatment,* 145.
9. Ibid.
10. Fingarette, H. *The Meaning of Criminal Insanity,* 126.
11. Bean, P. *Compulsory Admission to Mental Hospitals,* 67.
12. "Treating teens in trouble." *Newsweek,* January 20, 1986, 52–54.
13. Sussman, N. and S. E. Hyler. "Factitious disorders," in Kaplan, *CTP-III,* 2:2002.
14. Ibid.
15. Ibid.

16. Porter, S. "Mental health care tab being assumed by more employers." *Syracuse Herald-Journal,* January 10, 1986, B-7.

17. "For you and your family—A hospital cash plan that . . ." Special offering to Chase Manhattan Visa Card Holders (Philadelphia: Insurance Company of North America, 1985).

18. Vaillant, G. E. and J. C. Perry. "Personality disorders," in Kaplan, *CTP-III,* 2:1562.

19. Ibid.

20. Ibid.

21. Ibid.

22. Ibid.

23. Ibid.

24. Ibid., 1569.

25. Jaspers, K. *General Psychopathology,* 8.

26. Thurber, J. "A unicorn in the garden," in Thurber, J., *The Thurber Carnival,* 2d ed., 268–69.

27. Landers, A. "Dear Ann Landers." *Syracuse Herald-Journal,* June 27, 1985, D-8.

28. Ibid.

29. Ibid.

30. Macaulay, T. Quoted in Dunham, E. *Man Against Myth,* 430.

31. Ibid.

32. "Mental patient taken to movie, escapes." *Syracuse Herald-Journal,* October 9, 1985, A-7.

33. Casano, K. "Reaction mixed to Senate state mental hospital report." *Clinical Psychiatry News* 13 (June 1985): 7.

34. "Psychiatric centers fail to report patient crimes, State panel says." *New York Times,* December 22, 1985, 33.

35. Ibid.

36. Borzecki, M. A. and J. S. Wormith. "The criminalization of psychiatrically ill people." *The Psychiatric Journal of the University of Ottawa* 10 (December 1985): 241–247.

37. See Szasz, T. S. *Heresies.*

38. See generally, Klein, J. *Paternalism,* and Sartorius, R., ed. *Paternalism.*

39. McCullough, L. B. and S. Wear. "Respect for autonomy and medical paternalism reconsidered." *Theoretical Medicine* 6 (1985): 295–308, 295.

40. Ibid., 303.

41. Pellegrino, E. and D. C. Thomasma. *A Philosophical Basis of Medical Practice,* 214.

42. Freedman, D. X. "Presidential address: Science in the service of the ill." *American Journal of Psychiatry* 139 (September 1982): 1087–1095, 1092.

43. Bean, P. *Compulsory Admission to Mental Hospitals*, 122.

44. Freedman, D. X. "Presidential address," 1087.

45. "Team MDs call for mandatory drug tests." *American Medical News*, March 14, 1986, 1.

46. Herrington, B. S. "Outpatient commitment." *Psychiatric News* 21 (February 7, 1986): 7, 25.

47. Ibid.

48. "Demonstration Against Psychiatric Oppression." Mimeographed flier, 1983.

49. Laing, R. D. *Wisdom, Madness, and Folly*, x.

50. Breggin, P. "The shame of my life." *AHP Perspective* (August–September 1985): 9.

51. Hobbes, T. *Leviathan*, 164.

52. Szasz, T. S. *Karl Kraus and the Soul-Doctors*, 157.

53. Rabiner, C. J. "Hospital treatment of the problem patient." *Highland Highlights;* Fall 1985 (Ashville, N.C.: Highland Hospital) 2.

54. Lamb, H. R. "Keeping the mentally ill out of jail." *Hospital and Community Psychiatry* 32 (April 1981): 255–258, 258.

55. Koch, E. Quoted in Barbanel, J. "Walking wounded: Koch's new policy on the mentally ill." *New York Times*, November 22, 1985, A-17.

CHAPTER 5: MENTAL ILLNESS AS METAPHOR

1. Aristotle *Poetics*, 1459a; in McKeon, R., ed. *The Basic Works of Aristotle*, 1479.

2. Kety, S. "From rationalization to reason." *American Journal of Psychiatry*, 131 (September 1974): 957–963, 961.

3. Justin, St. Quoted in Strauss, M. B., ed. *Familiar Medical Quotations*, 94–95.

4. Aristotle. *Poetics*, 1459b; in McKeon, R., ed. *The Basic Works of Aristotle*, 1476.

5. See Turbayne, C. M. *The Myth of Metaphor*.

6. Ibid., 14.

7. Ibid., 17.

8. Hobbes, T. *Leviathan*, 37.

9. Ibid., 442.

10. Lewis, C. S. *The Pilgrim's Regress*, 145.

11. Freud, S. "The claims of psycho-analysis to scientific interest" (1913), in *SE*, 13:172.

12. Freud, S. *The Psychopathology of Everyday Life* (1901), in *SE*, 6.

13. Freud, Sophie (Loewenstein). "Freud's metapsychology revisited," *Social Casework* 66 (March 1985): 139–151, 150.

14. Lewis, C. S. *The Screwtape Letters*, 33.

15. Stern, F. "Fink shrinks." *New York Review of Books*, December 19, 1985, 49.

16. Laing, R. D. "Anti-psychiatry." *AHP Perspective*, December, 1985, 10.

17. Korzybski, A. *Science and Sanity*, x.

18. Korzybski, A. Quoted in Hayakawa, S. I., ed. *Language, Meaning, and Maturity*, 1.

19. Hobbes, T. *Leviathan*, 67–68.

20. Korzybski, A. *Science and Sanity*, 532–533.

21. See Rapoport, A. "What is semantics?" In Hayakawa, S. I. ed. *Language, Meaning, and Maturity*, 3–18.

22. Ibid., 16.

23. Rapoport, A. Quoted in Hayakawa, S. I., *Language, Meaning, and Maturity*, 293.

24. Plato. *Republic*, 405d; in Hamilton, E. and H. Cairns, eds. *The Collected Dialogues of Plato*, 650.

25. Ibid., 459d–e; 698–699.

26. Goethe, J. W. von. "Italienische Reise" (May 27, 1778), in *Gedenkausgabe*, 11:362; the translation is mine.

27. Embler, W. *Metaphor and Meaning*, 77.

28. Feuchtersleben, E. von. *Medical Psychology* (1845); quoted in Schreber, D. *Memoirs of My Nervous Illness*, 412.

29. Jacobi, M. Quoted in Pauleikhoff, B., *Das Menschenbild im Wandel der Zeit*, 2:168–169; the translation is mine.

30. Ibid.

31. Kraepelin, E. *Lectures on Clinical Psychiatry*, 1.

32. Bleuler, E. *Dementia Praecox*, 429.

33. Ibid.

34. See Szasz, T. S. *Schizophrenia*.

35. Bleuler, E. *Dementia Praecox*, 438.

36. Kety, S. "From rationalization to reason," 962.

37. Schoenfeld, C. G. "An analysis of the views of Thomas Szasz." *Journal of Psychiatry and Law* 4 (Summer 1976): 245–263, 250.

38. Roth, M. "Schizophrenia and the theories of Thomas Szasz," in Kerr, A. and P. Snaith, eds. *Contemporary Issues in Schizophrenia*, 104.

39. Ibid., 105.

40. Ibid., 113.

41. Ibid., 114.

42. Krauthammer, C. "The myth of Thomas Szasz: Libertarianism gone mad," in Krauthammer, C. *Cutting Edges*, 75–81; 75.

43. Ibid., 76.

44. Ibid., 77.

45. Gostin., L. "The ideology of entitlement: The application of contemporary legal approaches to psychiatry," in Bean, P., ed. *Mental Illness,* 27–54, 37.

46. Klein, D. F. "A proposed definition," 62.

47. Ibid.

48. Schoenfeld, C. "Views of Thomas Szasz," 254.

49. Korson, S. M. "Amazing chutzpah." (Letters), *Arizona Republic,* November 16, 1985, 16.

50. Laor, N. "Hobbesian principles in Szasz's writings." *Clio Medica,* 19 (1984): 32–39, 32.

51. Ibid.

52. Laor, N. "Procrustean psychiatry." *Philosophy and Social Sciences* 15 (1985): 337–347, 337.

53. Guze, S. B. "Nature of psychiatric illness: Why psychiatry is a branch of medicine." *Comprehensive Psychiatry* 19 (1978): 295–307, 298.

54. See Szasz, T. S. *The Myth of Psychotherapy.*

55. Karasu, B. T. Quoted in "Economic realities force psychiatrists to reevaluate all kinds of psychotherapies." *Clinical Psychiatry News* (February 1986): 1.

56. *Mills et al. v. Rogers,* Brief for the American College of Neuropsychopharmacology as Amicus Curiae, in the Supreme Court of the United States, Mark Mills, et al., Petitioners v. Rubie Rogers, et al., Respondents. On Writ of Certiorari to the United States Court of Appeals for the First Circuit, No. 80-1417, October, 1980.

57. Fingarette, H. *The Meaning of Criminal Insanity,* 20.

58. Ibid., 249.

59. Turner, J. *Without God,* 4.

60. Russell, M. "Sue 'em!" *Syracuse Herald-Journal,* April 4, 1986, A-13.

61. See Ryle, G. *The Concept of Mind.*

CHAPTER 6: MENTAL ILLNESS AND THE PROBLEM OF IMITATION

1. Swift, J. *Gulliver's Travels,* 275.

2. Eissler, K. R. "Malingering," in Wilbur, G. B. and W. V. Muensterberger, eds. *Psychoanalysis and Culture,* 252–253.

3. Hay, G. G. "Feigned psychosis: A review of the simulation of mental illness," in Kerr, A. and P. Snaith, eds. *Contemporary Issues in Schizophrenia,* 194.

4. Rosen, G. "Psychic epidemics in Europe and the United States," in Rosen, G., *Madness in Society,* 195–225, 202.

5. Molière. *A Doctor in Spite of Himself* (1666), in Molière, *The Misanthrope and Other Plays,* 179.

6. See Szasz, T. S., *Sex By Prescription.*

7. Molière. *The Imaginary Invalid* (1673), in Molière, *The Misanthrope and Other Plays*, 273.

8. Molière. *A Doctor in Spite of Himself*, 184–85.

9. Ibid., 190.

10. Ibid., 196.

11. Guillain, G. *J.-M. Charcot*, 174.

12. See Szasz, T. S. *The Myth of Mental Illness*, Chap. 1.

13. Thomas, K. *Religion and the Decline of Magic*, 480.

14. See, for example, Gilman, S. *Seeing the Insane*.

15. Munthe, A. *The Story of San Michele*, 296.

16. Batchelor, I. R. C. *Henderson and Gillespie's Textbook of Psychiatry*, 10th ed., 156.

17. Maloney, M. P. "Malingering," in Corsini, R., ed. *Encyclopedia of Psychology*, 2:329.

18. Bleuler, E. *Dementia Praecox*, 220.

19. Coleridge, S. T. Quoted in Strauss, M. B., ed. *Familiar Medical Quotations*, 354.

20. Rosenhan, D. "Being sane in insane places." *Science* 179 (1973): 250–258.

21. Ibid.

22. Berger, P. L. and T. Luckmann. *The Social Construction of Reality*, 177.

23. Thomas, K. *Religion and the Decline of Magic*, 483–484.

24. Ibid., 459.

25. Ibid.

26. Ibid., 483.

27. Ibid.

28. Hobbes, T. *Leviathan*, 445.

29. Ibid., 442.

30. Bok, S. *Lying*, 236.

31. Rush, B. *Medical Inquiries*, 265.

32. Rush, B. *Letters*, 2: 1090.

33. Rush, B. *Medical Inquiries*, 109.

34. Ibid., 110.

35. Shainess, N. "Ethics and sex research." (Letters), *Psychiatric News* 13 (June 2 1978): 2.

36. Naftulin, D., et al. "The Doctor Fox lecture: A paradigm of educational seduction." *Journal of Medical Education* 48 (July 1973): 630–635, 631.

37. Ibid., 634.

38. Ibid., 635.

39. Ibid.

40. Dunham, B. *Man Against Myth*, 304.

41. Ibid.

42. Franklin, B. Quoted in Randi, J. "Be healed in the name of God!" *Free Inquiry* 6 (Spring 1986): 8–23, 10.

43. Goldsmith, M. *Franz Anton Mesmer*, 153.

44. Franklin, B. Quoted in Buranelli, V. *The Wizard from Vienna*, 165.

45. See Haldipur, C. V. "The meanings of psychotherapy." *Psychological Medicine*, 15 (1985): 727–732.

46. Proust, M. Quoted in Strauss, M. B., ed. *Familiar Medical Quotations*, 319.

47. Sartre, J. -P. *Being and Nothingness*, 51.

48. Guze, S. B. "Mental disease classification." *Hospital Practice* (August 1980): 77–81.

49. Ibid.

50. Meadow, R. "Fictitious epilepsy." *The Lancet* (July 7, 1985): 25–28, 26–27.

51. Ibid., 27.

52. Meropol, N. J., C. V. Ford, and R. M. Zaner. "Factitious illness: An exploration in ethics." *Perspectives in Biology and Medicine* 28 (Winter 1985): 269–281.

53. Ibid., 270.

54. Chapman, J. S. "Peregrinating problem patients: Münchausen's syndrome." *Journal of the American Medical Association* 165 (1957): 927–933, 933.

55. *DSM-III*, 287.

56. Ibid.

57. Nazario, S. L. "Medical malady that resists cure: One of 50 doctors an impostor." *Wall Street Journal*, April 2, 1986, 21.

58. Lynn, E. J. and M. Belza. "Factitious posttraumatic stress disorder: The veteran who never got to Vietnam." *Hospital and Community Psychiatry* 35 (July 1984): 697–701, 697.

59. Ibid.

60. Ibid., 700.

61. See "Man who lied about Vietnam to be tried." *New York Times*, June 7, 1985, B-2.

62. "'Son of Sam' killer Berkowitz says 'urge to kill,' not demons, drove him." *Washington Post*, February 23, 1979, A-3.

63. "Doctor refutes Berkowitz." *Syracuse Herald-Journal*, March 6, 1979, 4.

64. Buyer, B. "Berkowitz claims he feigned insanity to justify slayings." *Buffalo Evening News*, August 1, 1980, 1, 4.

65. Ibid.

66. Ibid.

67. Buyer, B. "Claims for disability benefits authorized, Berkowitz says." *Buffalo Evening News*, August 3, 1980, A-1, A-10.

68. Edmonds, R. "Son of Sam taps Uncle Sam." *Daily News* (New York), June 5, 1980, 4.

69. Buyer, B. "Berkowitz claims."

70. Wooden, K. *The Children of Jonestown*, 59.

71. Ibid., 61–62.

72. Ibid., 103.

73. Ibid., 103–04.

74. Buchanan, P. J. Quoted in Szasz, T. S. "Jim Jones as Jesus." *The Therapeutic State*, 179–81.

75. Ungerleider, T. Quoted in Szasz, T. S. "The freedom abusers." *The Therapeutic State*, 182–186, 184–185.

76. Poussaint, A. Quoted in ibid., 185.

77. Reston, J. Quoted in ibid., 184.

78. Lane, M. Quoted in ibid., 183.

79. Garry, C. Quoted in ibid.

80. Wooden, K. *The Children of Jonestown*, 112.

81. Ibid., 141.

82. See Szasz, T. *The Therapeutic State*, 182.

83. Canon 1101, in Coriden, J. A., et al. *The Code of Canon Law*, 784.

84. Ibid.

85. See, for example, Scheff, T. *Being Mentally Ill.*

86. Lewis, C. S. *The Screwtape Letters and Screwtape Proposes a Toast*, 46.

CHAPTER 7: MENTAL ILLNESS AND THE PROBLEM OF INTENTIONALITY

1. Kramer, H. and J. Sprenger. *The Malleus Maleficarum*, 131-32.

2. *DSM-III*, 62.

3. Ibid., 63–64.

4. Koch, E. Quoted in "Officials say arsonists set Grand Central fire." *Syracuse Herald-Journal*, August 29, 1985, B-1.

5. *DSM-III*, 294.

6. See, for example, "Creativity and madness linked, study says." *New York Times*, September 23, 1984, 63.

7. Plato. *Phaedus*, 245a; in Hamilton, E. and H. Cairns, eds. *The Collected Dialogues of Plato*, 492.

8. Plato, *Laws*, 719e; in ibid., 1310.

9. Aristotle. Quoted in Heschel, A. J. *The Prophets*, 392.

10. Plato. Quoted in ibid.

11. Seneca. Quoted in ibid., 391.

12. Cicero. Quoted in ibid.

13. Goethe, J. W. von. Quoted in ibid., 382–383.
14. Arendt, H. *The Human Condition,* 167.
15. Langer, S. *Philosophy in a New Key,* 75.
16. Freud, S. "The claims of psycho-analysis to scientific interest," in *SE,* 13: 187.
17. Freud, S., "Leonardo da Vinci and a memory of his childhood," in *SE,* 11: 68.
18. Freud, S. "The Moses of Michelangelo," in *SE,* 13: 212.
19. Ibid.
20. Ibid.
21. See, for example, Arens, R. *Make Mad the Guilty.*
22. Bazelon, D. "The dilemma of punishment," in Blom-Cooper, L., ed. *The Literature of the Law,* 388–408.
23. Marshall, J. *Intention in Law and Society,* 70.
24. Ibid., 81.
25. Ibid., 83.
26. Ibid., 99.
27. See Burnham, J. *The Suicide of the West.*
28. "Supreme Court roundup: Confessions and insanity." *New York Times,* January 14, 1985, A-13; see also "Court considers use of confessions of mentally ill." *Psychiatric News* 21 (March 7 1986): 1, 15.
29. Eckholm, E. "In the natural world, deceit found pervasive." *New York Times,* January 14, 1986, C-1, C-3.
30. Ibid.
31. See Lieberman, E. J. *Acts of Will,* and Szasz, T. S. "The pretensions of the Freudian cult." *The Spectator* (London), October 5, 1985, 32.
32. See Wilson, C. *New Pathways in Psychology.*
33. Ibid., 240.
34. Maslow, A. Quoted in ibid., 15.
35. Laing, R. D. *Wisdom, Madness, and Folly,* 6.
36. Schowalter, E. "R. D. Laing's ideas." *New York Times Book Review,* November 17, 1985, 43.
37. Wilson, C. *New Pathways,* 224.
38. Ibid., 225.
39. Ibid., 229.
40. Ibid.
41. Ibid., 223–224.
42. Ibid., 242.
43. Rajneesh, B. S. Quoted in "Embittered Bhagwan vows to stay in India." *Syracuse Herald-Journal,* November 18, 1985, A-5.
44. Mansfield, Sir J. Quoted in Collison, G. D. *A Treatise on the Law* (1812), 1: 671.
45. Heinroth, J. C. *Textbook of Disturbances of Mental Life* (1818), 21.

CHAPTER 8: MENTAL ILLNESS AND THE PROBLEM OF RESPONSIBILITY

1. Twain, M. "A new crime," in *The Writings of Mark Twain*, 19: 244.
2. See, for example, Moran, R. "The origin of insanity as a special verdict." *Law and Society Review*, 19 (1985): 487–519.
3. Pinel, P. Quoted in Smith, R. *Trial by Medicine*, 36.
4. Smith, R. *Trial by Medicine*, 125.
5. Ibid.
6. See, for example, Lewin, T. H. D. "Psychiatric evidence in criminal cases for purposes other than the defense of insanity." *Syracuse Law Review* 26 (Fall 1975): 1051–1115.
7. Wynter, A. Quoted in Skultans, V. *Madness and Morals*, 129.
8. Maudsley, H. *Responsibility in Mental Disease*, 133.
9. Ibid., 163–164.
10. Ibid., viii.
11. Charney, M. Quoted in "Calls for an active antismoking role for psychiatrists." *Clinical Psychiatry News*, 14 (March 1986): 9.
12. Freud, S. *The Psychopathology of Everyday Life* (1901), in *SE*, 6: 253–254.
13. Ibid., 254.
14. Freud, S., *Introductory Lectures on Psycho-Analysis* (1916–1917), in *SE*, 15: 106.
15. Trueblood, D. E. "Contemporary psychiatry and the concept of responsibility," in Schoeck, H. and J. W. Wiggins, eds. *Psychiatry and Responsibility*, 19–37, 21.
16. See Szasz, T. S. *The Ethics of Psychoanalysis*.
17. Maclagan, W. G. "Respect for persons as a moral principle." Parts I and II, *Philosophy* 35 (July & October 1960): 193–217, 289–305.
18. Moore, M. S. *Law and Psychiatry*, 244.
19. Ibid., 245.
20. See, Szasz, T. S. and G. J. Alexander. "Mental illness as an excuse for civil wrongs." *Journal of Nervous and Mental Disease* 147 (1968): 113–123.
21. Canon 1095, in Coriden, J., et al. *The Code of Canon Law*, 775.
22. Spencer, H. *Social Statics*, 309.
23. See Szasz, T. S. *Psychiatric Justice*.
24. See *Jackson v. Indiana*, 406 U.S. 715, 1971.
25. Moore, M. S. *Law and Psychiatry*, 373.
26. Hinckley, J. W., Jr. "The insanity defense and me." *Newsweek*, September 20, 1982, 30.
27. "Judge orders hospital to free patient in slaying of husband." *New York Times*, August 1, 1980, B-2.
28. Moore, M. S. "Some myths about 'mental illness.'" *Archives of General Psychiatry* 32 (December 1975): 1483–1497, 1495.

29. Hinckley, Jack and J. A. Hinckley." Illness is the culprit." *Reader's Digest,* March 1983, 77, 78, 81.

30. Shakespeare, W. *Hamlet,* Act 5, Scene 2, lines 219–226.

31. Hinckley, J. W., Sr. and J. A. Hinckley. Quoted in Evans, C. "Hinckleys cling to hope of normal life for son." *Fort Worth Star Telegraph,* June 1, 1985, 21A.

32. "Two charged with trespass on hospital psychiatric ward." *Burlington (Vermont) Free Press,* August 7, 1985, 3–B.

33. Lewin, T. H. D. "Psychiatric evidence," 1054.

34. Mercier, C. Quoted in Skultans, V. *Madness,* 132.

35. Smith, R. *Trial by Medicine,* 40.

36. Ibid., 140.

37. Waggoner, D. "A remorseless murderer goes free . . . ." *People,* September 23, 1985, 61–65, 61.

38. Ibid.

39. Ibid., 65.

40. Britt, H. Quoted in Farrell, D. and S. F. Rubenstein. "Reaction to the death of Dan White." *San Francisco Chronicle,* October 22, 1985, 2.

41. Schmidt, D. Quoted in Sward, S. and M. Z. Barabek. "Hose hooked to car exhaust: S. F. Mayor's killer dies in his garage." *San Francisco Chronicle,* October 22, 1985, 1.

42. Blinder, M. Quoted in Butler, K. and Z. Maitland. "Psychiatrists speak out: Suicide 'confirmed trial diagnosis.'" *San Francisco Chronicle,* October 22, 1985, 2.

43. See Szasz, T. S. "How Dan White got away with murder," in Szasz, T. S., *The Therapeutic State,* 137–146.

44. "Catholic Church says it won't 'judge' White." *San Francisco Chronicle,* October 22, 1985, 3.

45. Anonymous. "A new theory of schizophrenia." *Journal of Abnormal and Social Psychology* 57 (1958): 226–236, 227.

46. See Church, G. J. "Sorry, your policy is cancelled." *Time,* March 24, 1986, 16–26.

47. Keyes, D. *The Minds of Billy Milligan.*

48. See *Leland v. Oregon,* 343 U.S. 790, 1952; cited in, and discussed by, Lewin, T. H. D., "Psychiatric evidence." 1078.

49. Moore, M. S. *Law and Psychiatry,* 244–245.

50. Hobbes, T. *Leviathan,* p. 244.

51. "Victim sues over release of patient." *American Medical News,* October 4, 1985, 22.

52. Zane, M. and T. G. Keane. "Fired day worker kills ex-boss, dies in gunbattle." *San Francisco Chronicle,* January 7, 1986, 1, 16.

53. "'I'm sick, I'm sick, and I have no one.'" (Editorial), *New York Times*, October 25, 1985, A-26; see also "Accused subway assailant was in mental hospital." *Syracuse Herald-Journal*, October 24, 1985, A-10.

54. Brody, M. "The high cost of *not* institutionalizing psychiatric patients." (Letters), *New York Times*, November 15, 1985, A-34.

55. Twain, M. "A new crime," 245.

56. Shaw, G. B. Quoted in Stevenson, B., ed. *The MacMillan Book of Proverbs*, 1389.

57. Szasz, T. S. *Psychiatric Slavery*, Chap. 8; see also Szasz, T. S., ed. *The Age of Madness*.

58. Morse, S. J. "Excusing the crazy: The insanity defense reconsidered." *Southern California Law Review* 58 (March 1985): 777–836, 793.

59. Ibid., 789.

60. Ibid., 836.

61. Jeunesse, W. L. "Under orders: Suit by 5 mentally ill spurs ruling state care must improve for all." *Arizona Republic* October 1, 1985, A-1, A-2.

62. Ibid.

63. See *United States Department of Treasury, Bureau of Alcohol, Tobacco, and Firearms v. Anthony J. Galioto*, Brief of Amicus Curiae in the Supreme Court of the United States, October Term, 1985, mimeographed, 20 (Richard E. Gardiner and Robert Dowleut, Counsels).

64. Ibid., 12.

65. Ibid., 18.

66. See *Tarasoff v. Regents of University of California*, 529 P.2d 553, 118 Cal. Rptr. 129, 1974.

67. See Stone, A. A. "Vermont adopts *Tarasoff*: A real barn-burner." *American Journal of Psychiatry*, 143 (March 1986): 352–355.

CHAPTER 9: MENTAL ILLNESS AS STRATEGY

1. Lewis, C. S. *The Screwtape Letters and Screwtape Proposes a Toast*, 162.

2. Group for the Advancement of Psychiatry. *Criminal Responsibility and Psychiatric Expert Testimony*, 8.

3. Kolb, L. C. *Noyes' Modern Clinical Psychiatry*, 7th ed., 407.

4. Ibid., 408.

5. Ibid., 376.

6. Ibid.

7. Ibid.

8. Ibid., 379–380.

9. Brody, M. "The high cost," (Letters), *New York Times*, November 15, 1985, A-34.

10. "The devil made him do it." *Syracuse Herald-Journal,* April 29, 1974, 1.

11. Clendinen, D. "Defendant in a murder trial puts the devil on trial." *New York Times,* March 23, 1981, B-1, B-6.

12. Ibid.

13. Ibid.

14. "Vietnam syndrome frees vet." *Detroit News,* September 21, 1980, A-1, A-3.

15. *Durham v. United States,* 214 F.2d, 862 (D.C. Circuit), 1954.

16. Blackstone, W. *Commentaries on the Laws of England,* 212.

17. Thornton, M. "Death row said to drive killer insane." *Washington Post,* November 11, 1985, A-6.

18. "Comprehensive exam, review of defense reports required to determine competency to be executed, APA says in brief." *Psychiatric News* 21 (March 7, 1986): 3, 5.

19. "Assessing mental competency of prisoners needs standardization." *Psychiatric News,* December 6, 1985, 14.

20. "Comprehensive exam."

21. Shakespeare, W. *Macbeth,* Act 5, Scene 3, lines 39–44.

22. Ibid., lines 45–46.

23. See "5000 legal abortions done in California in 9 months." *Hospital Tribune,* November 18, 1968, 3.

24. See Szasz, T. S. *Ceremonial Chemistry.*

25. Fagen, C. R. and Messing, P. "Angels stalk mad slasher." *New York Post,* November 13, 1980, 1, 3.

26. "Cops hunt psycho in slaying of two in Buffalo." *Syracuse Post-Standard,* October 10, 1980, 1.

27. King, W. "Disturbed suspect is sought in seven ritualistic killings of Coast hikers." *New York Times,* December 2, 1980, A-16.

28. Ibid.

29. "Disease fear." *Parade,* February 13, 1966, 14.

30. See Dannhauser, W. J. "Religion and the conservatives." *Commentary,* December 1985, 51–55.

31. "Hinckley's parents honored." *New York Times,* April 4, 1986, D-19.

32. Hobbes, T. *Leviathan,* 494, 497.

33. Ibid., 495.

CHAPTER 10: MENTAL ILLNESS AS JUSTIFICATION

1. Cartwright, S. A. "Report on the diseases and physical pecularities of the negro race." *New Orleans Medical and Surgical Journal,* 7 (1851): 691–715; references are to Szasz, T. S. "The sane slave." *American Journal of Psychotherapy,* 25 (April 1971): 228–239, 233.

2. Werblowsky, R. J. and G. Wigoder, eds. *The Encyclopedia of the Jewish Religion*, 97.

3. Finkelstein, L. *The Jews*, 1741.

4. Radhakrishan. *The Hindu View of Life*, 40.

5. See Filmer, R. *Patriarcha* (1640); quoted in Schochet, G. J. *Patriarchalism in Political Thought;* all references to Filmer are from this source.

6. Schochet, *Patriarchalism*, 45.

7. Ibid., 15.

8. Maine, Sir H. *Ancient Law*, 250.

9. Hobbes, T. *Leviathan*, 362.

10. Berlin, I. *Four Essays on Liberty*, 19–20.

11. Jefferson, T. "Notes on the State of Virginia" (1781), in Koch, A., and W. Peden, eds. *The Life and Selected Writings of Thomas Jefferson*, 276–277.

12. Madison, J. "Memorial and remembrance against religious assessments" (1785), in Meyers, M., ed., *The Mind of the Founder*, 10.

13. Lewis, C. S. *The Screwtape Letters and Screwtape Proposes a Toast*, 69–70.

14. Lewis, C. S. "The humanitarian theory of punishment," *Res Judicatae.* (Melbourne, Australia: Melbourne University), 6 (1953) 225–239, 229.

15. See Cartwright, S. "Report."

16. Ibid., 229–234.

17. Holmes, O. W. Quoted in Levy, L. W. *Treason Against God*, x.

18. Jefferson, T. "Letter to Thomas Jefferson Randolph." November 24, 1808, in *Jefferson's Letters*, 249.

19. Levy, L. W. *Treason*, 208.

20. Ibid., xii.

21. *DSM-III*, 62.

22. Ibid., 67.

23. Ibid., 176.

24. Ibid., 291.

25. Ibid., 261.

26. Ibid., 266–267.

27. Ibid., 11.

28. Luther, M. Quoted in Levy, L. W. *Treason*, 127.

29. Ibid.

30. Ibid.

31. See Szasz, T. S. *Law, Liberty, and Psychiatry* and *Psychiatric Slavery.*

32. Jefferson, T. "Letter to John Adams." June 15, 1813, in *Jefferson's Letters*, 286.

33. Roth, L. Quoted in Byrne, G. "Refusing treatment in mental institutions: Values in conflict." *Hospital and Community Psychiatry*, 32 (April 1981): 255–258, 258.

34. Jefferson, T. "Virginia statute of religious liberty" (1786), in Syrett, H. C., ed. *American Historical Documents*, 95.

CHAPTER 11: MENTAL ILLNESS AS LEGAL FICTION

1. *Warner v. Packer*, 139 App. Div. 207, 123 N.Y. Supp. 725 (2d Dept. 1910); quoted in Warren, O. L. *Negligence in the New York Courts*, 20: 768.
2. Black, H. C. *Black's Law Dictionary*, 751.
3. Muller, H. J. *Freedom in the Western World*, 40–41.
4. Fuller, L. L. *Legal Fictions*, 53.
5. Quoted in Fingarette, H. *The Meaning of Criminal Insanity*, 25.
6. Hobbes, T. Quoted in, Hall, D. "A fear of metaphors." *New York Times Magazine*, July 14, 1985, 6–7, 6.
7. Locke, J. Quoted in ibid.
8. Bentham, J. Quoted in Fuller, L. L. *Legal Fictions*, 2.
9. Hall, D. A. "A fear of metaphors," 6.
10. Cohen, F. S. "Transcendental nonsense and the functional approach," in Hayakawa, S. I., ed., *Language, Meaning, and Maturity*, 184–214, 198.
11. Ibid.
12. Blackstone, W. Quoted in Fuller, L. L. *Legal Fictions*, 2.
13. Ibid., 3.
14. See Noonan, J. T., Jr. *Persons and Masks of the Law*.
15. Ibid., ix.
16. Ibid.
17. Ibid., 6.
18. Sullivan, H. S. *The Interpersonal Theory of Psychiatry*, 19.
19. Noonan, J. T., Jr. *Persons*, 11.
20. Ibid.
21. Ibid., 57.
22. Ibid., 58.
23. Ibid., 20.
24. See Gogol, N. *Dead Souls* (1842).
25. Ibid., 60–61.
26. Ibid., 276, 278.
27. Jefferson, T. "Notes on the State of Virginia" (1781), in Koch, A. and W. Peden, eds. *The Life and Selected Writings of Thomas Jefferson*, 279.
28. See *Robinson v. California*, 370 U.S. 660, 1962.
29. Ibid., 666.
30. Ibid., 674.
31. Ibid.

32. See Sherman, D. E. "Geriatic profile of Thomas Jefferson (1743–1826)," *Journal of the American Geriatric Society* 25 (1977): 112–117.

33. Lewis, C. S. *The Business of Heaven*, 54.

34. Noonan, J. T., Jr. *Persons*, 39.

35. Locke, J. *Two Treatises on Government*, 60.

36. Noonan, J. T., Jr. *Persons*, 41.

37. Ibid.

38. See Szasz, T. S. *Psychiatric Slavery*.

39. Szasz, T. S. *The Myth of Mental Illness*, and *Law, Liberty, and Psychiatry*.

40. Blackstone, W. *Commentaries on the Laws of England*; quoted in Noonan, J. T., Jr. *Persons*, 47.

41. Ibid.

42. Ibid.

43. Montesquieu. Quoted in ibid., 48.

44. Ibid.

45. Schraiber, R. "Care for the mentally ill." (Letters), *Newsweek*, January 27, 1986, 12.

46. Noonan, J. T., Jr. *Persons*, 51.

47. Ibid., 54.

48. Ibid.

49. Ibid.

50. Coriden, J. A., et al., eds. *The Code of Canon Law*, 541.

51. Ibid.

52. Ibid., 542.

53. Ibid., 775.

54. Ibid.

55. Ibid., 777.

56. Ibid.

57. Ibid.

58. Ibid., 778.

59. Black, H. C. *Black's Law Dictionary*, 751.

60. Byrne, E. "After 'mental illness' what?," in Bradie, M. and M. Brand, eds. *Action and Responsibility*, 122.

61. Lewin, T. H. D. "Psychiatric evidence in criminal cases for purposes other than the defense of insanity." *Syracuse Law Review* 26 (Fall 1975): 1051–1115, 1071.

62. Morris, N. "Mental illness and the criminal law," in Bean, P., ed. *Mental Illness*, 1–26.

63. Fingarette, H. "Insanity and responsibility." *Inquiry* 15 (1972): 6–29, 7.

64. Shakespeare, W. *Henry VI, Part Two*, Act 4, Scene 2, line 83.

65. Fingarette, H. "Insanity and responsibility," 27.

66. Fingarette, H. *The Meaning of Criminal Insanity,* 249.

67. Morse, S. J. "Excusing the crazy: The insanity defense reconsidered." *Southern California Law Review,* 58 (March 1985): 777–836, 822.

68. Ibid., 823.

69. Ibid., 827.

70. See Batlett, K. "Diabolic dealings: Psychiatrist tells of meeting Satan during exorcism." *Arizona Republic,* December 15, 1985, AA-12, AA-13.

71. See Minogue, K. *Alien Powers.*

CHAPTER 12: MENTAL ILLNESS AS EXPLANATION

1. Kierkegaard, S. Quoted in Jaspers, K. *General Psychopathology,* 425.

2. Wilson, C. *New Pathways in Psychology,* 47.

3. Peckham, M. *Explanation and Power,* 58–59.

4. Ibid., 60.

5. Franklin, J. "The mind fixers." *The Baltimore Evening Sun,* July 23–31, 1984; a special reprint.

6. Ibid.

7. Ibid.

8. Ibid., 10.

9. Berg, C. *Deep Analysis,* 190.

10. Gruber, A. Quoted in Schmeck, H. M. "Brain defects seen in those who repeat violent acts." *New York Times,* September 17, 1985, C-1, C-3.

11. Elliot, T. Quoted in ibid.

12. Restak, R. "Is free will a fraud?" *Science Digest,* October 1983, 50–53.

13. "Six-year old killed in hospital rampage." *Syracuse Herald-Journal,* June 24, 1980, A-4.

14. Carriere, V. "Victim got killer out of hospital, jury told." *The Globe and Mail* [Toronto], June 27, 1980, 5.

15. Winch, P. *The Idea of a Social Science,* 52–53.

16. Carlyle, T. *Sartor Resartus,* 280.

17. Moore, M. *Law and Psychiatry,* 197.

18. "All-white job setting ordered." *New York Times,* June 8, 1985, 28.

19. Hobbes, T. *Leviathan,* 97.

20. Branch, C. H. H. "Psychiatric education of physicians: What are our goals?" *American Journal of Psychiatry,* 125 (August 1968): 133–137, 135.

21. Voltaire. Quoted in Stevenson, B., ed. *The Macmillan Book of Proverbs,* 975.

22. Peckham, M. *Explanation and Power,* 2.

23. Ibid., ix.

24. Ibid., 65.

25. Ibid.

26. Ibid., 269.

27. Jefferson, T. "Letter to Nicholas Dufief," April 19, 1814, in Koch, A. and W. Peden, eds. *The Life and Selected Writings of Thomas Jefferson,* 636.

28. Johnson, S. Quoted in Stevenson, B., ed. *The Macmillan Book of Proverbs,* 2388.

BIBLIOGRAPHY

Alexander, F., *The Medical Value of Psychoanalysis* (Philadelphia: Saunders, 1968).

American Psychiatric Association, *Diagnostic and Statistical Manual of Mental Disorders*, 3rd ed. (Washington, D.C.: American Psychiatric Association, 1980).

Arens, R., *Make Mad the Guilty: The Insanity Defense in the District of Columbia* (Springfield, IL: Charles C. Thomas, 1969).

Arieti, S., *Understanding and Helping the Schizophrenic: A Guide for Family and Friends* (New York: Basic Books, 1979).

Bartlett, J., ed., *Familiar Quotations*, 12th ed. (Boston: Little, Brown, 1951).

Batchelor, I. R. C., *Henderson and Gillespie's Textbook of Psychiatry*, 10th ed. (London: Oxford University Press, 1969).

Bayer, R., *Homosexuality and American Psychiatry* (New York: Basic Books, 1981).

Bean, P., *Compulsory Admission to Mental Hospitals* (Chichester: Wiley, 1980).

Bean, P., ed., *Mental Illness: Changes and Trends* (Chichester: Wiley, 1983).

Beethoven, L. von, *Beethoven: Letters, Journals and Conversations*, ed. and trans. by M. Hamburger (Garden City, NY: Doubleday Anchor, 1960).

Berg, C., *Deep Analysis* (London: Allen & Unwin, 1946).

Berger, P. L. and T. Luckmann, *The Social Construction of Reality: A Treatise in the Sociology of Knowledge* (New York: Doubleday Anchor, 1967).

Berlin, I., *Four Essays on Liberty* (London: Oxford University Press, 1969).

Black, H. C., *Black's Law Dictionary*, rev. 4th ed. (St. Paul, MN: West, 1968).

Blackstone, W., *Commentaries on the Laws of England: Of Public Wrongs* (1755–1765) (Boston: Beacon Press, 1962).

Bleuler, E., *Dementia Praecox, or the Group of Schizophrenias* (1911), trans. by J. Zinkin (New York: International Universities Press, 1950).

Blom-Cooper, L., ed., *The Literature of the Law* (New York: Macmillan, 1965).

Bok, S., *Lying: Moral Choice in Public and Private Life* (New York: Vintage, 1979).

Bowker, J., *Problems of Suffering in Religions of the World* (Cambridge: Cambridge University Press, 1970).

Bradie, M. and M. Brand, eds., *Action and Responsibility* (Bowling Green, OH: Bowling Green State University Press, 1980).

Buranelli, V., *The Wizard from Vienna* (New York: Coward, McCann and Geoghegan, 1975).

Burnham, J., *Suicide of the West: An Essay on the Meaning and Destiny of Liberalism* (New Rochelle, NY: Arlington House, 1964).

Carlyle, T., *Sartor Resartus* (New York: Home Book, 1890).

Carroll, J. B., ed., *Language, Thought, and Reality: Selected Writings of Benjamin Lee Whorf* (New York: Wiley, 1956).

Chesen, E. S., *Religion May Be Hazardous to Your Health* (New York: Macmillan/ Collier, 1972).

Collison, G. D., *A Treatise on the Law, Concerning Idiots, Lunatics, and Other Persons Non Compotes Mentis* (2 vols.; London: W. Reed, 1812).

Coriden, J. A., et al., *The Code of Canon Law: A Text and Commentary* (New York: Paulist Press, 1985).

Corsini, R. J., ed., *Encyclopedia of Psychology* (4 vols.; New York: Wiley, 1984).

Darnton, R., *Mesmerism and the End of the Enlightenment in France* (Cambridge: Harvard University Press, 1968).

De Assis, M., *The Psychiatrist and Other Stories*, trans. by W. L. Grossman and H. Caldwell (Berkeley: University of California Press, 1963).

Dostoyevsky, F., *The Brothers Karamazov* (1880), trans. by C. Garnett (New York: Random House, 1950).

Dubovsky, S. L. and M. P. Weissberg, *Clinical Psychiatry in Primary Care* (Baltimore: Williams and Wilkins, 1978).

Dunham, B., *Man Against Myth* (New York: Hill & Wang, 1962).

Edelson, M., *The Idea of Mental Illness* (New Haven: Yale University Press, 1971).

Embler, W., *Metaphor and Meaning* (Deland, FL: Everett/Edwards, 1966).

Fingarette, H., *The Meaning of Criminal Insanity* (Berkeley: University of California Press, 1972).

Finkelstein, L., *The Jews: Their History, Culture, and Religion*, 3rd ed. (New York: Harper & Row, 1960).

Freud, S., *The Standard Edition of the Complete Psychological Works of Sigmund Freud* (24 vols.; London: Hogarth Press, 1953–1974).

Fuller, L. L., *Legal Fictions* (Stanford, CA: Stanford University Press, 1976).

Gilman, S. L., *Seeing the Insane* (New York: Wiley, 1982).

Goethe, J. W. von, *Gedenkausgabe der Werke, Briefe und Gespräche* (27 vols.; Zürich and Stuttgart: Artemis Verlag, 1962).

Gogol, N., *Dead Souls,* trans. by A. R. MacAndrew (New York: Signet, 1961).

Goldsmith, M., *Franz Anton Mesmer: A History of Mesmerism* (New York: Doubleday, 1934).

Group for the Advancement of Psychiatry, *Criminal Responsibility and Psychiatric Expert Testimony,* Report 26 (New York: GAP, 1954).

Guillain, G., *J.-M. Charcot, 1825–1893: His Life—His Work,* trans. by P. Bailey (New York: Hoeber, 1959).

Hamilton, E. and H. Cairns, eds., *The Collected Dialogues of Plato, Including the Letters* (Princeton: Princeton University Press, 1973).

Hayakawa, S. I., ed., *Language, Meaning, and Maturity* (New York: Harper & Brothers, 1954).

Heinroth, J. C., *Textbook of Disturbances of Mental Life, or Disturbances of the Soul and Their Treatment* (1818), trans. by J. Schmorak (2 vols.; Baltimore: Johns Hopkins University Press, 1975).

Henderson, Sir D. and I. R. C. Batchelor, *Henderson's and Gillespie's Textbook of Psychiatry,* 9th ed. (London: Oxford University Press, 1962).

Heschel, A. J., *The Prophets* (New York: Harper & Row, 1962).

Hobbes, T., *Leviathan* (1651), ed. by M. Oakeshott (New York: Macmillan/Collier, 1962).

Hoffer, A. and H. Osmond, *What You Should Know About Schizophrenia* (Ann Arbor, MI: American Schizophrenia Foundation, 1965).

Hunter, R., and I. Macalpine, *Three Hundred Years of Psychiatry, 1535–1860: A History Presented in Selected English Texts* (New York: Oxford University Press, 1963).

Isselbacher, K. J., et al., eds., *Harrison's Principles of Internal Medicine,* 9th ed. (New York: McGraw-Hill, 1980).

Jahoda, M., *Current Concepts of Positive Mental Health* (New York: Basic Books, 1958).

Jaspers, K., *General Psychopathology,* (1923), trans. by J. Hoenig and M. W. Hamilton (Chicago: The University of Chicago Press, 1963).

Jefferson, T., *Jefferson's Letters,* arranged by W. Whitman (Eau Claire, WI: E. M. Hale & Co., n.d.).

Jefferson, T., *The Political Writings of Thomas Jefferson,* ed. by E. Dumbauld (Indianapolis: Bobbs-Merrill, 1955).

Jung, C. G., *Memories, Dreams, Reflections,* ed. by Aniela Jaffé, trans. by R. and C. Winston (New York: Pantheon, 1963).

Kaplan, H. I., A. M. Freedman, and B. J. Sadock, eds., *Comprehensive Textbook of Psychiatry/III,* 3rd ed. (3 vols.; Baltimore: Williams and Wilkins, 1980).

Kenny, A. J. P., et al., *The Nature of Mind* (Edinburgh: University Press, 1972).

Kenny, A. J. P., et al., *The Development of Mind* (Edinburgh: University Press, 1973).

Kerr, A., and P. Snaith, eds., *Contemporary Issues in Schizophrenia* (London: Gaskell, 1986).

Keyes, D., *The Minds of Billy Milligan* (New York: Random House, 1981).

Kissane, J. M., ed., *Anderson's Pathology,* 8th ed. (2 vols.; St. Louis: Mosby, 1985).

Kleinig, J., *Paternalism* (Totowa, NJ: Rowman and Allanheld, 1984).

Koch, A. and W. Peden, eds., *The Life and Selected Writings of Thomas Jefferson* (New York: Modern Library, 1944).

Kolb, L. C., *Noyes' Modern Clinical Psychiatry,* 7th ed. (Philadelphia: Saunders, 1968).

Korzybski, A., *Science and Sanity: An Introduction to Non-Aristotelian Systems and General Semantics* (1933), 3rd ed. (Lakeville, CT: International Non-Aristotelian Library Publishing Company, 1950).

Kraepelin, E., *Einführung in die Psychiatrische Klinik* (Leipzig: Johann Ambrosius Barth, 1901).

Kraepelin, E., *Lectures on Clinical Psychiatry* (1901) (New York: Hafner, 1968).

Kramer, H. and J. Sprenger, *The Malleus Maleficarum,* (1486), trans. by Rev. M. Summers (New York: Dover, 1972).

Krauthammer, C., *Cutting Edges: Making Sense of the Eighties* (New York: Random House, 1986).

Laing, R. D., *Wisdom, Madness, and Folly: The Making of a Psychiatrist* (New York: McGraw-Hill, 1985).

Langer, S. K., *Philosophy in a New Key* (New York: Mentor, 1953).

Levy, L. W., *Treason Against God: A History of the Offense of Blasphemy* (New York: Schocken, 1981).

Lewis, C. S., *The Abolition of Man* (New York: Macmillan, 1947).

Lewis, C. S., *The Business of Heaven,* ed. by W. Hooper (New York: Harvest, 1984).

Lewis, C. S., *The Pilgrim's Regress* (New York: Bantam, 1981).

Lewis, C. S., *The Screwtape Letters and Screwtape Proposes a Toast* (New York: Macmillan, 1961).

Lieberman, E. J., *Acts of Will: The Life and Work of Otto Rank* (New York: Free Press, 1985).

Locke, J., *Two Treatises on Government* (1690) (New York: Mentor, 1960).

Maine, H., *Ancient Law* (London: J. M. Dent & Sons, 1861).

Marshall, J., *Intention in Law and Society* (New York: Minerva Press, 1968).

Maudsley, H., *Responsibility in Mental Disease,* 4th ed. (London: Kegan Paul, Trench & Co., 1885).

McKeon, R., ed., *The Basic Works of Aristotle* (New York: Random House, 1941).

Menninger, K., *The Vital Balance: The Life Process in Mental Health and Illness* (New York: Viking, 1963).

Meyers, M., ed., *The Mind of the Founder: Sources of the Political Thought of James Madison* (Indianapolis: Bobbs-Merrill, 1973).

Minogue, K., *Alien Powers: The Pure Theory of Ideology* (New York: St. Martin's, 1985).

Minogue, K., *The Liberal Mind* (London: Methuen, 1963).

Molière, *The Misanthrope and Other Plays*, trans. by J. Wood (Baltimore: Penguin, 1959).

Moore, M. S., *Law and Psychiatry: Rethinking the Relationship* (New York: Cambridge University Press, 1984).

Munthe, A., *The Story of San Michele* (1929) (New York: Dutton, 1957).

Noonan, J. T. Jr., *Persons and Masks of the Law* (New York: Farrar, Straus and Giroux, 1976).

Pauleikhoff, B., *Das Menschenbild im Wandel der Zeit* (2 vols.; Hurtgenwald: Guido Pressler Verlag, 1983).

Peckham, M., *Explanation and Power: The Control of Human Behavior* (New York: Seabury Press/Continuum, 1979).

Pellegrino, E. D. and D. C. Thomasma, *A Philosophical Basis of Medical Practice* (New York: Oxford University Press, 1981).

Petersdorf, R. G., et al., eds., *Harrison's Principles of Internal Medicine*, 10th ed. (New York: McGraw-Hill, 1983).

Radhakrishan, *The Hindu View of Life* (New York: Macmillan, 1962).

Rinkel, M., ed., *Biological Treatment of Mental Illness* (New York: L. C. Page, 1966).

Robbins, S. L., *Pathologic Basis of Disease*, 1st ed. (Philadelphia: Saunders, 1974).

Robbins, S. L., et al., eds., *Pathologic Basis of Disease*, 3rd ed. (Philadelphia: Saunders, 1984).

Rosen, G., *Madness in Society: Chapters in the Historical Sociology of Mental Illness* (Chicago: The University of Chicago Press, 1968).

Rush, B., *Letters of Benjamin Rush*, ed. by L. H. Butterfield (2 vols.; Princeton: Princeton University Press, 1951).

Rush, B., *Medical Inquiries and Observations upon the Diseases of the Mind* (1812) (New York: Hafner, 1962).

Ryle, G., *The Concept of Mind* (London: Hutchinson's University Library, 1949).

Sartorius, R., ed., *Paternalism* (Minneapolis: University of Minnesota Press, 1983).

Sartre, J.-P., *Being and Nothingness: An Essay on Phenomenological Ontology*, trans. by H. Barnes (New York: Philosophical Library, 1956).

Scheff, T. J., *Being Mentally Ill: A Sociological Theory* (Chicago: Aldine, 1966).

Schochet, G. J., *Patriarchalism in Political Thought* (New York: Basic Books, 1975).

Schoeck, H. and J. W. Wiggins, eds., *Psychiatry and Responsibility* (New York: Van Nostrand, 1962).

Schreber, D., *Memoirs of My Nervous Illness*, trans. by I. MacAlpine and R. Hunter (London: William Dawson and Sons, 1955).

Skultans, V., *Madness and Morals: Ideas on Insanity in the Nineteenth Century* (London: Routledge and Kegan Paul, 1975).

Smith, R., *Trial By Medicine: Insanity and Responsibility in Victorian Trials* (Edinburgh: Edinburgh University Press, 1981).

Sodeman, W. M., Jr. and T. M. Sodeman, *Sodeman's Pathologic Physiology: Mechanisms of Disease*, 7th ed. (Philadelphia: Saunders, 1985).

Spencer, H., *Social Statics* (New York: D. Appleton & Co., 1888).

Spitzer, R. L. and D. F. Klein, eds., *Critical Issues In Psychiatric Diagnosis* (New York: Raven Press, 1978).

Stansbury, J. B., et al., eds., *The Metabolic Basis of Inherited Diseases*, 5th ed. (New York: McGraw-Hill, 1983).

Stedman's Medical Dictionary, 21st ed. (Baltimore: Williams and Wilkins, 1966).

Stephen, J. F., *Liberty, Equality, Fraternity* (1873) (Cambridge: Cambridge University Press, 1967).

Stevenson, B., ed., *The Macmillan Book of Proverbs, Maxims, and Famous Phrases* (New York: Macmillan, 1948).

Strauss, M. B., ed., *Familiar Medical Quotations* (Boston: Little, Brown, 1968).

Sullivan, H. S., *The Interpersonal Theory of Psychiatry*, ed. by H. S. Perry and M. L. Gawell (New York: Norton, 1953).

Swift, J., *Gulliver's Travels* (1726) (New York: Signet, 1960).

Syrett, H. C., ed., *American Historical Documents* (New York: Barnes & Noble, 1960).

Szasz, T. S., ed., *The Age of Madness: A History of Involuntary Mental Hospitalization Presented in Selected Texts* (Garden City, NY: Doubleday Anchor, 1973).

Szasz, T. S., *Ceremonial Chemistry: The Ritual Persecution of Drugs, Addicts, and Pushers* (Garden City, NY: Doubleday Anchor, 1976).

Szasz, T. S., *The Ethics of Psychoanalysis: The Theory and Method of Autonomous Psychotherapy* (New York: Basic Books, 1965).

Szasz, T. S., *Heresies* (Garden City, NY: Doubleday Anchor, 1976).

Szasz, T. S., *Ideology and Insanity: Essays on the Psychiatric Dehumanization of Man* (Garden City, NY: Doubleday Anchor, 1970).

Szasz, T. S., *Karl Kraus and the Soul-Doctors: A Pioneer Critic and His Criticism of Psychiatry and Psychoanalysis* (Baton Rouge: Louisiana State University Press, 1976).

Szasz, T. S., *Law, Liberty, and Psychiatry: An Inquiry into the Social Uses of Mental Health Practices* (New York: Macmillan, 1963).

Szasz, T. S., *The Manufacture of Madness: A Comparative Study of the Inquisition and the Mental Health Movement* (New York: Harper & Row, 1970).

Szasz, T. S., *The Myth of Mental Illness: Foundations of a Theory of Personal Conduct* (New York: Hoeber-Harper, 1961), rev. ed. (New York: Harper & Row, 1974).

Szasz, T. S., *The Myth of Psychotherapy: Mental Healing as Religion, Rhetoric, and Repression* (Garden City, NY: Doubleday Anchor, 1978).

Szasz, T. S., *Psychiatric Justice* (New York: Macmillan, 1965).

Szasz, T. S., *Psychiatric Slavery: When Confinement and Coercion Masquerade as Cure* (New York: Free Press, 1977).

Szasz, T. S., *Schizophrenia: The Sacred Symbol of Psychiatry* (New York: Basic Books, 1976).

Szasz, T. S., *Sex By Prescription* (Garden City, NY: Doubleday Anchor, 1980).

Szasz, T. S., *The Therapeutic State: Psychiatry in the Mirror of Current Events* (Buffalo, NY: Prometheus Books, 1984).

Thomas, K., *Religion and the Decline of Magic* (London: Weidenfeld and Nicolson, 1971).

Thurber, J., *The Thurber Carnival*, 2nd ed. (New York: Harper & Brothers, 1945).

Turbayne, C. M., *The Myth of Metaphor*, rev. ed. (Columbia: University of South Carolina Press, 1970).

Turner, J., *Without God, Without Creed: The Origins of Unbelief in America* (Baltimore: Johns Hopkins University Press, 1985).

Twain, M., *Authorized Edition of the Complete Works of Mark Twain* (23 vols.; New York: Harper & Brothers, 1923).

Twain, M., *Pudd'nhead Wilson* (1884) (New York: Signet, 1964).

Warren, O. L., *Negligence in the New York Courts*, 3rd ed. (New York: Matthew Bender, 1978).

Weaver, R., *Ideas Have Consequences* (Chicago: Phoenix Books, 1962).

Werblowsky, R. J. and G. Wigoder, eds., *The Encyclopedia of the Jewish Religion* (New York: Holt, Rinehart and Winston, 1965).

Wiener, P. P., ed., *Dictionary of the History of Ideas: Studies of Selected Pivotal Ideas* (5 vols.; New York: Scribner's, 1973).

Wilbur, G. B. and W. Muensterberger, eds., *Psychoanalysis and Culture* (New York: International Universities Press, 1951).

Wilson, C., *New Pathways in Psychology* (New York: Taplinger, 1972).

Winch, P., *The Idea of a Social Science* (London: Routledge and Kegan Paul, 1958).

Wooden, K., *The Children of Jonestown* (New York: McGraw-Hill, 1981).

Wyngaarden, J. B. and L. H. Smith, eds., *Cecil's Textbook of Medicine*, 17th ed. (2 vols.; Philadelphia: Saunders, 1985).

NAME INDEX

SUBJECT INDEX